APPLICATIONS OF
Good Psychiatric Management for Borderline Personality Disorder

A PRACTICAL GUIDE

T0176384

APPLICATIONS OF
Good Psychiatric Management for Borderline Personality Disorder
A PRACTICAL GUIDE

Edited by

Lois W. Choi-Kain, M.D., M.Ed.
John G. Gunderson, M.D.

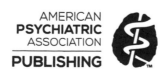

AMERICAN
PSYCHIATRIC
ASSOCIATION
PUBLISHING

Copyright © 2019 American Psychiatric Association Publishing

ALL RIGHTS RESERVED

First Edition

Manufactured in the United States of America on acid-free paper

23 22 21 20 19   5 4 3 2 1

American Psychiatric Association Publishing
800 Maine Avenue SW
Suite 900
Washington, DC 20024-2812
www.appi.org

Library of Congress Cataloging-in-Publication Data

Names: Choi-Kain, Lois W., editor. | Gunderson, John G., 1942–2019 editor. | American Psychiatric Association Publishing, issuing body.
Title: Applications of good psychiatric management for borderline personality disorder : a practical guide / edited by Lois W. Choi-Kain, John G. Gunderson.
Description: Washington, D.C. : American Psychiatric Association Publishing, [2019] | Includes bibliographical references and index.
Identifiers: LCCN 2018061676 (print) | LCCN 2019000444 (ebook) | ISBN 9781615372539 (eb) | ISBN 9781615372256 (pbk. : alk. paper)
Subjects: | MESH: Borderline Personality Disorder | Psychotherapy—methods
Classification: LCC RC569.5.B67 (ebook) | LCC RC569.5.B67 (print) | NLM WM 190.5.B5 | DDC 616.85/852--dc23
LC record available at https://lccn.loc.gov/2018061676

British Library Cataloguing in Publication Data

A CIP record is available from the British Library.

This book is dedicated to the legacy of John Gunderson, whose pioneering work over more than four decades legitimized borderline personality disorder (BPD) as a psychiatric illness. John's insistent effort to improve our understanding and treatment of patients with BPD has transformed the field as well as the lives of millions of patients and families. John's spirit will live on in Good Psychiatric Management and all who apply its pragmatic principles in their care of patients

Contents

PART I
Clinical Services

PART II
Providers

PART III

Implementation and Integration

PART IV
Conclusion

Contributors

Karen A. Adler, M.D.
Instructor in Psychiatry, Harvard Medical School, Boston; Per Diem Psychiatrist, McLean Hospital, Belmont, Massachusetts

Claire Brickell, M.D.
Instructor, Harvard Medical School; Attending Psychiatrist, Outpatient Psychiatry Services, Boston Children's Hospital, Boston, Massachusetts

Patrick Charbon, M.D.
Psychiatrist, Cabinet d'un á monde l'autre, Lausanne, Switzerland

Lois W. Choi-Kain, M.D., M.Ed.
Medical and Program Director, Gunderson Residence, McLean Hospital, Belmont; Director, McLean Hospital Adult Borderline Center and Training Institute, McLean Hospital, Belmont; Assistant Professor in Psychiatry, Department of Psychiatry, Harvard Medical School, Boston, Massachusetts

Jessica Droz, M.D.
Chief Resident, Section Karl Jaspers of General Psychiatry Service, Department of Psychiatry, University Hospital Center, University of Lausanne, Lausanne, Switzerland

Robert P. Drozek, M.S.W., LICSW
Staff Therapist, Adult Center for Borderline Personality Disorder and Training Institute; Teaching Associate in Psychiatry, Harvard Medical School, Cambridge, Massachusetts

Ellen F. Finch, B.A.
Ph.D. Candidate, Department of Psychology, Harvard University, Cambridge, Massachusetts

John G. Gunderson, M.D.
Professor of Psychiatry, Emeritus, Harvard Medical School, Boston; Consultant in Psychiatry, McLean Hospital, Belmont, Massachusetts

Richard G. Hersh, M.D.
Special Lecturer, Columbia University Medical Center; Adjunct Faculty, New York University School of Medicine; Faculty, Columbia Center for Psychoanalytic Training and Research, New York, New York

Victor Hong, M.D.
Clinical Assistant Professor, Department of Psychiatry, University of Michigan, Ann Arbor, Michigan

Gabrielle Ilagan, B.A.
Clinical Research Assistant, Adult Borderline Center and Training Institute, McLean Hospital, Belmont, Massachusetts

Evan A. Iliakis, B.A.
Clinical Research Assistant, Gunderson Programs, McLean Hospital, Belmont, Massachusetts

James A. Jenkins, M.D.
Instructor in Psychiatry, Harvard Medical School, Boston; Medical Director, 3East Cambridge Residence, McLean Hospital, Belmont; Staff Psychiatrist, Gunderson Residence, McLean Hospital, Belmont, Massachusetts

Stéphane Kolly, M.D.
Psychiatrist, General Psychiatry Service, Department of Psychiatry, University of Lausanne, Lausanne, Switzerland

Ueli Kramer, Ph.D.
Private Lecturer, Adjunct Psychologist, General Psychiatric Services, University of Lausanne; Research Project Director; Private Lecturer, Section Karl Jaspers and University Psychotherapy Institute, Department of Psychiatry, University Hospital Center, University of Lausanne, Lausanne, Switzerland

Paul S. Links, M.D., M.Sc., FRCPC
Professor, Department of Psychiatry and Behavioural Neurosciences, McMaster University, Hamilton, Ontario, Canada

Deanna Mercer, M.D., FRCPC
Assistant Professor, Department of Psychiatry, University of Ottawa; Borderline Personality Disorder Clinic, Canadian Mental Health Association, Ottawa, Ontario, Canada

Brian A. Palmer, M.D., M.P.H.
Assistant Professor of Psychiatry, Department of Psychiatry and Psychology, and Vice Chair, Education, Department of Psychiatry and Psychology, Mayo Clinic, Rochester, Minnesota

Daniel G. Price, M.D.
Assistant Professor of Psychiatry, Tufts University School of Medicine; Director of Residency Training, Department of Psychiatry, Maine Medical Center, Tufts University, Portland, Maine

Ana M. Rodriguez-Villa, M.D., M.B.A.
M.D. Candidate, Geisel School of Medicine, Dartmouth and M.B.A. Candidate, Tuck School of Business, Dartmouth, Hanover, New Hampshire

Anne K.I. Sonley, M.D., J.D.
Psychiatry Resident, University of Toronto, Borderline Personality Disorders Clinic, Center for Addiction and Mental Health, Toronto, Ontario, Canada

Brandon T. Unruh, M.D.
Medical Director, Mentalization-Based Treatment Clinic, Assistant Medical Director, Gunderson Residence, Assistant Director, Borderline Personality Disorder Training Institute, McLean Hospital, Belmont, and Instructor in Psychiatry, Harvard Medical School, Cambridge, Massachusetts

Igor Weinberg, Ph.D.
Assistant Professor of Psychology, Harvard Medical School, Boston; Associate Psychologist, Adult Outpatient Services, McLean Hospital, Belmont, Massachusetts

Disclosure of Competing Interests

The following contributors to this book have indicated a financial interest in or other affiliation with a commercial supporter, a manufacturer of a commercial product, a provider of a commercial service, a nongovernmental organization, and/or a government agency, as listed below:

Lois W. Choi-Kain, M.D., M.Ed.—*Royalties*: HMS Continuing Education, Course Director; Springer, author/coeditor

John G. Gunderson, M.D.—*Royalties*: From American Psychiatric Association Publishing for *Handbook of Good Psychiatric Management for Borderline Personality Disorder*

The following contributors to this book have indicated no competing interests to disclose:

Karen A. Adler, M.D.
Claire Brickell, M.D.
Patrick Charbon, M.D.
Robert P. Drozek, M.S.W., LICSW
Richard G. Hersh, M.D.
Victor Hong, M.D.
James A. Jenkins, M.D.
Brian A. Palmer, M.D., M.P.H.
Daniel G. Price, M.D.
Ana M. Rodriguez-Villa, M.D., M.B.A.
Brandon T. Unruh, M.D.

Preface

For the past 5 years, John Gunderson and I have argued about what the "G" in "GPM" signifies. John embraced the idea that his approach is *good* psychiatric management (GPM) of patients with borderline personality disorder (BPD). I believe this is because of John's roots: he was a Midwesterner by nature, with a tendency to be modest despite his paradigm-shifting contributions to our field. GPM indeed is a *good* treatment, shown to be as effective as the veritable giant of all BPD treatments, dialectical behavior therapy (DBT; McMain et al. 2009, 2012). In addition, having been trained as a psychoanalyst, with a deep appreciation for developmental perspectives, John aimed for a treatment that is *good enough*, using the term coined by pediatrician and psychoanalyst Donald Winnicott. Winnicott used this phrase, *good enough*, to describe the way that mothers begin to respond less and less perfectly to babies as they grow, allowing them to experience moderate levels of frustration in order to appreciate the difference between their needs and reality (Winnicott 1953). Reality, rather than caretaking in the most idealized forms, involves a world in which others will not always respond exactly in the most immediate or optimal way for any given human being (Winnicott 1971). GPM centrally incorporates the idea that its practitioners are available in a caring but limited way. By design, GPM does not incorporate a large team, lengthy groups, or around-the-clock coaching because it is realistic and attuned to the idea that a large majority of patients with BPD do not die by suicide and eventually achieve symptomatic remission over time. John said to me specifically, "GPM is not an ambitious treatment, but it is good enough for most." As described in all the chapters written by our family of GPM experts, GPM emphasizes the idea that the clinician is there as a steady source of understanding and encouragement for patients with BPD, so they can not only survive but, more importantly, function to build a life that provides self-esteem and structure. That is what most parents basically aim for in the endeavor of raising their children. It is also what most clinical professionals want for their patients.

For me, despite my appreciation for these foundations of all the good in GPM, I assert that the "G" in GPM stands for *generalist*. I deeply appreciate the empirical foundations for GPM established by Shelly McMain and Paul Links, who with a large team of collaborators converted John's seminal textbook *Borderline Personality Disorder: A Clinical Guide* (Gunderson 1984, 2001; Gunderson and Links 2008) into a manualized treatment and then tested it against well-run DBT in the largest outpatient trial of manualized psychotherapy for BPD to date (McMain et al. 2009, 2012). McMain and Links independently developed the term *generalist* because they wanted to test whether DBT outstripped a well-informed structured approach to clinical management of BPD by psychiatrists, psychologists, master's-level clinicians, and nurses with at least 1 year of experience in treating BPD (McMain et al. 2009). Their findings—that GPM matched DBT in all outcomes at 12 and 36 months—created a paradigm shift in itself, leading us to consider the question of what in *general* can health professionals who are not experts or specialists do when encountering a patient with BPD?

This book is dedicated to the *general* practitioner—the pharmacologist, the social worker, the primary care provider, the inpatient attending physician, the nurse, the emergency department personnel, the consultation-liaison psychiatrist, the supervising attending physician, and the resident in psychiatry—who is devoted to the *general* care of patients. As discussed throughout the book, patients with BPD actively seek help from health professionals. They show up in abundance; they occupy primary care provider's offices, emergency departments, acute care, and outpatient treatment at levels 10- to 20-fold more than their prevalence in the community at large.

Finally, I believe GPM to be a *general* model that well-meaning health care professionals can utilize in order to understand and guide care for a number of psychiatric disorders. GPM's recipe constitutes *good* basic care. Diagnosing problems, educating patients about their illness, expecting patients to be responsible for themselves with their vulnerabilities, and encouraging everyday function as well as life outside of treatment is just *good* care. Health care professionals routinely diagnose common problems such as hypertension, diabetes, and infection. They teach their patients what they should know to take care of whatever ailments they suffer. They also prepare human beings for different developmental phases from infancy to old age.

Our colleague Eric Plakun has been an important critic of the evidence-based treatment groundswell. At the annual meeting of the North American Society for the Study of Personality Disorders in 2017, he delivered a plenary address in which he challenged the requirement for randomized controlled trials as a singular standard for determining clinical guidelines. Plakun pointed to the fact that a majority of joint cardiovascular practice guidelines of the American College of Cardiology and the American Heart Association have been driven by expert opinion or low levels of evidence, not randomized controlled trials (Tricoci et al. 2009). Randomized controlled trials objectively demonstrate what works and what works *less well*. These studies take enormous expertise, manpower, and money to run. It is important to balance what is generally known about psychiatric care and BPD with evidence from trials to implement *good general* care.

A recent meta-analysis, whose first author was a postdoctoral fellow at Macquarie University in Australia, quantifies the cost savings of treating BPD (Meuldijk et al. 2017). Her analysis of financial expenditures in published randomized controlled trials of psychotherapies for BPD estimates the cost offset from providing an evidence-based treatment for BPD when comparing expenditures from the year before treatment to the year after is three dollars a year per patient. In the United States alone, this would save the country several billion dollars a year even if only a fraction of patients with BPD sought treatment, especially if treatment were more accessible and available. The worldwide implications are more staggering.

In the past 5 years, we (John, our chapter authors, and I) toured the country and the world to attempt to make GPM a feasible standard of care. Made possible by an anonymous gift to us at McLean Hospital from a grateful patient who wanted to spread good general care beyond those who could afford treatment with specialists, as well as a matching fund donated by other grateful families of those who recovered from BPD in our service, we held numerous *training-the-trainer* trainings for faculty of U.S. psychiatry residency programs who teach our future psychiatrists. We sent tens of thousands of GPM manuals (Gunderson and Links 2014) to psychiatry residents across the United States. This is how we came to know those who wrote chapters of this book; they are our first GPM trainers. This project was fun and meaningful but also draining because it took me away from my small children and husband (i.e., work before love). Because GPM taught me not to be an idealized martyr to my work, I decided to stop spreading myself too thin to be helpful.

To broaden our scope, using this generous donation by the families we have worked with in the Gunderson Residence program, we are providing free online GPM trainings for the next 2 years on the Harvard Medical School online continuing education website (http://hms.harvard.edu/BPD) for continuing education credits. (See also Appendix A, "Additional Resources.") We hope this endeavor will extend the scope of *good enough* or *generalist* evidence-based care so it becomes the standard of care worldwide. I hope the "G" in GPM comes to stand for *generic* BPD care, which implies that any system or patient can obtain this care at low cost. Although generic treatments alter the financial gain of brand name treatments, they are basic to providing the public with accessible health care.

These efforts to spread access to care for patients with BPD have been work as well as a labor of love. John Gunderson has left a legacy of converting sophisticated cutting-edge treatment into practical medical management. While he has left me the charge to move GPM into the future, I face some healthy doubts. John has occupied a position within the circle of BPD experts and researchers as an arbiter—that is, an appreciator and critic—of all evidence-based treatments for BPD (Gunderson et al. 2018). For me, I value that position of being an arbiter over being the face of a specific brand name. What I aim to focus on in the next phase of BPD treatment is the spreading of *good* and *general* care to most patients and their health care providers. This goal is just as ambitious as forging the cutting edge of treatment innovation that turned the tide of stigma against BPD as a so-called wastebasket diagnosis (Knight 1953) or untreatable illness to one of hope and recovery. Those who revolutionized attitudes toward BPD through building its specialty evidence-based treatment leveled a plausible foundation for us to understand the basic mechanisms for what works and then package it in a globally deliverable way. Basically, they developed the brand name treatments, and we are aiming to make the generic version that essentially has comparable ingredients and efficacy.

When John Gunderson started his residency training, there was no such thing as borderline personality disorder. There was a group of patients on the borderline of other diagnoses that nobody understood or knew how to handle. Most thought that these patients were simply untreatable. John did not believe this. John tried to understand these patients, describe them more clearly, and pave the way to better outcomes in their care. Just a few years after graduating from residency, John boiled down a complex psychoanalytic literature on borderline patients into a pragmatic set of defining features. Along with the development of methods to reliably diagnose borderline patients, John's work led to the incorporation of borderline personality disorder into DSM. Over the last four decades, with the publication of more than 300 papers and 12 books, John worked systematically to legitimize the BPD diagnosis. With many collaborators, John discriminated BPD from psychotic, mood, and trauma-related disorders; elucidated its longitudinal course; and assessed genetic and familial contributions.

In the last stretch of his career, John developed GPM to improve access to care. Whereas John's early contributions challenged the notion patients with BPD were not treatable, GPM challenges the notion that patients with BPD can only be treated by specialists or in intensive outpatient psychotherapies. With optimism that most patients with BPD can get well and that most clinicians can provide good care, John and I gathered a team of GPM trainers to write this book to provide practical guidance. We hope it changes beliefs that patients with BPD cannot be treated in acute or nonspecialized settings

Lois W. Choi-Kain, M.D., M.Ed.

References

Gunderson JG: Borderline Personality Disorder. Washington, DC, American Psychiatric Press, 1984

Gunderson JG: Borderline Personality Disorder: A Clinical Guide. Washington, DC, American Psychiatric Publishing, 2001

Gunderson JG, Links PS: Borderline Personality Disorder: A Clinical Guide, 2nd Edition. Washington, DC, American Psychiatric Publishing, 2008

Gunderson JG, Links PS: Handbook of Good Psychiatric Management for Borderline Personality Disorder. Washington, DC, American Psychiatric Publishing, 2014

Gunderson JG, Fruzzetti A, Unruh B, Choi-Kain L: Competing theories of borderline personality disorder. J Pers Disord 32(2):148–167, 2018 29561723

Knight RP: Borderline states. Bull Menninger Clin 17(1):1–12, 1953 13009379

McMain SF, Links PS, Gnam WH, et al: A randomized trial of dialectical behavior therapy versus general psychiatric management for borderline personality disorder. Am J Psychiatry 166(12):1365–1374, 2009 19755574

McMain SF, Guimond T, Streiner DL, et al: Dialectical behavior therapy compared with general psychiatric management for borderline personality disorder: clinical outcomes and functioning over a 2-year follow-up. Am J Psychiatry 169(6):650–661, 2012 22581157

Meuldijk D, McCarthy A, Bourke ME, et al: The value of psychological treatment for borderline personality disorder: systematic review and cost offset analysis of economic evaluations. PLoS One 12(3):e0171592, 2017 28249032

Tricoci P, Allen JM, Kramer JM, et al: Scientific evidence underlying the ACC/AHA clinical practice guidelines. JAMA 301(8):831–841, 2009 19244190
Winnicott DW: Transitional objects and transitional phenomena: a study of the first not-me possession. Int J Psychoanal 34(2):89–97, 1953 13061115
Winnicott DW: Playing and Reality. New York, Psychology Press, 1971

Acknowledgments

John Gunderson and I (L.C.K.) acknowledge and thank the many people who made this book and the work represented in it possible. Much of what we have done in our work together in the past 5 years grew out of numerous philanthropic gifts made to us through the Development Office at McLean Hospital in Belmont, Massachusetts. The Gunderson Residence, founded at the hospital in 2009 through a large anonymous gift and developed by me and my dear friend and partner Karen Jacob, has provided the clinical ground where we have tried to implement a blend of the best evidence-based treatments for borderline personality disorder (BPD) in a rigorous and informed way. Out of this, we have built lifelong relationships with patients and families who have joined our cause to advance research and treatment for BPD and other severe personality disorders.

These patients and their families have multiplied the reach of our efforts. Their support through philanthropy has allowed our center to grow a training institute so we can teach other professionals what we know as well as what our expert friends have to teach us. This philanthropic support has also allowed us to proliferate more practical versions of this gold standard to environments where there are limited clinical resources. Importantly, we could not do this without the Development Office staff, particularly the late Cathie Cook, Lori Etringer, and Jeff Smith. Also, it is important that we thank the leaders of McLean Hospital—Scott Rauch, Joe Gold, Shelly Greenfield, and Phil Levendusky—for their support and collaboration in building the Gunderson Residence, the Borderline Personality Disorder Training Institute (BPDTI), and the national and international training efforts we do in addition to our clinical duties.

We received a game-changing anonymous gift from one grateful patient and family who, despite ample financial resources and motivation, could not find definitive treatment because the diagnosis of BPD was delayed until late into the patient's adult life. Out of this heart-wrenching experience, our project to improve access to care for BPD was born to promote greater awareness of, earlier diagnosis of, and more access to care for BPD. A matching campaign launched by our development officers produced another sizable donation made by multiple families, which increased our resources considerably. This project focused on the proliferation of general or good psychiatric management (GPM) as a standard of care among adult psychiatry programs in the United States. Through these efforts, we have trained more than 90 residency directors and faculty to be trainers of future psychiatrists in GPM. We supplied every program in the country with the GPM manual and held courses to train clinicians and faculty to both do and train others to do GPM all over the United States, training more than 4,000 mental health professionals for free or low cost. We also partnered specifically with Maine Medical Center and the charismatic but down-to-earth director of residency training and outpatient psychiatry, Dan Price. Maine Medical Center, located in our region, is founded on a more organized public health care system, not self-pay services. The grant for this project also funded Sara Masland to partner with Dan and his team to build a group curriculum and study the effects of introducing GPM in a larger service system.

The cadre of GPM trainers born out of this effort helped us to write this book. They include world experts or well-known researchers on BPD, core faculty training future mental health professionals in GPM, and local clinical experts who specialize in BPD treatment. In particular, we thank Brian Palmer, Richard Hersh, and Dan Price, who have done extensive teaching and travel with us. Brian integrated GPM trainings into the offerings from Mayo Clinic's continuing education program and also organized well-attended residents' workshops at the annual meetings of the American Psychiatric Association. We thank all our GPM-dedicated trainers who have incorporated it as the essential approach to BPD for trainees in their programs across the country and the world. Their work has helped us and, more importantly, their students and their patients.

On a more personal note, we thank all our dear friends and colleagues who have worked side by side with us in our clinical, teaching, and research endeavors at McLean Hospital. This list includes but is not limited to Amy Gagliardi, Karen Jacob, Brandon Unruh, George Smith, Betsy

Ressler, and Joe Flores. We especially thank Chris Palmer and his office at McLean's Department of Postgaduate and Continuing Education for the many collaborations with the BPDTI because they would not have occurred without his guidance and partnership. Kerry Ressler has also been a wonderful partner in keeping our research program alive and growing. Last but most certainly not least are our ground soldiers, the administrative and research assisting staff of the BPDTI. Ana Rodriguez-Villa, Jenna Adams, Liz Albert, Ellen Finch, and now Gabs Ilagan and Evan Iliakis did much of the heavy lifting of the BPDTI's courses, projects, and grants. Most of them were instrumental in finishing this book.

For me (L.C.K.), it is important to thank those who have helped me grow as a professional. My husband Mike and daughters Emma and Abbie have had to give up much time with me for my "work before love" affliction. Also, I want to thank my teachers and others who were so influential in shaping my career: Salman Akhtar, Glen Gabbard, Anthony Bateman, Peter Fonagy, and Steven Cooper. Finally, I thank my coeditor, John Gunderson, who passed away January 11, 2019, in the course of publishing this book. For his investment in me as a person and a psychiatrist, I am deeply grateful.

Chapter 1

An Overview of Good Psychiatric Management

ORIGINS AND DIRECTIONS

John G. Gunderson, M.D.
Lois W. Choi-Kain, M.D., M.Ed.

We developed this book because most clinicians will need to treat patients with borderline personality disorder (BPD) and can use help in doing so. Patients with BPD represent about 1 in every 4–5 psychiatric hospitalizations and a similar fraction of outpatient clinic visits (Chanen et al. 2008; Korzekwa et al. 2008; Zimmerman et al. 2008), about 1 in 10 visits in

1

the emergency department (Chaput and Lebel 2007; Tomko et al. 2014), and 1 in 20 visits to primary care providers (Gross et al. 2002). Not only are these patients a major presence in virtually all clinical care sites, but they are frequently experienced as impatient, needy, and burdensome, especially when they perceive that their particular needs are not being addressed. This book is intended to provide helpful how-to advice and wisdom about how their care can best be managed. The word *managed* is key: This book is not about lengthy intensive interventions; it is about management strategies, such as calming, encouraging, advising, and otherwise facilitating getting your patients with BPD in a position to pursue productive lives.

This book's management perspective contrasts with that of the majority of books about the treatment of patients with BPD, which emphasize lengthy complex psychotherapies aimed at bringing about deep psychological changes. Such therapies are for specialists. In this book, our focus is on the majority of patients who are not seeking such psychotherapies and on the majority of clinicians who are not primarily psychotherapists or BPD specialists. This book is addressed to health professionals who simply want to take better care of the patients with BPD who come under their care, with the goal of helping these patients move on with their lives.

To make this book readable, understandable, and most of all useful, our authors have included case vignettes in most chapters to illustrate common problems that clinicians can expect to encounter in usual practice. Each vignette is interrupted with "decision points," demonstrating occasions within the therapy in which a clinician is faced with making an intervention and often needs to consider a variety of options. We provide options that occur to us and then discuss and rate their relative merits. We want readers to consider and rate these options alongside us. Instead of aiming for readers to learn the right answer, this is an exercise in active learning. Decisions made in clinical reality rarely fit the supposedly clear answers provided as multiple-choice options. Do not be surprised if you disagree with our ratings or if you think of other options that might be preferable. We will not be. We want you to learn how to think in good psychiatric management (GPM) terms—that is, practical, thoughtful, and realistic ways—about the care of patients with BPD. We do not aim to create followers who remain tightly adherent to our ideas.

There is strong reason to believe that with shorter-term, less demanding interventions, the majority of patients with BPD can and will get better, as well as or nearly as well as those patients who receive their care from specialists (Choi-Kain et al. 2017; Gunderson 2016). Longitudinal studies of the past 20 years convincingly show that most patients with BPD go on to remission or even to recovery in the absence of intensive specialized evidence-based treatments (Gunderson et al. 2011; Zanarini et al. 2012). There is still growing evidence establishing the value of less intensive nonspecialist interventions (Gunderson 2016). Just as GPM established its value in a comparison to dialectical behavior therapy (DBT), a similar once-weekly model called structured clinical management (Bateman and Krawitz 2013) established its value against standard mentalization-based treatment (MBT) (Bateman and Fonagy 2009). Thus, structured clinical management (SCM) and GPM, less-intensive generalist treatments developed expressly for BPD, have proven effective in two large randomized controlled trials (Bateman and Fonagy 2009; McMain et al. 2009). Specifically, SCM proved effective in reducing BPD symptoms—most notably self-harm—within the first 6 months of treatment but was outpaced by MBT at 18 months (Bateman and Fonagy 2009). GPM performed as well as DBT across a range of outcomes, spanning BPD symptoms, interpersonal functioning, anger, and depression (McMain et al. 2009). As important as the GPM and structured clinical management findings are the results of the DBT-dismantling study, which showed that its group component seems to carry much of the effectiveness (Linehan et al. 2015). Notably, the onerous requirement of around-the-clock, over-the-weekend coverage seems to be dispensable. In addition to these studies, a large psychopharmacological trial (Crawford et al. 2018) recently demonstrated that although lamotrigine failed to show an advantage over placebo, both arms of the study had robust clinically significant improvements—larger than would be expected from treatment as usual. The obvious conclusion to be drawn from findings of Crawford et al. (2018) is that the regular attention of motivated psychiatrists to monitoring changes in signs and symptoms of BPD had a powerful and positive effect on outcome (Gunderson and Choi-Kain 2018).

This book's unspoken mandate for clinicians to use GPM can be criticized on the basis that the empirical support for this model of treatment rests on only one study (McMain et al. 2009, 2012). That study was a well-designed, large, multisite study in which GPM proved to be the equivalent to what was acknowledged to be high-quality DBT, conducted under the supervision of the study's primary investigator. However, it is worth noting that the vast majority of scientific findings are not investigated further in replication studies, with an estimated 1.07% overall replication rate in the field of psychology, for instance (Makel et al. 2012). In other words, the truth is that such a replication, which would be considered significant in the world of research, is unlikely to occur in the present research environment. We believe that the usage of GPM's model really does not and should not depend on the completion of such a study. Its usage depends on the cumulative research cited here. Moreover, the rationale for learning GPM derives from the absence of any reasonable alternative. Patients with BPD keep arriving in our offices, our clinics, our emergency departments, and our hospitals. These patients deserve to expect that every clinician has been taught how to provide them with basic services from which they have a reasonably good chance of benefiting. GPM meets this need.

GPM developed from clinical experience. Unlike the other evidence-based treatments for BPD, GPM was not preceded by a theory (Gunderson et al. 2018). It evolved gradually over many years since its first iteration in 1984 (Gunderson 1984). What followed were refinements integrated into the American Psychiatric Association's guidelines for the treatment of BPD (American Psychiatric Association Practice Guidelines 2001), culminating in the manualization of the treatment with the help of Paul Links (Gunderson and Links 2014). GPM's evolution was influenced by all the best BPD psychotherapies. Otto Kernberg's object relations theory (Kernberg 1967), Marsha Linehan's cognitive-behavioral paradigm (Linehan 1993), and Peter Fonagy and Anthony Bateman's developmental perspectives (Fonagy and Bateman 2008) all influenced the GPM approach. It first became identified as a distinctive model of therapy in a case report in *The American Journal of Psychiatry*, in which it served to provide a foil against which interventions directed by Kernberg's transference-focused psychotherapy (Clarkin et al. 2007) and Bateman and Fonagy's MBT (Bateman and Fonagy 2006) could be compared (Gunderson et al. 2007). The editor of the journal, Bob Michaels, suggested that the pragmatic eclectic treatment that I (J.G.G.) was providing actually represented a third form of treatment. It turns out he was right, but GPM's claims to legitimacy as a bona fide model for treating BPD needed to wait until GPM integrated BPD's genetic contribution, elaborated a theory of interpersonal hypersensitivity (Gunderson and Lyons-Ruth 2008), and, most importantly, received empirical support from McMain et al. (2009). GPM as it currently stands also integrates medication management. This is done with full recognition that the actual benefits from medications are questionable, although we also recognize that in the prevailing health care systems, almost all patients with BPD will be given medications. It is pragmatic then to do what is possible to make these medications useful rather than to have their prescribing be uninformed or conducted by independent providers.

The specificity of GPM for BPD has two major advantages. The first is that it does not get unduly distracted by signs and symptoms such as impulsive acts or emotional outbursts. Rather, it maintains a focus on the core personality disorder issues related to interpersonal relationships. The centrality of interpersonal relationships in BPD has been recognized in most of the clinical literature. Similarly, the centrality of interpersonal relationships to personality disorders is now usefully recognized in the alternative proposal for personality disorder diagnosis in DSM-5 (American Psychiatric Association 2013). BPD's characteristically troubled and unstable interpersonal relationships best distinguish this disorder from all others (Gunderson and Lyons-Ruth 2008). A second advantage is that treatments for BPD require a focus on its symptoms as a basis for treating other comorbidities instead of vice versa. The history of BPD has been one in which treatments designed for other disorders—for example, psychoanalysis for neuroses, antidepressants for depression, and mood stabilizers for bipolar disorder—have been given to patients with BPD but with harmful results.

GPM began with a utilitarian once-weekly individual-session format meant specifically for adult patients with BPD. It then became apparent that GPM was well suited for use as an initial intervention at the early stages of the development of BPD, and therefore the use of more intensive specialist care could be reserved for nonresponders (see Appendix B, "Stepped Care Model" [Choi-Kain et al. 2016]). It has been rewarding to learn about the development of other applications of GPM. Those applications populate this book. The first part of this book considers the applications of GPM to general hospital as well as psychiatric inpatient and outpatient treatment settings. The second part considers the use of GPM by different psychiatric and nonpsychiatric providers. The third part considers GPM's implementation in brief format and for narcissistic personality disorder as well as in integration with other evidence-based therapies for BPD. The range of applications described in this book means that you will not necessarily read this book from start to finish. Rather, some chapters will have immediate relevance to your clinical work, whereas others can rest as reserve resources to be read as clinical exposure changes. Our goal is that you will find this book useful and entertaining. We hope it will lend confidence, structure, and specificity to your care of patients with BPD so that your efforts feel rewarding. If that occurs, we predict that the reluctance and usual anxieties many clinicians have when working with patients with BPD will eventually diminish and be replaced with the sort of general good concern you have for any other patient who needs and deserves your care.

References

American Psychiatric Association: Diagnostic and Statistical Manual of Mental Disorders, 5th Edition. Arlington, VA, American Psychiatric Association, 2013

American Psychiatric Association Practice Guidelines: Practice guideline for the treatment of patients with borderline personality disorder. Am J Psychiatry 158 (10 suppl):1–52, 2001 11665545

Batemen A, Fonagy P: Mentalization-Based Treatment for Borderline Personality Disorder: A Practical Guide. New York, Oxford University Press, 2016

Bateman A, Fonagy P: Randomized controlled trial of outpatient mentalization-based treatment versus structured clinical management for borderline personality disorder. Am J Psychiatry 166(12):1355–1364, 2009 19833787

Bateman AW, Krawitz R (eds): Borderline Personality Disorder: An Evidence-Based Guide for Generalist Mental Health Professionals. Oxford, UK, Oxford University Press, 2013

Chanen AM, Jovev M, Djaja D, et al: Screening for borderline personality disorder in outpatient youth. J Pers Disord 22(4):353–364, 2008 18684049

Chaput YJA, Lebel MJ: Demographic and clinical profiles of patients who make multiple visits to psychiatric emergency services. Psychiatr Serv 58(3):335–341, 2007 17325106

Choi-Kain LW, Albert EB, Gunderson JG: Evidence-based treatments for borderline personality disorder: implementation, integration, and stepped care. Harv Rev Psychiatry 24(5):342–356, 2016 27603742

Choi-Kain LW, Finch EF, Masland SR, et al: What works in the treatment of borderline personality disorder. Curr Behav Neurosci Rep 4(1):21–30, 2017 28331780

Clarkin JF, Levy KN, Lenzenweger MF, Kernberg OF: Evaluating three treatments for borderline personality disorder: a multiwave study. Am J Psychiatry 164(6):922–928, 2007 17541052

Crawford MJ, Sanatinia R, Barrett B, et al: The clinical effectiveness and cost-effectiveness of lamotrigine in borderline personality disorder: a randomized placebo-controlled trial. Am J Psychiatry 175(8):756–764, 2018 29621901

Fonagy P, Bateman A: The development of borderline personality disorder—a mentalizing model. J Pers Disord 22(1):4–21, 2008 18312120

Gross R, Olfson M, Gameroff M, et al: Borderline personality disorder in primary care. Arch Intern Med 162(1):53–60, 2002 11784220

Gunderson JG: Borderline Personality Disorder. Washington DC, American Psychiatric Press, 1984

Gunderson JG: The emergence of a generalist model to meet public health needs for patients with borderline personality disorder. Am J Psychiatry 173(5):452–458, 2016 27133405

Gunderson JG, Choi-Kain LW: Medication management for patients with borderline personality disorder. Am J Psychiatry 175(8):709–711, 2018 30064243

Gunderson JG, Links P: Handbook of Good Psychiatric Management for Borderline Personality Disorder. Washington, DC, American Psychiatric Publishing, 2014

Gunderson JG, Lyons-Ruth K: BPD's interpersonal hypersensitivity phenotype: a gene-environment-developmental model. J Pers Disord 22(1):22–41, 2008 18312121

Gunderson JG, Bateman A, Kernberg O: Alternative perspectives on psychodynamic psychotherapy of borderline personality disorder: the case of "Ellen." Am J Psychiatry 164(9):1333–1339, 2007 17728417

Gunderson JG, Stout RL, McGlashan TH, et al: Ten-year course of borderline personality disorder: psychopathology and function from the Collaborative Longitudinal Personality Disorders Study. Arch Gen Psychiatry 68(8):827–837, 2011 21464343

Gunderson JG, Fruzzetti A, Unruh B, et al: Competing theories of borderline personality disorder. J Pers Disord 32(2):148–167, 2018 29561723

Kernberg O: Borderline personality organization. J Am Psychoanal Assoc 15(3):641–685, 1967 4861171

Korzekwa MI, Dell PF, Links PS, et al: Estimating the prevalence of borderline personality disorder in psychiatric outpatients using a two-phase procedure. Compr Psychiatry 49(4):380–386, 2008 18555059

Linehan M: Cognitive-Behavioral Treatment of Borderline Personality Disorder. New York, Guilford, 1993

Linehan MM, Korslund KE, Harned MS, et al: Dialectical behavior therapy for high suicide risk in individuals with borderline personality disorder: a randomized clinical trial and component analysis. JAMA Psychiatry 72(5):475–482, 2015 25806661

Makel MC, Plucker JA, Hegarty B: Replications in psychology research: how often do they really occur? Perspect Psychol Sci 7(6):537–542, 2012 26168110

McMain SF, Links PS, Gnam WH, et al: A randomized trial of dialectical behavior therapy versus general psychiatric management for borderline personality disorder. Am J Psychiatry 166(12):1365–1374, 2009 19755574

McMain SF, Guimond T, Streiner DL, et al: Dialectical behavior therapy compared with general psychiatric management for borderline personality disorder: clinical outcomes and functioning over a 2-year follow-up. Am J Psychiatry 169(6):650–661, 2012 22581157

Tomko RL, Trull TJ, Wood PK, et al: Characteristics of borderline personality disorder in a community sample: comorbidity, treatment utilization, and general functioning. J Pers Disord 28(5):734–750, 2014 25248122

Zanarini MC, Frankenburg FR, Reich DB, et al: Attainment and stability of sustained symptomatic remission and recovery among patients with borderline personality disorder and Axis II comparison subjects: a 16-year prospective follow-up study. Am J Psychiatry 169(5):476–483, 2012 22737693

Zimmerman M, Chelminski I, Young D: The frequency of personality disorders in psychiatric patients. Psychiatr Clin North Am 31(3):405–420, vi, 2008 18638643

PART I
Clinical Services

Chapter 2

Inpatient Psychiatric Units

John G. Gunderson, M.D.
Brian A. Palmer, M.D., M.P.H.

Because patients with borderline personality disorder (BPD) constitute about 20%–25% of all psychiatric admissions, they represent a very costly component of mental health services (Soeteman et al. 2008; Zimmerman et al. 2008). They constitute 9% of all emergency department visits and 50% of all recurrently suicidal patients in emergency departments (Hong 2016). Their hospitalizations rarely occur as single episodes. Patients with BPD have an average of 14.3 weeks of hospitalization, compared with 2.4 weeks for patients with major depressive disorder, and they have nearly five times as many hospitalizations (Bender et al. 2001). More than two-thirds are rehospitalized by 2 years, and two-thirds of those will have had multiple intervening hospitalizations (Zanarini et al. 2004). The severe depression, recurrent suicide attempts, and/or self-endangering acts that trigger most BPD admissions are not responsive to medication control. Ironically, many of these patients will eventually remit, and once this occurs the disorder rarely relapses and their hospitalizations become increasingly rare.

The prevailing and persistent wisdom about hospital care for patients with BPD includes avoiding hospitalization when possible and making stays as brief as possible (Gunderson and Links 2008; Quaytman and Sharfstein 1997; Sederer and Thorbeck 1986). This practice is driven by the knowledge that poorly managed hospitalizations can be harmful to patients with BPD and disruptive for other patients (Knight 1953). The primary and universal value of hospitalizations involves its holding function, which dramatically improves the safety and limits the self-endangering behaviors of all patients. This function is not therapeutic in a positive sense; it is used to prevent "unsafe" action from occurring. Feeling held explains why patients with BPD who have high levels of depression at hospital admission improve more dramatically than depressed patients without BPD (Yoshimatsu et al. 2015). Decreasing suicidality and depression can obviously benefit patients with BPD, and often repeatedly, with subsequent hospitalizations. The caveat is that the containment function of hospitalization is often concretely interpreted by patients with BPD as lifesaving, and thus hospital care can become an addictive solution to basic survival. Containment also causes the hospital to serve as an asylum—a respite from life's stressors. The asylum function means that hospitalization can offer the appealing secondary gain of escaping unwanted responsibilities. Because hospitalizations for patients with BPD have these potentials to be harmful, it is more important that inpatient units offer services that are explicitly designed to serve their particular needs than it is for other diagnostic groups (Gunderson 1978). For patients with BPD, successful hospitalizations depend on hospitals performing their positive functions as container and asylum while actively minimizing the detrimental potential inherent in these functions.

Patients with BPD often enter mental health care through admissions to inpatient care. It is our impression that what then happens within psychiatric hospitals can greatly influence the subsequent course for patients with BPD, including their rates of readmission and their time to remission. Hospitalization not only can impact the course of BPD but also can have a significant effect on establishing mental health professionals' attitudes about this disorder. For many of these professionals, their primary exposure to this disorder often occurs in this context.

TABLE 2–1.	Principles to ensure effective hospital stays for patients with borderline personality disorder
Psychoeducation	Provide diagnostic disclosure.
	Explain interpersonal hypersensitivity model.
	Explain limited benefit of medications.
Structure	Provide structure through psychoeducation, goal setting, multiple hours of daily groups, homework, etc.
	Avoid unstructured milieus, which can be actively harmful.
Focusing on patient's life stressors	Be proactive in identifying these stressors.
	Involve family and/or romantic partners.
	Address stressors in groups, too.
Aftercare planning	Schedule planning, including safety planning, for first week after discharge.
	Involve patient in a group (i.e., Alcoholics Anonymous, church, structured outpatient therapy).

In this chapter, we first describe the uses and misuses of hospitals and then describe the application of good psychiatric management (GPM; Gunderson and Links 2014) for a usual course of hospitalization (typically from 3 to 10 days). We propose specific ways in which inpatient milieus can provide positive and even enduring benefits while minimizing the hospital's potential for harmful effects on the patients with BPD or on others.

How to Make Hospitalizations Effective

In this section, we discuss four principles that can assure that hospital stays will be helpful for patients with BPD. These principles, summarized in Table 2–1, are psychoeducation, structure, focusing on the patient's life stressors, and aftercare planning.

Psychoeducation

All hospitalized patients with BPD stand to benefit from psychoeducation about their disorder. An unapologetic disclosure of the diagnosis should be a standard aspect of initiating hospital treatment for all patients with BPD. Psychoeducation begins with the BPD diagnosis, followed by an explanation of the handicaps of interpersonal hypersensitivity and the limited role of medications (for psychoeducational scripts, see Gunderson and Links 2014).

Disclosure of the diagnosis can comfortably be done by reviewing DSM-5 (American Psychiatric Association 2013). After reviewing the individual criteria of BPD, a narrative explanation can enhance the patient's understanding of the diagnosis (Figure 2–1). This task involves the patient and is usually a validating experience for patients with BPD. Disclosure of the diagnosis should not be delayed for stabilization of co-occurring disorders (Case et al. 2007; Morey et al. 2010). Patients and families are reassured by knowing that they are not alone and that there exists a large body of knowledge about this disorder. They are enlightened by an education about the origins of BPD (specifically recognition of its heritability), its usual course (the fact that most remit and do not relapse), and its treatability. This psychoeducation diminishes the patients' sense of alienation and aloneness, offers more hope for their future, encourages trust in the clinician's ability to help, and improves their compliance with proposed treatments. In other words, the benefits for patients with BPD are immediate, broad, and impressive.

Inpatient physicians frequently diagnose a mood or anxiety disorder as the primary diagnosis on admission of a patient with BPD. Although mood and anxiety disorders are frequently comorbid, they are very rarely the reason a patient with BPD is admitted to the hospital. Focusing on these diagnoses sets up a hospitalization that inappropriately emphasizes medications. Worse, deemphasizing BPD deprives patients of the benefits they deserve and prevents the appropriate focus on interpersonal hypersensitivity, emotion regulation skills, and life stressors outside of the hospital—including active and robust discharge planning. Most problematically, the diagnosis of a mood or anxiety disorder rather than BPD frames the solution as external as opposed to internal to the patient; that is, an undue focus is placed on medications and the prescriber, while the patient's responsibility to take care of himself or herself more effectively with better coping skills is neglected. Identifying BPD as the primary diagnosis and developing a treatment plan specific to BPD care is an essential first step. BPD can absolutely be made as a primary hospital diagnosis. In fact, for Medicare patients, BPD falls under DRG 883 (diagnosis-related group for disorders of personality and impulse control), which is reimbursed at a higher rate than DRG 885 (diagnosis-related group for psychoses), the category that includes major depressive disorder.

All patients with BPD will also benefit from psychoeducation about how their interpersonal hypersensitivity is a central symptom of their dis-

People with BPD are born with a genetic disposition to be highly sensitive and reactive to their caretakers. They are more apt to attribute rejection or anger to parental behaviors than are other children. They have usually grown up feeling that they were unfairly treated and that they did not get the attention or care they needed. They resent this and, as young adults, they hope to establish a relationship with someone who can make up to them for what they feel is missing. The desired relationship is exclusive, setting in motion intense reactions to real or perceived slights, rejections, or separations. Predictably, both their unrealistic expectations and their intense reactions cause such relationships to fail. When this happens, people with BPD will feel rejected or abandoned, and they cannot resolve their anger about being treated unfairly and their fear that they are bad and deserved the rejection. Both conclusions can lead them to become self-destructive. Their anger about being mistreated or their shame about being bad or their self-destructive behaviors can evoke guilty or protective feelings in others. Such guilt or rescuing responses from others validate the borderline person's unrealistically negative perceptions of mistreatment and sustain their unrealistically high expectations of having their needs met. Thus, the cycle is apt to repeat itself.

FIGURE 2–1. Script for diagnostic disclosure for borderline personality disorder (BPD).

Source. Excerpt from Gunderson JG, Links PS: *Handbook of Good Psychiatric Management for Borderline Personality Disorder.* Washington, DC, American Psychiatric Publishing, 2014, pp. 23–24. Copyright © 2014 American Psychiatric Publishing. Used with permission.

order (Gunderson and Lyons-Ruth 2008). Receiving this education early in the hospitalization process helps keep patients focused on the interpersonal stresses they need to address (discussed later), while also providing a marker for their understanding of the problematic interactions they predictably will have as inpatients. Interpersonal hypersensitivity explains why patients with BPD get such rapid symptom relief from being held and why the prospect of moving out of the hospital reactivates their symptoms. It predicts their excessive reactivity to even modest signals of disappointment, irritation, or rejection. It also predicts their efforts to find exclusive relationships within which they hope to avoid such experiences. Staff can then explain that the patients' efforts to attain such exclusive relationships are unrealistic and that such efforts foreclose the possibility of stable and satisfactory partnerships. This information does not by any means solve the problem, but awareness of this issue is a necessary prelude to patients' making the necessary effort to change. It is helpful to patients, as well as their significant others, to consider that this interpersonal hypersensitivity may be genetically determined and thereby has made patients' interactions with caretakers exceptionally difficult from early in life. This awareness usefully diminishes parent blaming and the hostility it triggers from vilified parents.

A third essential component of the BPD patient's psychoeducation concerns explaining the limited benefits of medications. Patients often do not welcome this information because this message means that their getting well will depend on changing their relationships and learning self-control. One of the most common and pernicious errors in hospital treatments of patients with BPD is that additional medications are prescribed when the existing medications are not helping. Hospitalized patients with BPD who have already received psychiatric care as outpatients will typically have had prior treatment with antidepressants, anxiolytics, and mood stabilizers (Zanarini et al. 2004). After disclosing and consolidating the BPD diagnosis, inpatient physicians should inform patients that medications serve only an adjunctive role, a fact that will help explain why these medications have failed to be very helpful. A sequel to this discussion is to enlist the patient as a collaborator in reviewing his or her current medications and planning changes. (For example, patients should be weaned from antidepressants when they have proven ineffective for BPD depression and from benzodiazepines because they are usually harmfully disinhibiting and often addictive.)

Structure

As noted, the hospital milieu needs to be designed by the unit's leaders to maximize therapeutic potential for patients with BPD and minimize the potential for harmful effects. For patients with BPD, this means that the milieu needs to be highly structured. One of the earliest observations about inpatients with BPD was that they behave better with structure and worse in its absence (Knight 1953). Their reputation for being noncompliant, resistant to treatment, and intractable developed in large part from the horrors that occurred when the patients were given unstructured treatments. This same regressive phenomenon was evident in their lapses into paranoid or disengaged states when given unstructured psychological tests (Carr et al. 1979). Although structured proactive milieus are better for all psychiatric inpatients, they are more critical for patients with BPD because unstructured milieus are actively harmful to them (i.e., unstructured milieus unwittingly foster angry impulsive behavior or crises that harm others).

Structure offers a predictable organization of a patient's time and place. It is neither invasive nor neglectful—it is impersonal. Valuable ways to initiate structure in an inpatient program include the early psychoeducation as described and the establishment of goals. Although short-term goals within the hospital stay can be useful in the GPM model, these should follow *after* identifying and validating the BPD patient's predictably primary longer-term life goal of finding a stable and loving partner. Appreciating this primary goal will help the patient be motivated to work on shorter-term goals that will make this primary goal possible.

Other essential forms of structure are establishing a busy schedule, including 4 or more hours of group sessions daily with clear expectations about attendance and participation. The governing schedule and the governing expectations should be handed out to new admissions with visibly posted reminders. Other ways to increase structure include having clear rules and policies (e.g., a privilege system) with explicitly mandatory and prohibited social activities and regular homework (safety plans, self-assessments, autobiography, chain analyses).

A poster on the patient's wall identifying phases in his or her pathway of care, with behaviorally specific progress required to advance to the next phase, can be helpful. For example, phase 1 may include managing personal safety and following unit rules, phase 2 may include a thoughtful chain analysis of what led to the hospitalization, and phase 3 may include learning skills or strategies to address the problems identified in phase 2. Phase 4 can include establishing a schedule for the week after hospitalization, developing a crisis plan, and completing preparations for discharge (Figure 2–2).

Structures imposed by the milieu will expose a patient's problems with reliability and compliance. When such problems are identified, they should be discussed as maladaptive—*not* for the milieu, but for the patient's chances of attaining the partnerships he or she seeks. This deliberately and explicitly keeps the milieu's rules and expectations impersonal and helps establish the staff's focus on helping patients improve their lives outside the hospital. Again, the rationale for structure needs to be explicit. The rationale is not for the patient to be a "good patient." Instead, it is to help patients achieve more satisfactory lives.

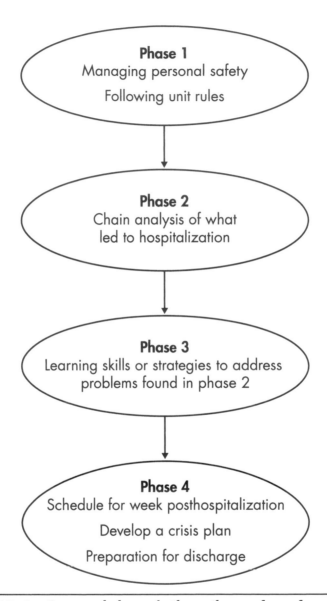

FIGURE 2–2.   Proposed phases in the pathway of care for a patient with borderline personality disorder.

Focus on Life Stressors

Sometimes, a focus on life stressors—for example, disclosure of sexual orientation, leaving an abusive partner, or finding less stressful work—can lead to early and lasting remissions (Gunderson et al. 2003). Maintaining the focus of patients with BPD on the problems in living that led to their admission—and that they will likely face again when they leave—is a second way (in addition to establishing structure) to delimit the potential harm of hospitals while enhancing their potential for positive effects. Maintaining focus on life stressors is often not easy. Typically, patients with BPD do not want to talk about real-life problems because these are associated with reminders of rejections or failures they would prefer to ignore. Getting patients to address their real-life problems requires initiative and commitment by the inpatient staff.

Inpatient staff should proactively engage patients with BPD in planning ways to diminish the stressors that prompted their admission. As noted in the introduction to this chapter, suicide attempts or other dangerous self-destructive behaviors usually precede admission. However, the stressors that trigger such behaviors are usually interpersonal experiences of real or perceived rejection or loss of interpersonal support (Brodsky et al. 2006; Yen et al. 2005). Adverse interpersonal events also trigger dissociation, devaluation, promiscuity, substance abuse, anger, depression, and panic attacks (Gunderson and Lyons-Ruth 2008). Therefore, whenever such symptoms emerge, recent interpersonal stressors can be assumed to have been present and should be actively identified by staff.

Inviting the involvement of the significant other(s) of the patient with BPD is a meaningful way to sustain a focus on the patient's life stressors. It is particularly important to involve anyone with whom the patient cohabitates, including romantic partners and parents. If patients object to such contacts, they should be told that the goal is to help their important others to better understand them and their BPD diagnosis. Patients should also be told they are welcome to participate in the meetings with significant others if they wish. If these clarifications do not placate the objections, then hospital staff may need to insist on such contacts. This insistence can be justified whenever the patient's hospitalization includes the issue of suicidality. Clinicians are often reluctant to use the intervention of involving significant other(s) because they are unaware of this possibility, are hoping to "build an alliance," or perhaps are just hoping to avoid the patient's predictably angry response. The alliance that hospital staff can establish with an inpatient with BPD within the usual 1–2 weeks of hospitalization is not the same as the alliance that a psychotherapist tries to develop. Clinicians in charge of overseeing inpatients with BPD can establish an alliance based in their displaying expertise (e.g., through psychoeducation), compassion, and good judgment, which can actually prove them to be helpful. An alliance cannot be expected to develop from being compliant with or validating the BPD patient's desires and feelings.

Another way to keep patients focused on their real-life problems is to emphasize these issues in the groups they are required to attend. As noted in the previous discussion on structure, 4 or more hours of group sessions a day should be required. Psychological growth is usually too lofty a goal within short-term hospital stays. Structured groups that focus on real-life issues are of most value. Self-assessment groups in which patients rotate discussing their current situational stressors are ideal. Another valuable type of group involves skills training. Attempting to teach all the components of dialectical behavior therapy (DBT) skills (Linehan 2015) is too much. Specific skills training in crisis management, safety planning, or self-soothing is particularly suitable. Other useful types of groups are those that focus on living situations, family issues, and school or vocational decisions. Because patients with BPD often prefer avoiding these issues, group leaders need to be active in selecting the topics, limiting digressions, enlisting and reinforcing active participation, and distributing attention. Additional privileges, such as off-unit status, should be contingent on meaningful engagement in group sessions. Groups can be so essential to making hospital care useful for patients with BPD that persistent nonparticipation should raise consideration of contingencies such as limiting access to phones, video games, or television; confining patients to their rooms; or even suspending hospitalization. This approach challenges patients who are using the hospital to avoid or escape life without engaging in treatment. A patient's hospitalization needs to either become effective or end; a patient's path to staying longer becomes contingent on meaningful participation in treatment.

Aftercare Planning

On average, a patient hospitalized for suicidal behaviors has a rate of suicide in the 3 months after hospitalization that is 200 times the global rate (Chung et al. 2017). Inadequate aftercare magnifies the likelihood of suicide, as well as relapse and readmission of discharged patients with BPD. It has already been emphasized that a hospital's therapeutic activities need not await extensive evaluations. The same is true for aftercare: plans for the patient's aftercare can and should begin with the intake interviews. Intake interviews should identify hypotheses about 1) who and what are the patient's major life stressors, 2) what additional social or therapeutic supports may be needed, and 3) how school or vocational reentry can be facilitated.

The hospital group program and individual work with the team should, at a minimum, ensure that every patient with BPD leaves with a schedule for the first week after hospitalization, as well as a written safety plan that includes specific skills that the patient can use. More will be said about this issue later in this section. Patients and families should be educated about the fact that patients with BPD tend to become more symptomatic during transitions, and therefore everyone needs to prepare for the transition home; far from being a honeymoon period that families and patients often desire, this is period of real risk that can and should be anticipated.

Developing an adequate outpatient treatment plan is an essential but challenging function that hospital staff provide. Sadly, most hospitalized patients with BPD will have had little, inconsistent, or inappropriate preexisting outpatient care. Identifying such limitations is often quite easy; however, resolving such limitations usually is not. Most clinicians dislike or are untrained in treating patients with BPD, and evidence-based therapies for BPD are rarely available. Finding acceptable providers is therefore often very difficult. It is valuable to know that experienced clinicians of all professions are likely to be satisfactory (Keuroghlian et al. 2016). Less experienced clinicians can do well if they are practical, are sensibly pragmatic, and have supervisory support. Using a hospital outpatient service can be useful. Unfortunately, many outpatient clinics place patients with BPD in a psychotherapy clinic, where they receive unstructured psychodynamic therapies, or in a mood disorder clinic, where they receive medication management. Both of these placements are likely to be harmful. Red flags should be waved for the following: clinicians who disagree with the BPD diagnosis, who believe such patients need intensive psychotherapy, who want to treat the comorbid disorder and avoid "BPD issues," or who require that an unfeasible team (e.g., a family therapist and psychoanalyst) be added.

Because doing so is easy, referring a discharged patient with BPD back to his or her prior provider has obvious appeal to busy hospital clinicians. Still, returning a patient to a prior treater who has not been helpful should be done with caution. Primary care providers have become comfortable managing major depression with medications, but BPD management necessarily relies on strategies that deemphasize the primacy of medications while insisting on adherence when they are used. Sometimes, giving outpatient providers the correct diagnosis in a nonaccusatory or noncritical way will help them become more effective. Most primary care physicians will be appreciative of information about the BPD diagnosis and ways the knowledge can guide their work.

A particularly valuable outpatient strategy is to involve the patient with BPD in a community-based self-help group, such as Alcoholics Anonymous, or any structured outpatient group therapy. Groups based on shared interests or values, such as volunteer activities, meetups, religious organizations, and continued education can also provide structured local support. If the hospital has an outpatient clinic, the hospital should establish a policy that all patients with BPD are required to participate in groups.

The major strategies for improving aftercare have already been embedded in the prior descriptions of good hospital care. Involving and educating patients with BPD and their significant others is a critical step as part of aftercare support. Parents and significant others should be enrolled in online educational or support websites or, better yet, attend parent groups or seek parent guidance or coaching (for resources, see www.borderlinepersonalitydisorder.com or www.borderlinepersonality disorder.org/family-connections/). A second strategy has been to identify the outpatient stressors and actively help the patient find ways to diminish these. Foremost in aftercare planning is helping the patient arrange structures and activities in daily life that are likely to be satisfying and in which they are likely to succeed; for example, taking one or a few classes or doing volunteer work are often incremental steps that should precede full employment or school.

A basic message is that patients with BPD and their families need to be collaborators in developing and evaluating aftercare options. It does them no favors for providers to uncritically support aftercare options because of accessibility and feasibility. Helping patients and families understand the limitations of available aftercare options is a far more valuable lesson than encouraging false hopes.

As indicated earlier, a safety plan should be prepared as discharge approaches. The plan should address four key areas: 1) identifying when the plan will be used (the provider should work with the patient to help identify markers that he or she is in crisis); 2) identifying skills that will be used, ideally skills that the patient has learned and practiced in the hospital; 3) identifying who the patient or significant others will call if efforts to use learned skills do not sufficiently mitigate the crisis (the list should include the National Suicide Prevention Lifeline phone number: 800-273-8255); and 4) identifying when and how the patient or significant others will access a medical professional if prior efforts have not been sufficient. In addition to the creation of a safety plan, the following are two easily structured inpatient group activities: 1) the development of a list of reasons for living and 2) the creation of a "hope box" or "survival kit" that can assist the patient in managing safety after discharge.

Case Vignette

The following case description includes decision points, each of which has several alternate responses listed at the end of the case. The reader will rate each response in terms of its level of helpfulness. Discussions of alternative responses follow.

Marsha is a 26-year-old single white female who is admitted to the psychiatric unit of a general hospital for her third time in the past year. She is admitted from the emergency department at 11 P.M. after a Prozac overdose of modest dangerousness. As the on-call resident, you initiate the intake interview upon Marsha's arrival on the inpatient unit. Marsha, who appears only mildly upset, asks whether she could first get something to eat. You direct her to the kitchen, where fruit and cereal are available. After 10 minutes, you go to fetch her. When you remind her that she needs to complete the intake interview, she responds irritably, "You know I've been here before. Can't you just check my records?" You respond, "I can appreciate that this interview may not be welcome, but it is required of both of us. I will try to complete it as quickly as possible." In the interview, Marsha discloses recurrent depressions, angry outbursts, binge eating, and a history of erratic substance abuse, including both the anxiolytic and the stimulant prescribed by her primary care provider. She identifies the recent rejection by her boyfriend as the trigger for her overdose. The diagnoses of BPD and substance abuse that were made during her prior hospitalizations are thereby confirmed.

Shortly after completing the interview, Marsha approaches the nursing office and asks for a sleeping medicine. The nurse tells her this is an issue to be taken up at morning rounds. Marsha angrily stalks back to her room, where she is restless, complaining several times about the 15-minute checks, before eventually falling asleep. Morning rounds focus on management of Marsha's medication. [**Decision Point 1**]

In your initial treatment planning interview, you, as Marsha's inpatient psychiatrist, review the meaning of the BPD diagnosis, its genetic contributions, and its usual course. Though Marsha is comfortable with the BPD diagnosis, she is unfamiliar with and greatly interested in the information about its genetics and course. You then ask Marsha about her life outside the hospital. She indicates she has alternated living with her parents and her boyfriend until she and her boyfriend recently broke up. She complains, "Now I will need to live with my parents. I hate that!" Except for occasional babysitting jobs, she has been unemployed for 6 months. Before that, and despite having a junior college education, she had a variety of low-paying unskilled jobs. She says she has given "100% of myself to my boyfriend" and has had little other social life, adding, "I just want to get married." With respect to her treatment, she indicates that her primary care provider is "wonderful. He reviews my depression, answers my requests for medications, and seems to really care about me. We don't talk much about my life. He knows I hate my family, but he probably doesn't even know about my boyfriend." [**Decision Point 2**]

Within the day's scheduled group therapies, Marsha is quiet and guarded. When asked, she says she has never felt comfortable in group therapies. In contrast, and despite her lack of sleep, you observe that during her free times Marsha comfortably socializes with other patients. [**Decision Point 3**]

In a late afternoon meeting with the unit's social worker, Marsha becomes irritated and resists answering questions about her family. She complains that her father is weak and her mother is mean and reiterates that she hates having to live with them. When asked if she thought her mother loved her, she says, "That's what she says, but she never has anything nice to say about me!" She notes that her mother has disapproved of her recent boyfriend and all her previous boyfriends. About her boyfriend, she says, "I fell in love. He was so talented and charming. He claimed he loved me, but after a while we didn't talk much. Sometimes we did drugs together." It turned out that this boyfriend, whom she hoped to marry, was a musician who worked part-time at a filling station and had a serious drug habit. When asked, she denies permission for the social worker to contact her parents. This refusal is discussed at rounds the next morning. [**Decision Point 4**]

Marsha gives her consent to the social worker's contacting her parents after learning that its purpose is to help them understand BPD with the goal of trying to make their living together less stressful. She also agrees with her psychiatrist's suggestion that she taper off her anxiolytic and stimulant. On the other hand, despite having been advised of the importance of group participation, Marsha continues to remain quiet in her mandatory interpersonal, DBT, and arts/crafts groups. Worse, she sometimes disrupts these group therapies with whispered exchanges with another patient, Jennifer, with whom she has quickly developed a "best friend" relationship. [**Decision Point 5**]

Because of Marsha's ongoing problem with employment, a meeting with a vocational counselor is arranged. Marsha discusses this plan with a mental health worker, questioning how it might help. "I know I should find work if I'm going to be able to move out of my parents' house, but there's no job I want that anyone would hire me for." The mental health worker says, "Maybe it will be different this time." Marsha responds by changing the subject. [**Decision Point 6**] After further discussions, the inpatient staff and vocational counselor conclude that Marsha should start with a job that will not stress her and she might like work that involves taking care of people or animals.

By the fourth day, Marsha's participation in groups has improved. She voices insight into her fearfulness about becoming independent and is active in identifying ("exposing") this issue in other patients. She has also begun to talk more openly about her boyfriend, and when she gets feedback that he is "a real loser," she seems to appreciate how self-destructive that relationship has been. [**Decision Point 7**]

After the subject of leaving the hospital was initiated on her fifth day, Marsha voiced suicidal ideas and made an aborted effort to contact her ex-boyfriend. She also requested an increase in her Prozac. [**Decision Point 8**] Staff interpreted these as signs of her predictable fears about leaving the security and support of the hospital, and Marsha accepted their interpretation. This indicated that she had begun to incorporate the understanding of herself as someone who wants to be cared for and who fears more independence. Although she remained impatient and irritable with her mother, she could recognize that her parents were providing supports she needed. In response to learning about Marsha's illness (and its handicaps), her parents appeared to respond less critically to her and with conscious effort to validate her complaints. They enrolled in a parent support group. With the help of the social worker, Marsha made an appointment with a potential Alcoholics Anonymous sponsor and with a dog-walking agency. In other respects, her aftercare was unsettled. She wanted to continue with her primary care provider, and no other provider was identified.

Decision Points: Alternative Responses

Rate each response in terms of its level of helpfulness with a rating of 1 (will be helpful), 2 (possibly helpful, continuing reservations), or 3 (not helpful—or even harmful).

1. In the discussion of Marsha's medications at morning rounds, you, as the psychiatrist in charge of her care, should

   A. Try to find a medication that will help her sleep.
   B. Propose weaning her from the anxiolytic she is taking.
   C. Look to augment the Prozac she has been taking with another selective serotonin reuptake inhibitor (SSRI).
   D. Validate the nursing staff when they express apprehension about her likely noncompliance.
   E. Raise the question of whether medications can be helpful to her.

2. In response to Marsha's report about her outpatient life, you should

   A. Convey support for her current outpatient care.
   B. Tell Marsha that to fulfill her hopes for a future stable marital partnership, she will first need to take better care of herself.
   C. Ask Marsha whether she would like to change things about herself.
   D. Explain (psychoeducation) how attaining stable work can make her a better candidate for marriage.

3. How might you understand the disparity between Marsha's apparent sociability and her nonparticipation in group therapies?

 A. Marsha exaggerated her distress in order to get into the hospital, but she has little interest in therapy.
 B. Marsha does not understand that active participation in groups is expected and central to the value of her inpatient stay.
 C. Marsha's lack of a social support network is not because of social anxiety.
 D. Marsha's remitted depression symptoms are due to the hospital's containment and asylum functions.

4. After hearing the social worker's report of Marsha's family alienation and drug-abusing boyfriend, you should

 A. Suggest that the social worker needs to enlist the boyfriend's involvement.
 B. Propose that family therapy would be helpful.
 C. Reluctantly conclude that the parents cannot be involved despite knowing that their collaboration is important in establishing her aftercare plan.
 D. Explain that the purpose of meeting with her parents is to provide them with psychoeducation about BPD so that they might become less stressful to her.
 E. Advise Marsha (psychoeducation) about the predictably bad outcomes of exclusive relationships.

5. In response to Marsha's continued failure to constructively use the groups and her new relationship with Jennifer, staff should

 A. Tell Marsha she will be confined to her room during scheduled groups unless she makes better use of them.
 B. Support Marsha's new friendship with Jennifer as one of the benefits that the unit takes pride in encouraging.
 C. Consider whether the types of groups being offered are well suited for patients like Marsha.
 D. Tell Marsha that the scheduled visit by her parents will be canceled unless she participates better in groups.
 E. Advise Marsha that the friendship she is forming with Jennifer follows the pattern of exclusivity that, like her relationships with past boyfriends, is self-destructive and will end unsuccessfully.

6. In response to Marsha's discouraged or uninterested response to seeing a vocational counselor, staff should

   A. Validate her recognition that work is needed so she can stop living with her parents.
   B. Help her identify a type of work that is best suited to her interests and abilities.
   C. Appreciate that seeking work will be stressful.
   D. Remind her that employment is a source of structure and self-esteem that will enhance her becoming a good partner for someone.

7. In response to Marsha's insights into her fears of independence and her improved participation in groups, you should

   A. Tell her that her insights and participation are signs of progress.
   B. Suggest that her insights into her fears of independence will prevent the issue from being activated when she leaves the hospital.
   C. Underscore how useful a group therapy can be in her aftercare.
   D. Remind her that her fears about increased independence will get activated when she leaves the hospital.

8. In response to Marsha's suicidal ideas, effort to contact her boyfriend, and request for more Prozac, you should

   A. Interpret these as regressive symptoms in response to the impending discharge.
   B. Delay the discharge plan.
   C. Remind her that fears of independence will recur whenever she leaves a supportive environment.
   D. Encourage the parents to provide a "welcome home."
   E. Contact the boyfriend and advise him to become reinvolved during Marsha's transition from the hospital.
   F. Discuss the potential placebo benefit of increasing her dose of Prozac.

Decision Points: Discussion

Numbers within brackets indicate level of helpfulness ratings.

1. In the discussion of Marsha's medications at morning rounds, you, as the psychiatrist in charge of her care, should

A. Try to find a medication that will help her sleep. [3] (It is unclear how much her insomnia is a sustained issue. Even if it is, her substance abuse should limit consideration of a hypnotic. Inpatient units are excellent places to teach sleep skills.)

B. Propose weaning her from the anxiolytic she is taking. [1] (Anxiolytics are relatively contraindicated for patients with BPD. These medications are disinhibiting and habit forming.)

C. Look to augment the Prozac she has been taking with another SSRI. [3] (The value of SSRIs is uncertain for BPD. There is no support for augmentation, and doing this adds the risks of side effects while reinforcing the patient's unrealistic expectations.)

D. Validate the nursing staff when they express apprehension about her likely noncompliance. [2] (It is true that Marsha is not likely to be reliably compliant. Still, the negative attitude of the nursing staff may signal a more basic hostility toward patients with BPD that will be harmful.)

E. Raise the question of whether medications can be helpful to her. [1] (All inpatient staff should be taught that medications have inconsistent and modest effectiveness for patients with BPD. The discussion of Marsha's medications should start from this base.)

2. In response to Marsha's report about her outpatient life, you should

A. Convey support for her current outpatient care. [3] (You certainly do not want to disparage her primary care physician, but you recognize that unmonitored medications are not helpful to Marsha. Indeed, she has gone downhill in terms of hospital use and social functioning.)

B. Tell Marsha that to fulfill her hopes for a future stable marital partnership, she will first need to take better care of herself. [1] (This is true, and Marsha needs to know it.)

C. Ask Marsha whether she would like to change things about herself. [2] (This is a good question. Should she say no, this may not mean too much. Her answer is likely to change when she is less stressed and more allied with the interviewer.)

D. Explain (psychoeducation) how attaining stable work can make her a better candidate for marriage. [1] (Yes, linking her short-term tasks, such as attaining work, to her long-term goals—a stable partnership—is invaluable incentivization. It also shows your respect for her potential.)

3. How might you understand the disparity between Marsha's apparent sociability and her nonparticipation in group therapies?

   A. Marsha exaggerated her distress in order to get into the hospital, but she has little interest in therapy. [3] (She may or may not be interested in group therapies, and she may or may not have exaggerated her distress to get hospitalized, but this perspective is hostile and pejorative. It does not appreciate Marsha's need for help and the legitimate bleakness of her life.)
   B. Marsha does not understand that active participation in groups is expected and central to the value of her inpatient stay. [1] (Unless the inpatient unit makes this explicit and/or an existing patient culture conveys this, many patients with BPD will neither expect nor understand how significant group therapies are to making their hospital stay useful.)
   C. Marsha's lack of a social support network is not because of social anxiety. [2] (We do not know. Being in a holding environment with other identifiably mentally ill peers can diminish social anxieties.)
   D. Marsha's remitted depression symptoms are due to the hospital's containment and asylum functions. [1] (Yes. This is predictable. And it is just as predictable that depressive [and anxious] symptoms will reappear as Marsha leaves this protected environment.)

4. After hearing the social worker's report of Marsha's family alienation and drug-abusing boyfriend, you should

   A. Suggest that the social worker needs to enlist the boyfriend's involvement. [2] (It seems unlikely that the boyfriend will be a constructive part of Marsha's future. Inviting his involvement could be helpful if it will help her get perspective on him or help her terminate the relationship.)
   B. Propose that family therapy would be helpful. [3] (Family therapy might be helpful after Marsha and her parents have an alliance with the treatment and after they have established an ability to see things from the other's point of view. At present, Marsha's alienation and hostility indicates that she is not ready. The parents need to be evaluated.)
   C. Reluctantly conclude that the parents cannot be involved despite knowing that their collaboration is important in establish-

ing her aftercare plan. [3] (No, it is possible that Marsha will conclude that it is in her interest to have her parents involved. Moreover, you can use her overdose to override her objection. It is very important to enlist the parents' collaboration in establishing Marsha's aftercare plan.)

D. Explain that the purpose of meeting with her parents is to provide them with psychoeducation about BPD so that they might become less stressful to her. [1] (Yes, this message is often very satisfactory. Patients with BPD often fear that you will ally with parents against them.)

E. Advise Marsha (psychoeducation) about the predictably bad outcomes of exclusive relationships. [1] (This is an essential message. It will not make the wish for such a relationship go away, but forewarned is forearmed, and most patients with BPD will know this is true. They just do not want to think about it.)

5. In response to Marsha's continued failure to constructively use the groups and her new relationship to Jennifer, staff should

A. Tell Marsha she will be confined to her room during scheduled groups unless she makes better use of them. [2] (Worth considering, but she might welcome this as an avoidance strategy.)

B. Support Marsha's new friendship with Jennifer as one of the benefits that the unit takes pride in encouraging. [3] (It is possible for short-term hospitalizations to foster friendships, but these are unlikely to be more than transient. In this case, the "friendship" is contaminated by its alienating and distracting effects.)

C. Consider whether the types of groups being offered are well suited for patients like Marsha. [1] (Yes, interpersonal, DBT, and arts/crafts groups do not focus attention on Marsha's real-life problems with social isolation, employment, and family.)

D. Tell Marsha that the scheduled visit by her parents will be canceled unless she participates better in groups. [3] (Because she is ambivalent about involving her parents, and it is very important to involve them, this strategy would be counterproductive.)

E. Advise Marsha that the friendship she is forming with Jennifer follows the pattern of exclusivity that, like her relationships with past boyfriends, is self-destructive and will end unsuccessfully. [1] (Yes, that friendship is interfering with her using the hospital and will potentially end unsuccessfully. Having this self-destructive relationship pattern activated within the milieu provides a potentially powerful learning opportunity.)

6. In response to Marsha's discouraged or uninterested response to seeing a vocational counselor, staff should

   A. Validate her recognition that work is needed so she can stop living with her parents. [1] (Yes.)
   B. Help her identify a type of work that is best suited to her interests and abilities. [1] (Although a vocational counselor will bring added skills and knowledge to vocational issues, mental health workers should be comfortable and accustomed to helping patients consider their options. Staff should consider this a basic component of what they can do. Coming from peer counselors who are themselves working underscores its importance.)
   C. Reassure Marsha that seeking work need not be stressful. [3] (This overlooks her fears of becoming independent and her past failures to find work satisfying. Validating the difficulty she will encounter will be helpful. "You can do it" reassurances are likely to irritate or shame patients with BPD.)
   D. Remind her that employment is a source of structure and self-esteem that will enhance her becoming a good partner for someone. [1] (Yes, this message is one that all inpatient staff should be familiar and comfortable with.)

7. In response to Marsha's insights into her fears of independence and her improved participation in groups, you should

   A. Tell her that her insights and participation are signs of progress. [1] (Encourage her to understand that such self-examination and disclosure are important steps toward establishing friends and better social supports.)
   B. Suggest that her insights into her fears of independence will prevent the issue from being activated when she leaves the hospital. [3] (No. This response will interfere with her ability to use staff to manage the fears constructively, such as by getting supports and planning ways to moderate these expectations.)
   C. Underscore how useful a group therapy can be in her aftercare. [1] (Marsha should be urged to include a group therapy component to her aftercare. Recognizing the value of such therapy during her hospitalization helps makes this happen.)

    D. Remind her that her fears about increased independence will get activated when she leaves the hospital. [1] (Helping her anticipate and apply her new insights in an effective intervention.)

8. In response to Marsha's suicidal ideas, effort to contact her boyfriend, and request for more Prozac, you should

    A. Interpret these as regressive symptoms in response to the impending discharge. [1] (Yes.)

    B. Delay the discharge plan. [3] (This could become necessary, but this is overreactive. A calm, thoughtful "think first" response is needed.)

    C. Remind her that fears of independence will recur whenever she leaves a supportive environment. [1] (Yes, connecting discharge discussions to her increase in symptoms should be grounded in your education about her interpersonal hypersensitivity. She has shown enough insight and curiosity that she may be able to make use of this education.)

    D. Encourage the parents to provide a "welcome home." [3] (This could be a good idea, *if* the parents feel this way; a more useful tactic will be helping the parents anticipate that she may be more symptomatic during the transition and that their efforts to provide a stable, reliable, predictable environment will be helpful.)

    E. Contact the boyfriend and advise him to become reinvolved during Marsha's transition from the hospital. [3] (Boyfriend is unlikely to be supportive of her aftercare. Involving him is probably contraindicated at this time.)

    F. Discuss the potential placebo benefit of increasing her dose of Prozac. [3] (This could be a discussion to have with Marsha but probably not at a time when she is feeling fearful about diminished support. Focusing on skills and structure is more likely to be helpful to her regardless.)

Conclusion

Table 2–1 (see section "How to Make Hospitalizations Effective") offers a summary of interventions that are suggested at the time of admission, during the patient's stay, and in preparing for discharge. These interventions might be placed in the chart for patients with BPD as a guide for staff and could even be used as a checklist by which to assess whether the hospital is following the desired protocol.

The following 10 guidelines summarize what constitutes "GPM-style" hospitalizations for BPD:

1. Keep hospitalizations as short as possible.
2. Accurately make the diagnosis of BPD and document it as the primary diagnosis when it is indeed primary.
3. Start with essential psychoeducation about the diagnosis, genetics, and course.
4. Begin therapeutic actions and aftercare planning with the initial evaluations.Identify and discuss interpersonal stressors in rounds.Then begin psychoeducation about interpersonal hypersensitivity.
5. Remember that milieus should be structured, clear, and focused on pragmatic issues of daily living, *not* on relationships within the hospital.
6. Review medications, including consideration of their limited role. Do *not* readily accept patients' wish to add medications.
7. Routinely include school (or vocational) evaluation and counseling.
8. Include patients and their families as collaborators in assessing aftercare options.
9. Challenge protests about family involvement or group participation.
10. In safety planning, anticipate the challenges associated with hospital discharge.

It bears repeating that patients with BPD have a unique potential to be harmed by services that do not take into consideration their special needs. This means that the leaders of inpatient psychiatric units need to be proactive in creating a therapeutic community suitable for patients with BPD. This effort begins by making sure that staff are well informed about the diagnosis and not governed by unfounded attitudes of pessimism and guardedness. Such negative or hostile attitudes are common and predictably harmful; this issue needs to be identified and then addressed. Unfortunately, because many clinicians still believe that BPD is an untreatable or intractable condition, they do not give the diagnosis or do so only as a last resort in frustration or futility for those patients with numerous readmissions and numerous failed medication trials.

Because optimism and compassion are uniformly helpful, these attitudes should be fostered. Education about BPD, including its genetics, course, and treatability, is the primary way to change attitudes. Sometimes such education is best provided by a consultant. Certainly, attending a GPM workshop can be effective (Keuroghlian et al. 2016). GPM is available online (see Appendix A, "Additional Resources"). Additionally, as indicated in this chapter, the unit needs to be structured and staff need to be directed to keep the attention of their patients with BPD on the interpersonal stressors that triggered their admission, those that recur within the hospital community, and those that will await them when they leave.

References

American Psychiatric Association: Diagnostic and Statistical Manual of Mental Disorders, 5th Edition. Arlington, VA, American Psychiatric Association, 2013

Bender DS, Dolan RT, Skodol AE, et al: Treatment utilization by patients with personality disorders. Am J Psychiatry 158(2):295–302, 2001 11156814

Brodsky BS, Groves SA, Oquendo MA, et al: Interpersonal precipitants and suicide attempts in borderline personality disorder. Suicide Life Threat Behav 36(3):313–322, 2006 16805659

Carr AC, Goldstein EG, Hunt HF, et al: Psychological tests and borderline patients. J Pers Assess 43(6):582–590, 1979 521887

Case BG, Biel MG, Peselow ED, et al: Reliability of personality disorder diagnosis during depression: the contribution of collateral informant reports. Acta Psychiatr Scand 115(6):487–491, 2007 17498161

Chung DT, Ryan CJ, Hadzi-Pavlovic D, et al: Suicide rates after discharge from psychiatric facilities: a systematic review and meta-analysis. JAMA Psychiatry 74(7):694–702, 2017 28564699

Gunderson JG: Defining the therapeutic processes in psychiatric milieus. Psychiatry 41(4):327–335, 1978 715093

Gunderson JG, Links PS: Borderline Personality Disorder: A Clinical Guide, 2nd Edition. Washington, DC, American Psychiatric Publishing, 2008

Gunderson JG, Links PS: Handbook of Good Psychiatric Management for Borderline Personality Disorder. Washington, DC, American Psychiatric Publishing, 2014

Gunderson JG, Lyons-Ruth K: BPD's interpersonal hypersensitivity phenotype: a gene-environment-developmental model. J Pers Disord 22(1):22–41, 2008 18312121

Gunderson JG, Bender D, Sanislow C, et al: Plausibility and possible determinants of sudden "remissions" in borderline patients. Psychiatry 66(2):111–119, 2003 12868289

Hong V: Borderline personality disorder in the emergency department: good psychiatric management. Harv Rev Psychiatry 24(5):357–366, 2016 27603743

Keuroghlian A, Palmer BA, Choi-Kain LW, et al: The effect of attending good psychiatric management (GPM) workshops on attitudes toward patients with borderline personality disorder. J Pers Disord 30(4):567–576, 2016 26111249

Knight RP: Management and psychotherapy of the borderline schizophrenic patient. Bull Menninger Clin 17(4):139–150, 1953 13066875

Linehan MM: DBT® Skills Training Manual, 2nd edition. New York, Guilford, 2015.

Morey LC, Shea MT, Markowitz JC, et al: State effects of major depression on the assessment of personality and personality disorder. Am J Psychiatry 167(5):528–535, 2010 20160004

Quaytman M, Sharfstein SS: Treatment for severe borderline personality disorder in 1987 and 1997. Am J Psychiatry 154(8):1139–1144, 1997 9247402

Sederer LI, Thorbeck J: First do no harm: short-term inpatient psychotherapy of the borderline patient. Hosp Community Psychiatry 37(7):692–697, 1986 3721435

Soeteman DI, Hakkaart-van Roijen L, Verheul R, et al: The economic burden of personality disorders in mental health care. J Clin Psychiatry 69(2):259–265, 2008 18363454

Yen S, Pagano ME, Shea MT, et al: Recent life events preceding suicide attempts in a personality disorder sample: findings from the Collaborative Longitudinal Personality Disorders Study. J Consult Clin Psychol 73(1):99–105, 2005 15709836

Yoshimatsu K, Rosen BH, Kung S, et al: Improvements in depression severity in hospitalized patients with and without borderline personality features. J Psychiatr Pract 21(3):208–213, 2015 25955263

Zanarini MC, Frankenburg FR, Hennen J, et al: Mental health service utilization by borderline personality disorder patients and Axis II comparison subjects followed prospectively for 6 years. J Clin Psychiatry 65(1):28–36, 2004 14744165

Zimmerman M, Chelminski I, Young D: The frequency of personality disorders in psychiatric patients. Psychiatr Clin North Am 31(3):405–420, vi, 2008 18638643

Chapter 3

Emergency Departments

Victor Hong, M.D.

Managing a patient with borderline personality disorder (BPD) in the emergency department (ED) setting presents unique challenges that demand a targeted, organized approach. For a cohort of patients, the ED serves less of a triage function and has become a more integral part of the overall treatment framework. Given their notable mood instability and their common suicidal and self-injurious threats and behaviors, patients with BPD frequently present to the ED (Pascual et al. 2007). The ED visit is an opportunity for providers to help the patient with BPD navigate crises, to cultivate patient insight in real time, and to offer meaningful psychoeducation. Too often, however, these opportunities are missed. Clinicians' limited understanding of how to manage BPD patients in crisis and their excessive countertransference reactions can undercut the effectiveness of the ED visit. The singular nature of patients with BPD in this setting, characterized by recurrent ED visits, increased disruptive behaviors compared with those with other diagnoses, and chronic suicide risk, warrants their consideration as a "special population" with specific treatment guidelines (Boggild et al. 2004; Chaput and Lebel 2007; Heap and Silk 2008). Furthermore, it behooves ED staff treating the patient with BPD to take great care to avoid iatrogenic harm, which occurs all too frequently in the high-pressured, fast-paced, varied, inconsistent, often crowded, and chaotic ED.

Although most ED staff are not trained in psychodynamic principles, their training should include the basic concepts of transference and counter-transference, given that the usual emotional reactions toward patients with BPD commonly lead to negative outcomes. Feelings of anger, frustration, anxiety, fear, and rescue fantasies may arise in clinicians and staff when managing patients with BPD, particularly in the high-pressure setting of the ED (Gabbard and Wilkinson 1994). Although these reactions are understandable, basing clinical responses on them is suboptimal. Providers under the influence of such reactions are likely to approach patients with BPD in a manner that patients will interpret as naïve, dismissive, or hostile, exacerbating the patients' sense of isolation and impeding the clinicians' ability to establish rapport and trust. Even seasoned clinicians may experience hopelessness based on the myth that patients with BPD do not recover and deepened by a confirmation bias that occurs after repeated negative experiences with patients with BPD, particularly with those who return to the ED again and again with seemingly the same presentation. Staff may unconsciously feel or explicitly state, "We have no hope of helping this treatment-resistant patient." If unrecognized and unmanaged, provider reactions and attitudes can color interactions with the patient and influence critically important clinical decision making. For better or worse, each clinical interaction with a patient with BPD, including brief contacts in the ED, can profoundly affect the patient's treatment course.

Clinicians are often pointed toward the use of dialectical behavior therapy (DBT) skills; however, few ED providers are trained in DBT or have even a basic facility in this modality. Good psychiatric management (GPM), with its straightforward principles and easy-to-apply guidelines, offers an alternative model that is better suited to serve ED clinicians of varying disciplines and experience levels.

Using GPM in the Emergency Department

The principles of GPM described in the handbook by Gunderson and Links (2014) largely relate to the outpatient setting, affording the clinician guidelines of how to initiate and manage ongoing treatment for BPD. The fact that these guidelines are generally geared toward longer-term treatment begs the question of how to apply GPM in the ultimate short-term treatment setting, the ED. On examination, the goodness of fit of several of the core GPM principles for use in the ED becomes clear. Given that a single patient with BPD may visit the ED multiple times or with great frequency, the ED setting becomes part of the tableau of ongoing outpatient treatment (Gunderson and Links 2014). That said, even a one-time ED visit is a good opportunity to implement effective GPM principles with the patient with BPD who is in crisis. The most relevant and helpful GPM principles applicable in the ED setting are focusing on understanding interpersonal hypersensitivity; adopting an active, authentic approach to patients; delivering psychoeducation to patients and their families; and practically managing suicidality and self-harm. A singular advantage of training ED staff in GPM principles versus other modalities is the brevity of the training itself. In a relatively brief workshop, ED staff can learn and rehearse core GPM principles and thereby increase their confidence in skillfully managing patients with BPD (Keuroghlian et al. 2016).

Diagnostic Disclosure

Diagnostic disclosure of BPD is not traditionally implemented in the ED setting; however, GPM's encouragement to do this is helpful. ED clinicians may hesitate to definitively affirm a previously undiagnosed disorder because, when in crisis, patients may demonstrate features and symptoms not characteristic of their baseline conditions. For example, many patients who do not have BPD can, while emotionally dysregulated and in an acute crisis, appear to meet the criteria for the disorder. Nonetheless, there are clear benefits to discussing a potential BPD diagnosis and sharing one's professional opinion about this possibility, particularly if multiple sources of collateral information are available and the patient's words, behaviors, and clinical history all suggest the presence of BPD. When a patient presents to the ED recurrently, affording a serial history, the diagnosis may become even clearer. Raising patients' awareness of the possibility that they have BPD while providing good psychoeducation about the disorder arms them with a set of expectations and information to discuss with their outpatient providers. Furthermore, in most cases, patients and their families are actually relieved to know of a diagnosis that is hopeful and can explain the ineffectiveness or poor outcomes of previous treatment approaches.

Psychoeducation

One of the most helpful GPM principles to apply in the ED setting is psychoeducation. On a micro level, psychoeducation can help to organize patients' thinking about their diagnosis and treatment and may help explain their feelings and behaviors. On a macro level, psychoeducation serves the public health goal of destigmatizing the disorder and minimizing myths and misperception. Learning the facts about BPD is a key step in patients' understanding of themselves and may even reduce acute symptoms (Zanarini and Frankenburg 2008). Finally, by offering people, including those in acute distress in the ED, evidence supporting the good prognosis of most patients with BPD, clinicians can realistically inspire a measure of hope for a better tomorrow.

Treatment Approach

Approaching the patient with BPD in an active, authentic manner is central to GPM, and clinicians adopting this style can be particularly effective in the ED setting. Given the high volume of patients in the ED and providers' need to expeditiously reach a sound disposition for each of them, the skilled emergency clinician must rapidly build rapport with and demonstrate trustworthiness to patients. Connecting with a patient with BPD in crisis is challenging, but this task is made easier when clinicians follow established guidelines. Intentionally demonstrating genuine concern and adopting an active interview style are important initial steps.

Given the probable interpersonal hypersensitivity of patients with BPD and the likelihood that they will meet multiple new people during their ED visit, clinicians must pay close attention to how they behave in the room. Because a more detached interpersonal style will be interpreted by patients with BPD as dismissive or rejecting, a passive approach by the clinician can impede the establishment of a therapeutic alliance and lengthen the ED stay. In contrast, when the provider is active and curious about what brought the patient with BPD to the ED, as well as what the patient's recent interpersonal experience has been and what the patient thinks about it, the provider is likely to expeditiously assist the patient through his or her crisis.

When treating patients with BPD in the ED, a provider may apologize when indicated or use humor to ease tension. By validating the high-stress situation, the frustration of a likely long wait time, and the intensity of the patient's emotions, the provider can display a sense of caring and potentially inspire more open and honest discourse about the patient's experience, the level of risk, and actions that could be most helpful.

When a patient with BPD is in the ED, the participation of the patient is crucial. However, patients may be reluctant to discuss their thoughts, may provide vague interpretations of their behaviors, or may refuse to participate in any treatment plan. Such stances may require active challenges by clinicians. Providers should consider stating frankly how their ability to help is obstructed without the patient's active cooperation. Providers can acknowledge and normalize how difficult it can be to share intimate experiences with someone unfamiliar, while, nonetheless, underscoring the importance of the patient's honest disclosure and active participation. Providers are well served to present themselves as "not knowing" and uncertain, thereby requiring the patient's assistance in filling in the gaps of missing knowledge.

Interpersonal Hypersensitivity

An important goal in any ED setting is *throughput*—that is, quickly reaching a conclusion about the appropriate treatment for the patient and assisting in arranging the necessary resources. Understanding GPM's focus on interpersonal hypersensitivity as the core experience for patients with BPD is vital in making this possible. Exploring the patient's interpersonal world, recent relationship stresses, and the role of these triggers in worsening symptoms can get to the heart of the patient's presentation to the ED and provide clues to the appropriate disposition. Such dispositions can sometimes be expedited by involving or avoiding a triggering person. With some patients, it may be helpful to discuss their interpersonal hypersensitivity in straightforward terms so as to explicitly connect their distress and behaviors to this phenomenon (see Appendix C, "Interpersonal Coherence Model"). Furthermore, this discussion can focus the visit on what led to the crisis, what may help to move the patient past it, and how to potentially avoid future crises. Depending on the patient's degree of insight, he or she may not be able to immediately identify these connections, but over the course of the discussion or over several visits to the ED, with repeated attempts, the patient's self-awareness may grow.

Managing Suicidality and Self-Harm

One of the most challenging aspects of managing patients with BPD in the ED setting is that the vast majority of the time, they present with suicidal thoughts and/or behaviors. The often chronic nature of these symptoms further complicates the evaluation process, making it difficult to discern the patient's true safety risk. In addition, provider fears of liability may trump objective clinical presentations and drive treatment decisions. Straightforward guidelines help clinicians organize their approach and avoid common iatrogenic problems when managing the safety of patients with BPD.

While exploring the issue of suicidal thoughts and behaviors, one must also consider the implications of self-injurious behaviors. ED staff may be unsure how to handle such behaviors and how to put them in perspective and may have more negative reactions to self-harm than providers in other settings (Commons Treloar and Lewis 2008). Self-injurious behavior may sometimes be conflated with suicidality, and providers may treat the two as if they are one and the same, or at least related, thinking that self-injury is a direct stepping stone to suicide. It is important to note that although it is true that patients with BPD who self-harm are at significantly increased risk of a completed suicide, the presence of self-harm is not a good indicator of acute risk of suicide (Wedig et al. 2012). Clinicians, patients, and patients' loved ones may cite self-injury as compelling inpatient hospitalization, but there is no significant evidence that inpatient hospitalization reduces such behaviors. All that said, it is important to note that a significant increase in the intensity or frequency of self-harming behaviors, or of self-injury that causes significant physical harm, is notable and may indicate an increase in other symptoms or problems that raise a patient's acute risk of suicide. In these cases, it is important to parse out the acute from the chronic risk factors and consider these accordingly.

One crucial model to adhere to in the ED setting is that of "acute on chronic" risk. It is well documented that the lifetime risk of suicide is elevated in BPD, and it can be challenging to assess for safety in the context of this chronic risk (Black et al. 2004). Focusing on acute risk factors and imminent warning signs is paramount because these variables are linked with the patient's immediate safety risk and may be addressed in an inpatient setting. On the other hand, responding only to a patient's chronic suicidal ideation, which may be at its baseline level, can lead to unnecessary hospitalizations and ultimately confuse the patient regarding when inpatient hospitalization is truly needed. It is important to note that recurrent hospitalizations in patients with BPD can foster dependence and may actually worsen their long-term course (Paris 2004).

Stressful interpersonal events, concurrent major depression, and ongoing substance abuse all increase a BPD patient's acute risk and should factor into decisions about what level of care is safe and appropriate (Black et al. 2004). With all patients, warning signs of imminent risk include an increase in suicidal thinking, suicidal plans or intent, lack of a reason for living, intense anxiety, insomnia, hopelessness, feeling trapped, social withdrawal, anger, recklessness, and significant mood changes (Tucker et al. 2015). For patients with BPD, because many of these symptoms may be present chronically, special attention should be paid to acute changes in the symptoms and deviations from the patient's baseline. When acute risk factors are significant and exceed the chronic risk factors for a patient with BPD, short-term inpatient hospitalization should be considered until the crisis passes or sufficiently diminishes.

Given the recurrent suicidal behavior (and risk of completed suicides) in patients with BPD, provider fears of liability are often front and center when designing a disposition from the ED. Recognizing how to mitigate liability risk can help clinicians avoid making treatment decisions based solely on conservative risk management. Included in the ways to mitigate liability risk are paying attention to excessive countertransference reactions to patients with BPD and not allowing them to influence emotionally charged treatment decisions. Good communication with patients and other stakeholders is another GPM guideline to help manage liability risk and certainly optimizes ED care. In fact, good communication in general should be considered an essential tenet of safely managing patients with BPD in the ED setting. Family members, social supports, outpatient providers, colleagues, and supervisors are all valuable sources of support and information and can all be part of the treatment plan. Even if the patient protests or resists when ED staff members seek to contact others, if safety is in question, ED providers are obliged to gather as much information as possible to conduct a comprehensive safety assessment. The most effective deterrent of liability issues is to involve a professional colleague to advise or consult about any decision or judgment that might involve risk. Slowing down to discuss the case with another clinician can provide useful perspective and support. Peer and/or supervisory consultation can assuage providers' anxiety and help them regulate their own emotions. In a calm and regulated state, providers will be more likely to make a sound, rational decision rather than one based on potentially clouded judgment. Opportunities for consultation are usually available in the ED setting.

Family members and other social supports may provide invaluable collateral information regarding the BPD patient's imminent risk of suicide and can also help illuminate the strengths or weaknesses of the patient's social support network. This is useful particularly for patients who are unwilling to provide such information themselves. Furthermore, given the interpersonal focus of many BPD crises, reaching out to a patient's social supports can sometimes initiate the resolution of the crisis.

The patient's outpatient providers are critical sources of information regarding current and past treatments and potential safety risks. Furthermore, understanding whether the outpatient clinician is willing or able to continue treatment with the patient is important information for the ED staff to consider when crafting a disposition. If a patient visits the ED recurrently, this may indicate that the outpatient treatment has been ineffective, and discussions with the outpatient providers regarding the past and future course of treatment can be useful.

When approaching the patient with suicidal thoughts and behaviors in the ED, the provider should keep in mind several key points. The first is that no matter how recurrent the behavior, the clinician must express genuine concern. When the provider adopts a dismissive or hostile attitude (which can occur when "compassion fatigue" sets in with a patient who is particularly disruptive or who presents to the ED repeatedly), the patient with BPD may feel judged and shut down or may "up the ante," claiming increasing levels of suicidality in order to coerce supportive or protective reactions. Such behaviors further complicate the evaluation and increase the likelihood of an inadequate safety assessment.

That said, overreaction on the part of the ED clinician may trigger unnecessary hospitalizations that are unlikely to meaningfully reduce the BPD patient's suicide risk and can reinforce the pattern of using suicidality to avoid interpersonal stressors. To navigate this fine line successfully, the clinician must take time to translate what the word *suicidal* means to the patient, because every situation may be different. Does the patient with BPD actually want and intend to die, or is the patient expressing feelings of loneliness, depression, and rejection? Questions such as these should be considered when evaluating the authentic suicide risk of a patient with BPD.

Engaging the patient in a "chain analysis" following a suicide attempt or uptick in self-injurious behavior is recommended to help the provider and the patient understand the "story" of how the patient may have arrived at this breaking point. This step-by-step analysis of the events leading up to the behavior can engage the patient in better understanding moments prior to full-blown crisis when he or she could have sought intervention earlier, and this analysis can help the clinician gauge the nature of the self-harm—whether it was impulsive or planned and whether it was directly influenced by an acute stressor or due to a gradual accumulation of problems over time (Lynch et al. 2006). If the patient is to be discharged to home, safety planning should include how to recognize warning signs, how to make the patient's environment safer by reducing access to lethal means, and whom to contact (and whom to avoid) when in crisis. ED staff can further mitigate risk in the days following discharge by placing follow-up phone calls to patients with BPD (Miller et al. 2017).

Psychopharmacology

Awareness of developments in the practice of medication management for the treatment of BPD can guide the clinician in good decision making.

In the ED, there are potential pitfalls to avoid when prescribing psychotropic medications to the patient with BPD. When compared with patients with other psychiatric diagnoses, those with BPD receive more medications when in the ED (Pascual et al. 2007). On one hand, this may make sense, given that patients with BPD often present in an emotionally dysregulated manner, with high anxiety, agitation at times, and disruptive behaviors. However, providers must balance the desire to quickly calm patients with BPD with the drawbacks of relying on medications for this purpose. In general, it is prudent for clinicians to take extra care to administer medications to patients with BPD in the ED only if there is acute agitation and/or anxiety endangering the patient or others or if the patient's symptoms render a thorough interview impossible.

The most common medications used for patients with BPD in the ED setting are benzodiazepines and antipsychotics (Pascual et al. 2007). As in treating all patients, in the absence of imminent safety risks, the clinician's initial foray into managing agitation and anxiety should be verbal de-escalation (Richmond et al. 2012). Patients with BPD often arrive at the ED desperate for soothing and eager to take a medication that will quickly sedate them or calm their nerves. Similarly, the ED staff may prefer to quickly de-escalate a heated situation through medication. It is important to recognize that by using medications as the first-line approach to agitation and anxiety, the staff may, in part, be treating their own anxieties and frustrations rather than implementing a meaningful, effective intervention. Providers must remember that medications are typically not associated with significant benefit in the core symptoms of BPD, and they are often associated with a high rate of adverse effects (Stoffers et al. 2010; Zanarini et al. 2015).

The downsides of regularly administering medications to patients with BPD in the ED are numerous. Given the general lack of evidence regarding significant and consistent efficacy of any medications in reducing BPD symptoms, prescribing clinicians are likely to be presenting a dubious solution—medications—as a potential cure for patients' troubles. In addition to sending the wrong message that medications are the answer to their problems, overmedicating patients with BPD reinforces the use of the ED as the place to go for rapid relief of unwanted emotions.

Additionally, the habit-forming nature of benzodiazepines must be considered in patients who may be particularly primed to become dependent on a fast-acting medication with sedating and calming properties. Given their emotional reactivity, intense reactions to stress, and affective instability, individuals with BPD may expect to be soothed by benzodiazepines and become strongly attached to a belief that they are the only effective medication to treat their symptoms. The BPD patient's possible ensuing dependence on benzodiazepines can become its own separate, iatrogenic problem. Furthermore, when reduction of agitation or anxiety is the desired effect, ED staff must consider that in some patients with BPD, benzodiazepine use may escalate the situation by leading to disinhibition.

If, after balanced consideration, the provider deems medication use in the ED necessary, care should be taken to explicitly explain to the patient the reason for its use. The prescriber should underscore that medications are not intended to be long-term treatments but rather are a way to move forward with the evaluation process at hand. Patients should be provided with psychoeducation about the limitations of medications in treating BPD and reminded that psychosocial interventions are the primary treatment for the disorder. Certainly, changing a medication regimen in the acute ED setting is generally not recommended, given how difficult it is to understand a patient's baseline symptoms when he or she presents in crisis. If any minor changes to medications are deemed necessary, outpatient providers should be contacted and included in that decision-making process. Despite the limited utility of medication use and the contraindications mentioned here, providers should expect that many patients with BPD will request medication changes when in the ED. This is a good opportunity to educate the patient and reinforce that the outpatient prescriber is best positioned for medication management.

Family Interventions

A key component of successfully managing patients with BPD in any setting is involving families and loved ones. Although including families in the evaluation process may seem like an obvious step, it is frequently not practiced in the ED. Seeking collateral information from the patient's family and friends can help maximize communication between all the important stakeholders involved with the patient with BPD. BPD symptoms can be diminished or exacerbated by families; this accentuates the importance of contact with them while a patient is in crisis.

Several family scenarios may exist and influence ED providers' options when evaluating patients with BPD. Certainly, a patient with chronic BPD may have sufficiently dysfunctional relationships such that there is no longer contact with his or her family. The patient can also report and feel that no relationship exists or that one is impossible, although the family may perceive otherwise. Often, families will be willing to help with safety planning and reengage in support even when the patient thinks this is unlikely. This prospect can at least be given a chance rather than being dismissed outright.

Some patients with likely BPD present to the ED with several diagnoses and a history of ineffective treatments. These patients may not improve or may even get worse. In these cases, families may desperately seek answers, feeling that no one has provided them with a road map of how to help. Psychoeducation about the diagnosis of BPD itself, its appropriate treatment, and ways the family may be able to help can be exceptionally useful here.

Finally, in another subset of patients, often early in their treatment course, milder BPD or even subsyndromal symptoms may be present. For these patients, early interventions can be pivotal in determining the course of the disorder. Families are essential in these scenarios, helping to avoid pitfalls that may exacerbate a patient's symptoms and learning how to tap into useful resources. Practical guidelines are easily accessible and can be either briefly reviewed or printed out for families visiting the ED (Gunderson and Berkowitz 2006). Relevant principles include having reasonable expectations, keeping things calm in the home environment, expressing concern about but not overreacting to crises, being consistent as a family unit, and setting fair limits.

Case Vignette

The following case description includes decision points, each of which has several alternative responses listed at the end of the case. The reader will rate each alternative response in terms of its level of helpfulness. Discussions of responses follow.

> Dorothy is a 26-year-old woman who has presented to the ED three times in the past year. You are the ED psychiatrist on duty, speaking with a different patient in an interview room when Dorothy arrives. As you are leaving the room, a nurse says to you, "She's back" and shakes her head. You wonder who the nurse is talking about and immediately worry that your shift will be a difficult one, especially because there are now three patients waiting to be seen. After evaluating the two other patients, the social worker reminds you that Dorothy has previously been challenging to work with, once cutting herself while in the ED and on another occasion requiring restraints. This time Dorothy presents after ingesting 10 pills of diphenhydramine, 5 pills of fluoxetine, and 8 pills of trazodone in an apparent suicide attempt. After taking the pills, she texted relatives to inform them of what she had done, which prompted numerous 911 calls. She arrives at the ED with the formal diagnoses of bipolar disorder and post-traumatic stress disorder. You note that the mention of "Cluster B traits" is also included in her medical record. As you review her chart, you hear a commotion in the waiting room. Dorothy is telling staff that she has been waiting too long and demanding they allow her to leave. You go to see her. [**Decision Point 1**]

She calms somewhat as you begin your interview. Dorothy explains that beginning shortly after waking this morning, she has had a terrible day, and she finally decided that she should "end it all." In a somewhat jarring manner, she then abruptly looks directly at you and says that she is "all better now" and wants to go home. She adds that she probably just needs her "bipolar meds" changed. You ask some questions intended to better understand what may have preceded her overdose, but she quickly and irritably says that "nothing happened." She adds that things are "always the same" in that "no one cares about me and I always am the one who makes sacrifices for others." Dorothy volunteers that she does not trust anyone, as people have always "stabbed me in the back" throughout her life. [**Decision Point 2**]

Dorothy reports that she has taken more than 15 different psychiatric medications over the years, and although some seemed to help for brief periods of time, she would always eventually become unstable again. She has heard of newer medications and would like to start taking one. You advise her that you first need to discuss her current crisis. After you inquire several times about her social network, she reluctantly says she has some friends and relatives who probably do care about her. Many have contacted her while she has been in the waiting room to make sure she is okay. Dorothy says she was initially angry that relatives called 911, but she now realizes they were trying to help. Regarding the overdose, she begins to share more about events leading up to taking the pills. Her partner broke up with her several weeks ago, she is having trouble paying her rent, and yesterday one of her friends claimed not to have the energy to be supportive of her any longer. She has been drinking more alcohol to escape from her frustration and sense of hopelessness. She says, "Wouldn't you want to kill yourself?" She had not been planning the overdose and says it was impulsive. She is not sure she really wanted to die but does know that she wanted her pain to go away. [**Decision Point 3**]

When you decline to change her medications, Dorothy becomes angry, saying, "I guess you really don't want to help." You explain that in the ED setting, major medication changes are not usually made, especially after an overdose. You raise questions about the utility of medications, given that so many have been ineffective for her in the past. In addition, you express your concern that there may be another diagnosis in play that could explain her long history of failed medications.

After meeting with Dorothy, you reach her father by phone, seeking another viewpoint on her recent behavior and safety risk. He reveals that he has worried about her lately, particularly given her increased alcohol use. He says she has always notified someone after suicide attempts, and he has perceived these behaviors as "cries for help." Dorothy's father willingly agrees to come to the ED and help with safety planning. The ED social worker contacts her outpatient therapist, who says that she has never been sure of Dorothy's diagnosis of bipolar disorder because she has never actually seen her in a manic state. The therapist adds that Dorothy's reactivity to stress, frequent mood changes, and chronic suicidal thoughts and behaviors have suggested BPD, but she has not been confident enough to tell the patient that diagnosis. [**Decision Point 4**]

When you return to speak with Dorothy, you discuss her diagnoses. After reviewing the criteria for bipolar disorder and BPD, you raise the possibility that bipolar disorder misses the mark. Dorothy appears somewhat irritated at this suggestion but admits that some of the BPD criteria do seem to fit her. Dorothy denies having a drinking problem and refuses any of the substance abuse resources your team provides. To her dismay, you make no medication changes at this ED visit. She feels calmer now that her father has arrived at the unit and friends have offered emotional support via text. Her father actively engages in safety planning, Dorothy will stay with him for the near future, and he will make sure she gets to her upcoming therapy appointment. In the days following the ED visit, staff call her to follow up and she reports that she is doing better and has no active suicidal thoughts or plans.

Decision Points: Alternative Responses

Rate each response in terms of its level of helpfulness with a rating of 1 (will be helpful), 2 (possibly helpful, continuing reservations), or 3 (not helpful—or even harmful).

1. You meet Dorothy and

   A. Offer a medication to calm her down.
   B. Inform her that she is scaring other patients and that the staff cannot tolerate her behavior.
   C. Note that she seems angry and you would like her to help you understand why.
   D. Apologize for the wait, saying that you want to understand what brought her into the ED today.

2. In response to Dorothy's description of her suicide attempt, you

   A. Say you are concerned and that, despite her feeling better, inpatient hospitalization is something to consider.
   B. Enter into a discussion about her diagnosis.
   C. Ask her about her "bipolar meds."
   D. Request that she talk more about her stressful relationships.
   E. Say that although it may seem to her that nothing triggered her attempt to kill herself, often there are precipitating stressors that you would like to help her examine.

3. With this new information in hand, you should

    A. Delve into her medication history to determine what would be a good "next step" medication.
    B. Use this opportunity to focus on her safety risk.
    C. Say that given her recent stressors, you understand how she could feel so upset.
    D. Request to speak to some of her social supports and her outpatient providers.

4. In an attempt to wrap up the case, you should

    A. Advise that she seek a different therapist because you are not sure of the level of expertise of her current one.
    B. Involve her father in safety planning.
    C. Offer the diagnosis of BPD as a possibility.
    D. Express concern about her alcohol use.

Decision Points: Discussion

Numbers within brackets indicate level of helpfulness ratings.

1. You meet Dorothy and

    A. Offer a medication to calm her down. [3] (A medication to treat Dorothy's agitation may be indicated if her behavior places herself or other(s) at risk or if it interferes with the interview, but offering it prior to an initial assessment of the patient is contraindicated.)
    B. Inform her that she is scaring other patients and that the staff cannot tolerate her behavior. [2] (Setting limits with a patient can often help to organize his or her behavior within boundaries, and this is sometimes needed if the patient is distressing other patients or families in the ED. However, this is not the way to start the interaction. Particularly for a patient with likely BPD, a direct foray into limit setting without an attempt to first establish some measure of rapport will cause a patient like Dorothy to feel unheard and rejected and likely exacerbate her angry protests. Moreover, saying that ED staff cannot tolerate her behavior will also amplify her complaints.)
    C. Note that she seems angry and you would like her to help you understand why. [1] (Validating a BPD patient's feelings is im-

portant and can help establish that you are a provider who cares. Sometimes angry patients with BPD will only get angrier if you identify the feeling, but it is still a good intervention. An attempt at verbal de-escalation may also unearth the issues that may be causing her escalation [e.g., that she is not getting the attention she feels she deserves].)

D. Apologize for the wait, saying that you want to understand what brought her into the ED today. [1] (It is reasonable to apologize appropriately when managing a patient in a crisis. This response can expedite the development of a therapeutic alliance and demonstrate your concern for the patient's frustration. You want to understand what caused Dorothy's visit, but she may be unwilling to discuss it unless there is first some acknowledgment of her having had to wait.)

2.   In response to Dorothy's description of her suicide attempt, you

A. Say you are concerned and that, despite her feeling better, inpatient hospitalization is something to consider. [3] (A common error in managing BPD in the acute crisis setting is to assume that any type of self-harm or suicidal behavior requires inpatient hospitalization. Before the question of hospitalization is raised, there needs to be a reasonable suicide risk assessment. Although Dorothy may ultimately need to be hospitalized, that has not yet been determined, and introducing this possibility at this early stage may derail assessing the reasons for her overdose and a meaningful dialogue regarding alternative treatment options.)

B. Enter into a discussion about her diagnosis. [2] (Diagnostic consideration is important. It should be apparent to you that BPD is likely given Dorothy's repeated overdoses, anger, and interpersonal hypersensitivity, as well as the countertransference reactions from staff. If Dorothy has a misdiagnosis (e.g., bipolar disorder), radical changes to her treatment may be required. It might be tempting to begin that discussion at this point, but the opportunity to delve into her probable interpersonal stressors should take precedence. Understanding these better will help with your assessment of acute suicide risk, who needs to be included in the safety plan, and indeed her likely diagnosis.)

C. Ask her about her "bipolar meds." [2] (Certainly, there is a time when providing guidance and psychoeducation about Dorothy's medications may be necessary, particularly if she is hoping for you to change her medications. However, at this point, it is more important to demonstrate curiosity about her life and relationships and to determine if together you can identify any notable events that may have triggered this crisis and her presentation to the ED.)

D. Request that she talk more about her stressful relationships. [1] (Getting to the core issue of Dorothy's interpersonal hypersensitivity may expedite the gathering of information you need to craft an appropriate disposition. She has opened a door by describing one-sided relationships where she gets betrayed. If you walk through it, you may learn valuable information about her stressors and social supports and thereby help her connect her behaviors and feelings to adverse interpersonal events.)

E. Say that although it may seem to her that nothing triggered her attempt to kill herself, often there are precipitating stressors that you would like to help her examine. [1] (Challenging her assertion that "nothing happened" is important because this is unlikely and she cannot gain mastery of her behaviors if she does not learn the ability to identify what makes her suicidal. Dorothy needs to actively participate in the interview and in treatment planning. Working with a patient with BPD to explore triggers [particularly interpersonal triggers] to a crisis is an essential element of the ED interview.)

3. With this new information in hand, you should

A. Delve into her medication history to determine what would be a good "next step" medication. [3] (The medication history is not the most relevant information to gather at this point, because it will not guide treatment decisions, and, as aforementioned, one should rarely change a BPD patient's medications mid crisis. Part of psychoeducation for patients with BPD is that medications are merely adjunctive treatments and secondary to psychotherapy and case management.)

B. Use this opportunity to focus on her safety risk. [2] (At some point, you must assess for the patient's suicide risk, but she has already told you a lot and given you a window into her risk profile, including describing her social network and saying that she texted these individuals after she had taken the overdose. She has also revealed her overdependence on her social supports and her use of alcohol. It is important that, although provider liability risks are a concern, one makes disposition decisions based on the true dangerousness of the situation. Given the equivocal nature of Dorothy's attempt, there may be an opportunity for a safe discharge, which would be desired given that inpatient hospitalization may not meaningfully reduce her suicide risk.)

C. Say that given her recent stressors, you understand how she could feel so upset. [1] (Validation can be used as a tool to imbue the interaction with caring, but in this case the interpersonal nature of her stressors would be emphasized. This is an opportunity to tell her how her disorder begins with excessive reactivity to feelings of rejection or abandonment. This is at the core of her issues, and these feelings can be addressed.)

D. Request to speak to some of her social supports and her outpatient providers. [1] (Communicating with others in the life of the patient with BPD is integral to good emergency care. Making these contacts can also reduce liability risk. Those in Dorothy's life can contribute valuable information about her recent behaviors, warning signs of suicide, and likelihood that she can follow through with a safety plan. Her outpatient providers can weigh in on her safety risk and the type of follow-up care that can be reasonably arranged. Conducting a comprehensive safety assessment in cases of elevated suicide risk requires information from outside sources, regardless of whether the patient has given permission.)

4. In an attempt to wrap up the case, you should

A. Advise that she seek a different therapist because you are not sure of the level of expertise of her current one. [3] (Although it is a good idea to reevaluate the efficacy of a given treatment, it is not your place to recommend that Dorothy stop seeing her current therapist. In any case, it is best to engage in that discussion with the therapist to determine his or her ability to tailor the treatment and more effectively manage the BPD.)

B. Involve her father in safety planning. [1] (Even though the patient is an adult, her father represents both a valuable source of information about her past suicidal behaviors and a potential ally in arranging a safe disposition. Assisting the father in learning how to help the patient manage her symptoms and how to avoid exacerbating them is a goal here, in addition to bolstering the strength of her support system.)

C. Offer the diagnosis of BPD as a possibility. [1] (There is an opportunity here to discuss your impressions of her likely diagnoses. Although bipolar disorder and posttraumatic stress disorder are her historical diagnoses, BPD symptoms are also prominent. You might say, in an exploratory manner, "Have you heard of BPD? What do you know about it? Have you ever wondered if you may have it?" Your professional opinion of the likelihood of BPD and relevant psychoeducation can be included in this discussion, along with pointing the patient to written or online resources.)

D. Express concern about her alcohol use. [1] (A discussion about the risks of alcohol use and its effects on mood, anxiety, impulsivity, and sleep is relevant and part of good psychoeducation and safety planning with a patient with BPD. This information will be most effective if stated in a matter-of-fact, nonjudgmental tone.)

Conclusion

Despite the brevity of clinician-patient interactions in the ED, GPM principles are quite well suited to use in the ED, assisting clinicians in avoiding iatrogenic harm. GPM's treatment approach and focus on interpersonal hypersensitivity can help expedite the evaluation and disposition planning. Adhering to GPM's cautious approach toward medications benefits ED clinicians in avoiding overprescribing and inadvertently setting the expectation that medications are the desired modality of treatment. GPM provides guidelines that help clinicians organize seemingly complex safety assessments into a more easily repeatable structure. Discussing the BPD diagnosis directly with the patient and providing psychoeducation about the disorder can and should start in the ED. ED staff can be more efficiently trained in GPM's central principles than in other evidence-based treatments for BPD. The primary aim of clinical professionals in the ED—to channel patients to effective definitive care—will begin with these interventions, so that needless, unproductive, and frustrating recurrent visits to the ED will diminish.

References

Black DW, Blum N, Pfohl B, et al: Suicidal behavior in borderline personality disorder: prevalence, risk factors, prediction, and prevention. J Pers Disord 18(3):226–239, 2004 15237043

Boggild AK, Heisel MJ, Links PS: Social, demographic, and clinical factors related to disruptive behaviour in hospital. Can J Psychiatry 49(2):114–118, 2004 15065745

Chaput YJ, Lebel MJ: Demographic and clinical profiles of patients who make multiple visits to psychiatric emergency services. Psychiatr Serv 58(3):335–341, 2007 17325106

Commons Treloar AJ, Lewis AJ: Professional attitudes towards deliberate self-harm in patients with borderline personality disorder. Aust NZJ Psychiatry 42(7):578–584, 2008 18612861

Gabbard GO, Wilkinson SM: Management of Countertransference With Borderline Patients. Washington, DC, American Psychiatric Press, 1994

Gunderson JG, Berkowitz C: Borderline Personality Disorder Family Guidelines. New York, National Education Alliance for Borderline Personality Disorder, 2006. Available at: http://www.borderlinepersonalitydisorder.com/family connections/family-guidelines. Accessed October 1, 2017.

Gunderson JG, Links PS: Handbook of Good Psychiatric Management for Borderline Personality Disorder. Washington, DC, American Psychiatric Publishing, 2014

Heap J, Silk KR: Personality disorders, in Emergency Psychiatry: Principles and Practice. Edited by Berlin JS, Fishkind A, Lipson Glick R, Zeller SL. Philadelphia, PA, Lippincott Williams & Wilkins, 2008, pp 265–276

Keuroghlian AS, Palmer BA, Choi-Kain LW, et al: The effect of attending good psychiatric management (GPM) workshops on attitudes toward patients with borderline personality disorder. J Pers Disord 30(4):567–576, 2016 26111249

Lynch TR, Chapman AL, Rosenthal MZ, et al: Mechanisms of change in dialectical behavior therapy: theoretical and empirical observations. J Clin Psychol 62(4):459–480, 2006 16470714

Miller IW, Camargo CA Jr, Arias SA, et al: Suicide prevention in an emergency department population: the ED-SAFE study. JAMA Psychiatry 74(6):563–570, 2017 28456130

Paris J: Is hospitalization useful for suicidal patients with borderline personality disorder? J Pers Disord 18(3):240–247, 2004 15237044

Pascual JC, Córcoles D, Castaño J, et al: Hospitalization and pharmacotherapy for borderline personality disorder in a psychiatric emergency service. Psychiatr Serv 58(9):1199–1204, 2007 17766566

Richmond JS, Berlin JS, Fishkind AB, et al: Verbal de-escalation of the agitated patient: consensus statement of the American Association for Emergency Psychiatry Project BETA De-escalation Workgroup. West J Emerg Med 13(1):17–25, 2012 22461917

Stoffers J, Völlm BA, Rücker G, et al: Pharmacological interventions for borderline personality disorder. Cochrane Database Syst Rev 6(6):CD005653, 2010 20556762

Tucker RP, Crowley KJ, Davidson CL, et al: Risk factors, warning signs, and drivers of suicide: what are they, how do they differ, and why does it matter? Suicide Life Threat Behav 45(6):679–689, 2015 25858332

Wedig MM, Silverman MH, Frankenburg FR, et al: Predictors of suicide attempts in patients with borderline personality disorder over 16 years of prospective follow-up. Psychol Med 42(11):2395–2404, 2012 22436619

Zanarini MC, Frankenburg FR: A preliminary, randomized trial of psychoeducation for women with borderline personality disorder. J Pers Disord 22(3):284–290, 2008 18540800

Zanarini MC, Frankenburg FR, Bradford Reich D, et al: Rates of psychotropic medication use reported by borderline patients and Axis II comparison subjects over 16 years of prospective follow-up. J Clin Psychopharmacol 35(1):63–67, 2015 25384261

Chapter 4

Consultation-Liaison Service

James A. Jenkins, M.D.

Evan A. Iliakis, B.A.

Lois W. Choi-Kain, M.D., M.Ed.

Patients with borderline personality disorder (BPD) have a disproportionately higher burden of medical illness when compared with matched cohorts and are therefore high utilizers not only of psychiatric resources but also of medical and surgical care. In a United Kingdom–based registry review (Fok et al. 2012), female and male patients with a personality disorder diagnosis had life expectancies of 63.3 years and 59.1 years, respectively. The decrease in life expectancy compared with that for matched peers was 18.7 years for females and 17.7 years for males. Notably, similar decreases have been observed, but more widely publicized, for patients with chronic psychotic disorders (Hjorthøj et al. 2017). It is not surprising that patients with BPD have adverse health outcomes related to their difficulties with impulsivity, substance abuse, vulnerability to psychiatric polypharmacy, and emotional reactivity. Difficulties with emotional reactivity can lead patients with BPD to avoid necessary treatment when under duress or, when they do present for care, to be met with condescension and prejudice from medical providers, which further hinders the patient's motivation to follow up.

In this chapter, we review the specific ways in which the psychiatric consultation-liaison (C-L) service can help improve the experience of medical and surgical hospitalization and the quality of psychiatric care while reducing the potential iatrogenic harm inflicted by physicians who have not been trained to manage BPD. Good psychiatric management (GPM) is an easily adaptable, low-resource intervention that the psychiatric consultant can readily learn and put into use to accomplish these goals.

Overlap of Borderline Personality Disorder and Medical Illness

In a systematic review of the literature (Dixon-Gordon et al. 2015), the most common medical comorbidities seen with BPD included sleep disorders, metabolic syndrome, chronic pain, migraines, and sequelae of long-term substance use (i.e., lung cancer, HIV; prevalence rates for select disorders are summarized in Tables 4–1 and 4–2). With regard to sleep disorders, 95.5% of patients with a primary BPD diagnosis self-reported being poor sleepers versus 12% of control subjects; this was independent of another psychiatric condition that could account for insomnia (Semiz et al. 2008). Up to 49% of patients with BPD also reported regular nightmares versus 7% of control subjects (Semiz et al. 2008). There is evidence to suggest that objective measurements of sleep dysfunction strongly correlate with the severity of BPD symptoms and that patients in remission from BPD experience lower levels of sleep dysfunction (Bastien et al. 2008). The increased nighttime interruptions, unfamiliar noises, and lack of clear day-night cues in the hospital ward present exceptional challenges to patients with BPD who already struggle with sleep. The psychiatric consultant should bear this in mind on evaluation.

Patients with BPD have much higher rates of obesity, metabolic syndrome, and cardiovascular events. Compared with a control population, for instance, patients with BPD were shown to have higher rates of obesity (64.7% vs. 19.4%; Sansone et al. 2001). Longitudinal studies have shown

TABLE 4–1. **Prevalence of select medical complaints in patients with borderline personality disorder (BPD) as opposed to general population**

Problem		Prevalence in general population	Prevalence in BPD
Sleep related	Poor sleep[a]	12%	95.5%
	Regular nightmares[a]	7%	49%
Metabolic	Obesity[b]	19.4%	64.7%
	Metabolic syndrome[c]	10.6%	23.3%
Medical	Functionally incapacitating headache days[d]	5.9 days	18.1 days
	Headache medication overuse[d]	62%	74%
	Positive headache treatment response[d]	14%	58%
	Polycystic ovaries[e]	6.9%	30.4%

Source. Data from [a]Semiz et al. 2008, [b]Sansone et al. 2001, [c]Kahl et al. 2013, [d]Rothrock et al. 2007, and [e]Roepke et al. 2010.

TABLE 4–2. **Odds ratios for various medical complaints given borderline personality disorder symptomatology**

Medical problem	Odds ratio
Arthritis[a]	2.67
HIV[b]	2.1
Opioid prescription for chronic pain[c]	18.61

Source. Data from [a]Powers and Oltmanns 2013, [b]Bennett et al. 2009, and [c]Breckenridge and Clark 2003.

that where severity of obesity and BPD were correlated, the percentage of obese patients with BPD at start and at 6 years follow-up rose from 17% to 28% (Frankenburg and Zanarini 2006). BPD is also overrepresented in prevalence studies examining the extremely obese category (body mass index >40; Dixon-Gordon et al. 2015). It is widely known that obesity causes devastating adverse health effects and is also stigmatized by health care professionals. Thus, patients with BPD who are also obese are left to navigate multiple levels of stigma. Often, they are confronted with implicit or explicit cues from medical providers suggesting to them that they are at fault for their own illness. The psychiatric consultant should be prepared to validate patients' reactions to having faced such stigma. At the same time, it is important that the consultant avoid devaluation of other medical staff by modifying the message that the patients are responsible for their well-being, despite it not being their fault they have a disease.

Given that patients with BPD struggle to tolerate physical or psychological distress, it is not surprising that they are higher utilizers of prescription pain medications. A study investigating whether patients presenting with lower back pain were being started on nonsteroidal anti-inflammatory drugs or opioid analgesics found that nearly all patients receiving opioid prescriptions qualified for the BPD diagnosis (odds ratio 18.61; Breckenridge and Clark 2003). Studies have also demonstrated that patients with BPD who experience migraines have three times the level of functional incapacitation as a non-BPD matched cohort (Rothrock et al. 2007). Patients with BPD will struggle in the hospital environment to tolerate the usual discomfort associated with invasive medical and surgical procedures, as well as with their own physical illness, and will often expect immediate resolution of symptoms. In reaction, the medical or surgical team may be overly aggressive with palliative medications or may misclassify patients with BPD as "drug-seekers" rather than as dysphoric, pain sensitive, and care seeking.

There are myriad other health disorders for which a diagnosis of BPD has been associated with higher prevalence rates and worse outcomes. Most of these disorders (e.g., HIV, lung cancer) have a strong behavioral determinant (Dixon-Gordon et al. 2015). For patients with BPD who also have one or several "preventable" disorders, medical intervention can be fraught with feelings of intense shame or guilt for having not been more proactive in their prevention.

Aims of Psychiatric Consultation

There are two established goals that the C-L psychiatry service aims to achieve. The first and more traditional goal is providing adequate assessment and recommendations to help the primary medical or surgical providers manage comorbid psychiatric illness. This is the *consultation* role and does not differ from the approach taken by other medical and surgical specialties. The second aim of the C-L psychiatry service is to provide education to the consultee, nurses, and other members of the treatment team about the affective, behavioral, and cognitive changes that can optimize medical or surgical treatment. When this educational function is carried out by the psychiatrist in a formal fashion by joining morning rounds, leading team meetings, educating about interpersonal dynamics, and offering validation and support to the consultee, it provides the *liaison* aspect of C-L psychiatry (Kontos et al. 2003; Ramchandani et al. 1997). For patients with BPD, both consultation and liaison are crucial. GPM provides guidelines that can be easily adapted to address both functions of consultation and liaison, setting it apart from other evidence-based treatments for BPD.

Approaching the Consultation

The consulting psychiatrist should be prepared to encounter misdiagnosis in the medical record and misleading consultation questions from the consultee. In one study of referrals to C-L psychiatry, only 53% of consultations with referral questions regarding depression were able to confirm that diagnosis and only 42.8% of consults for questions relating to bipolar disorder were able to confirm that diagnosis (Dilts et al. 2003). In a different study (Al-Huthail 2008), a personality disorder diagnosis was made in 16%–20% of all psychiatric consultations on medical and surgical wards, and 20% of depression and 38% of anxiety referrals were ultimately given a primary diagnosis of personality disorder by a consulting psychiatrist. These data suggest that referring physicians struggle to identify the diagnosis of a personality disorder and likely have difficulty formulating a consultation question. Common requests for consultation include suicidal ideation, management of agitation/aggression, depression, anxiety, psychosis, and noncompliance with recommendations.

During the initial consultation, the C-L psychiatrist should speak with the consultee directly to clarify concerns, expectations, and observations of the patient. Initial suspicion of BPD should be high for questions related to suicidal ideation, self-harm, and other volitional behavioral problems, regardless of the consultee's or recorded psychiatric diagnosis. The differential diagnosis for consultations related to mood and anxiety disorders should also always include a possible BPD diagnosis to ensure that the diagnosis is not missed.

The initial discussion with the consultee should also include questions to gauge whether the team could inadvertently make reactive decisions due to their own anxiety or frustration. These decisions can include, but are not limited to, prematurely discharging the patient prior to completion of treatment, use of mechanical restraints, or use of highly sedating medications. The GPM consultant can clarify the consultee's sense of urgency and validate the difficulty of working with such patients (Riddle et al. 2016). When the consultant makes these efforts, the consultee can feel supported to follow standard of care rather than his or her emotional reaction without feeling incompetent.

The Duties of the Consulting Psychiatrist

The psychiatric consultant has several duties to fulfill regarding a patient with BPD. First and foremost, the consultant has a duty to the patient to form a basic alliance, enhance the patient's understanding of and ability to communicate his or her problem or distress, and protect the patient from potential harms. Second, the consultant has an obligation to advocate for the patient's interest to the medical team, thus managing the patient's treatment environment to optimize care. Third, the consultant should labor to enhance patient wellness and functionality by encouraging pursuit of values and reducing risk of future hospitalization. Lastly, the consultant is responsible for medication management as outlined in the GPM model, keeping new medications to a minimum and avoiding psychiatric polypharmacy where possible (Gunderson and Links 2014).

Forming an Alliance

From the moment that the consultant greets the patient, the focus should be on establishing an alliance, possibly even at the expense of gathering a complete history (Knesper 2007). The GPM approach for building an alliance, which is easily adopted by the psychiatric consultant, includes 1) displaying concerned attention, 2) active listening, 3) validation of painful experiences, and 4) demonstrating one's helpfulness through providing effective and practical assistance. Measures that are actively discouraged by GPM include 1) overemphasis on rescuing a patient; 2) splitting, where part of the team is viewed as good and part of the team is viewed as bad; and 3) splitting, where part of the team views the patient as innocent and victimized, while other members of the team view the patient as problem-

TABLE 4–3.	Good psychiatric management in a consultation-liaison setting: managing interpersonal interactions with patient with borderline personality disorder
Recommended maneuvers	Display concerned attention
	Actively listen
	Validate painful experiences
	Set goals for hospitalization
	Demonstrate helpfulness by providing practical assistance to reach stated goals
Usual pitfalls to avoid	Avoid fragilizing patient and relieving patient of responsibilities (i.e., regarding patient as victim of poor treatment)
	Avoid "splitting" of team (i.e., viewing one side of team as good and other side of team as bad; or having part of team view patient as innocent and mistreated and other part of team view patient as causing drama and at fault)
Relating to the patient	Own one's mistakes
	Observe realistic limits about patient's expectations for any specific medical admission
	Show usual emotional reactions to patient behavior when appropriate

atic and at fault. The relationship should be approached as a real (dyadic) relationship and when necessary should include 1) owning one's mistakes, 2) limit setting around unrealistic expectations, and 3) using self-disclosure of one's emotional reactions to the patient's behavior when appropriate. Table 4–3 summarizes the GPM approach for building an alliance.

On the C-L service, the psychiatrist holds a particularly advantageous position to build an alliance by being the patient's advocate or diplomat to the primary treatment team. Alliance can be further developed by providing education about the BPD diagnosis and its accompanying feeling states and interpersonal patterns, while also holding the patient accountable to be an agent in his or her own treatment. Simple interventions that can be performed on the C-L service include mediating disputes between members of the primary treatment team, providing reading material, and assigning homework to the patient to be reviewed at follow-up visits. Homework is a simple intervention that demonstrates both an interest in the patient's experience and a desire to understand the patient's perspective.

Different forms of alliance develop during outpatient psychotherapy. For the consultant, the goal is to develop a contractual alliance. The indicators of a contractual alliance are that there is an established agreement between patient and therapist on goals and roles and that the patient demonstrates a willingness to follow advice, fueled by trust that the consultant has good intentions. With those patients who are recurrently hospitalized or have delayed discharge, it is possible to form a deeper alliance; in these situations, GPM on the C-L service will begin to more closely approximate outpatient treatment.

Of note, there is an understanding in GPM that sessions are offered only insofar as they are found to be helpful. The consulting psychiatrist can also take this stance with follow-up visits after the initial consultation. If a contractual alliance cannot be achieved, it is best to support the primary treatment team to assist in containing reactivity to the patient's difficult behaviors.

Managing the Environment to Optimize Care

Once BPD is established as being a primary contributor to a patient's dysfunction in the hospital, there are several interventions that can help the medical or surgical team adopt a proactive—rather than a reactive—stance. One intervention is for the consultant to provide the team with brief and targeted education about the patient's interpersonal hypersensitivity and vulnerability to feeling rejected. Another intervention, if time permits, is to illustrate the GPM model of interpersonal hypersensitivity using specific transactions between the patient and the treatment team as a source of reference (see Appendix C, "Interpersonal Coherence Model"). Interventions like these improve the primary treatment team's understanding of the fluctuations in BPD symptoms as they relate to the interpersonal interactions that occur in the hospital. The explicit message that these interventions send is that there is some predictability to the patient's more problematic behaviors.

The consultant may need to provide guidance and instruction to the team to go against their impulses to further withdraw and ignore the patient when crisis or help-rejecting behaviors emerge on the wards. This advice may be especially important to convey to the nursing staff (Eren and Şahin 2016). Alternatively, the consultant may need to warn the primary team about the risks of responding punitively to these behaviors as a means of countertransference enactment. By being available to the team to answer further questions, the consultant can also help limit reactivity and encourage more thoughtful responses by the primary team. As occurs in work with individual patients in GPM, the psychiatric consultant serves as an affective container for the polarization that arises in treating these patients and serves as a model to the team for their introjection (Groves 1975). In addition, the GPM-informed C-L psychiatrist can provide the helpful Behavioral Management Protocol (see Table 4–4). This template can be adjusted to individualize the directives for a specific patient while making them structured and predictable for both staff and patients.

When a patient is self-harming or discussing suicidal thoughts, the team should be encouraged to take these behaviors seriously but not to overreact to them. Often, the team will need guidance about initiating continuous monitoring (i.e., having a sitter), issuing a psychiatric hold, advocating involuntary commitment, or increasing the level of psychiatric care. In response to the consultant's availability, the team will feel more supported and will be better able to tolerate the distress that arises in these challenging and uncertain situations. Depending on the severity of the patient's symptoms, consultants may also want to consider making themselves available by pager between hospital days to further limit the potential for iatrogenic harm.

Enhancing Patient Wellness and Functionality

Patients should be encouraged to proactively seek functional interpersonal interactions with their treatment team during their time in the hospital. The team should set clear limits on behaviors that seem overly dependent, manipulative, aggressive, or self-destructive. Honest feedback should be given on how these maladaptive behaviors serve to distance the treatment team and contribute to the patient's worsening mood and increased anxiety. The consultant should guide medical and surgical teams on how to more skillfully interact with each other, the patient, and the patient's loved ones. It is also important to periodically remind patients of their life outside the hospital and aspects of their lives that are not connected to their role as patients. Finding ways to encourage patients to pursue their values while in the hospital and making plans to do so after discharge can serve as a means to limit the reinforcing aspect of medical or surgical hospitalization.

TABLE 4–4.   Behavior management protocol for borderline personality disorder

Patient: _____ Date: _____

MR#: _____ Unit: _____

The following behavior management protocol will be used to guide the successful management of patient _____. This protocol serves to minimize or prevent the possibility of harmful, ineffective, and emotionally driven responses that are likely to arise as the result of _____'s borderline personality disorder while he or she is in the hospital. Examples of the types of problems likely to arise include staff-splitting (encouraging divisions between MDs/nurses, specialty teams, etc.), engaging in power/control struggles, and emergence of regressive or manipulative behaviors.

There are four areas of focus to reduce and prevent these types of complications:

1. Communication

_____ needs to be told in a simple, straightforward, and truthful fashion what is to be done to and for him or her. Anticipate that this patient will prefer to interact with staff who are supportive, while devaluing those who challenge him or her. Such differences in the patient's valuation of staff are likely to lead to differences in the staff's valuation of the patient, i.e., valued staff will find the patient likable; devalued staff will find the patient unlikable.

Intervention

Have daily staff reviews/conferences to plan _____'s treatment (in the form of meds, studies, labs, family visits, groups, etc.) and reach *consensus* about what is to be told to him or her. All staff will need to familiarize themselves with this plan so that patient will receive *consistent* communication.

2. Consistent Personnel

A critical impairment in patients with borderline personality disorder is their fundamental insecurity related to interpersonal hypersensitivity. The sense of object constancy, which most individuals form in early childhood, provides the basis of a stable character; however, it appears to be lacking in these patients. As a result, _____ may appear to panic or become very frustrated and angry when he or she perceives lapses in those taking care of him or her. In an ideal world, we could designate the same person to provide all care and decisions for the patient. Because this is not possible, simply remain mindful that this area is one of constant internal struggle for the patient.

TABLE 4–4.	**Behavior management protocol for borderline personality disorder *(continued)***

Intervention

At the start of each new shift change (especially for RNs and MDs), providers should briefly familiarize themselves with the patient and his or her consensus treatment plan. That provider can ask how things are going with the patient, explain his or her role in the treatment, and offer a *clear time frame* for how long he or she is going to be on duty.

Important decisions, such as changes in the treatment (e.g., medications), schedule, or timing of medical/surgical interventions, should be made by *one* (consistently identifiable by the patient) primary provider, and the rest of the team *should defer* to that provider. Finally, the patient should be provided with consistent and timely advance notice of when his or her hospitalization is expected to end. This may be achieved by creating *well-defined goals*—ability to discuss life problems, stabilize medications, establish an aftercare plan, etc.—and then notifying patient that the goals of the hospitalization have clearly been met.

3. Entitlement

By far, this is the most difficult aspect of the patient's character for others to bear. It is easy for others to be annoyed by offensive deservedness. Do not confront the patient on his or her entitlement or imply that he or she is undeserving of things he or she requests. Staff need to see this as a symptom of why this patient fails in interpersonal relationships. At times, _____ can appear to be a bottomless pit of need that we feel hopeless to satisfy. Such complaints should be reframed: "We wish we could be more able to fulfill your needs."

Intervention

Recognize that there is reassurance in telling _____ that he or she is likely to recover from his or her problems and that much of this work will need to be completed in the outpatient psychiatry setting. Say over and over again that you understand what the patient is saying and that you feel he or she deserves the best possible care but that learning to take care of oneself is the key to recovery. When possible, allow _____ to air his or her own suggestions and acknowledge or even compliment the patient, even if these ideas are not ultimately followed by the team. When a decision needs to be made, it is usually possible to incorporate the patient's list of options.

TABLE 4–4.   Behavior management protocol for borderline personality disorder *(continued)*

---

4. Setting Limits

_____ makes a lot of demands, which are often conflicting or unreasonable; the patient is quick to become enraged when his or her perceived needs are not met and may even make staff feel at fault for somehow failing (even though that is clearly not the case). The patient may even attempt blackmail or other threatening behavior to get his or her way.

Intervention

Do not try to argue with _____'s demands. *Quietly but firmly set limits* on treatment-interfering behaviors. If the patient ups the ante by threatening destructive behaviors toward self or others, quietly assure him or her that such behavior cannot be tolerated and that physical restraint can ensue if the he or she tries to carry it out. Remind the patient that any behavior, positive or negative, has consequences for both oneself and others. Remind yourself that the patient has a right to make demands and complain, but *you need not tolerate any behaviors that are clearly harmful to the patient's welfare or the welfare of other patients within the treatment community.*

Signature: _____

Print Name: _____ Date and Time: _____

Note.   MR=medical record.

Source.   Adapted from Groves 1975, with permission of J.E. Groves. Copyright © 1975 by SAGE Publications. Reprinted by permission of SAGE Publications, Inc.

Given the limited time available to the psychiatric consultant, other services may be utilized to foster this goal; for example, hospital chaplaincy and volunteer services can further connect the patient to his or her values and life outside the hospital.

If the patient demonstrates reluctance to be discharged or escalates talk of suicidality as he or she further stabilizes medically, education around the destructive nature of avoidance of responsibility should be given to the patient. The consultant can discuss his or her own worries about the dangers of further hospitalization, including psychiatric hospitalization. Some patients may need psychiatric hospitalization after medical discharge to receive further case management and support in planning for life outside the hospital. This recommendation should be made only when appropriate and with concern expressed to the patient.

Managing Medications

Most medical and surgical professionals may not have received training in the potential pitfalls of psychiatric medication management. The consultant should inform both the primary team and the patient about the lack of U.S. Food and Drug Administration–approved medications for the treatment of BPD and the fact that many medications come with more risks than benefits. That being said, if there is evidence of psychotic-like symptoms (e.g., paranoia, extreme agitation, hallucinations), low-dose antipsychotics may be used for a short duration of time in the hospital. The consultant should inform the primary team that anxiolytic medications should be prescribed as standing orders rather than on an as-needed basis. The use of standing orders avoids reinforcing the ideas that distress is intolerable and that medications should be used as first-line interventions for distressing symptoms.

Non-habit-forming medications to promote sleep have some utility in reducing vulnerability factors when behavioral interventions have failed; however, they should be presented explicitly to the patient as a short-term intervention. Initiation of antidepressants and mood stabilizers by the psychiatric consultant should be avoided at all costs, unless there is clearly an untreated psychiatric comorbidity (e.g., mania). At the time of discharge, any medication used on a short-term basis should be discontinued if possible, to avoid psychiatric polypharmacy.

For patients who need analgesia after discharge, the consultant should educate the treatment team about the high risk of patients with BPD misusing these medications and potentially developing substance use disorders. The team should be encouraged to make referrals to structured pain management programs or expedited appointments with primary care providers as needed. The standard as-needed medications for mild symptoms such as constipation, nausea, indigestion, and headaches should not be given at discharge unless these symptoms are related to the underlying illness that required hospitalization.

For patients who will be hospitalized for an extended period of time, the consultant may want to coordinate with outpatient prescribers to begin tapers from benzodiazepines and any other medication that has failed to demonstrate efficacy on an outpatient basis. This will reduce the potential for drug-drug interactions and unnecessary side effects. If there is no time to taper benzodiazepines, the patient should be educated about the contraindication and risks of taking these substances when diagnosed with BPD—namely, the risk of further impulsivity, disinhibition, and completed suicide.

Case Vignette

The following case description includes decision points, each of which has several alternative responses listed at the end of the case. The reader will rate each alternative response in terms of its level of helpfulness. Discussions of responses follow.

George is a 32-year-old man who was admitted to the inpatient medical service for the management of a flare-up of his Crohn's disease. Over the course of his admission, he intermittently refuses to be evaluated by several of the medical residents, leaves the floor for up to an hour at a time to smoke cigarettes, and curses loudly when his roommate is assigned. The medical team calls you, the C-L psychiatrist, when they are unable to wean him off of intravenous pain medication and worry that he may have bipolar disorder requiring psychiatric admission. You briefly review George's medical record and the medical progress note for today, in which a reference is made to his cursing at a nurse on rounds this morning. You now feel ready to page the consultee.

The consultee returns your page and sounds exasperated when you ask for a clarification of the consultation question regarding bipolar disorder. She identifies herself as the intern on the team and states, "Please just come and see him. I have too many patients to take care of, and he doesn't even want to get better. If he wants to leave, he can leave. I am only calling you because my attending physician thinks he might be manic or something." [**Decision Point 1**]

You arrive on the medical floor to see a group of security guards standing outside the room of a screaming patient. The medical intern is standing behind the security guards trying to call her attending physician to get authorization for discharge orders. You ask the medical intern what her concerns are and what the risks of discharge at this point would include. She responds that the patient has not been violent, but that most of the other patients on the floor are afraid of him and his assigned nurse wants to search his room to see if he has any drugs that would justify the discharge. She states that he is still in the midst of a Crohn's flare-up and is having several episodes of bloody diarrhea per day and has not yet achieved stable volume status or oral intake. Also, a rise in his kidney function test on his 4 A.M. blood work suggests that he might be developing an acute kidney injury. You thank the intern for taking the time to discuss her concerns with you in the midst of the current chaos and ask if you can try to speak with the patient first, without security present. You also ask if the room search could be postponed for the current time until you can gather more information. She reluctantly agrees.

You enter the room and introduce yourself to George and explain that you have been asked to do a consultation. [**Decision Point 2**] After you have elaborated further on your role, George replies, "Oh, great. They sent a shrink to see me. I've seen so many of you shrinks, and you never help me. All you want to do is lock me up in the hospital, but this time I am not crazy! I know that bitch nurse is out to get me thrown out of here so that I die in my sleep! No one gives a damn about me." You respond with a warm, gentle smile and say with some irreverence, "Ouch! I hate being called a shrink. I would like to think I could be more useful than those others. In fact, I was hoping I could help you figure out how to help you get your point across to the medical team so they might start to listen to you better." George seems intrigued and calms down. He takes a seat on the bed and starts to engage in conversation with you. As he sits, his hospital sleeve falls back to reveal more than 20 horizontal, well-healed scars on his forearms. You take note of this but choose not to ask about it at this time.

As George calms down, you ask what has been upsetting him over the past several days. He states that he is very annoyed about being in the hospital and feels that he is trapped and being experimented on. He says, "I don't know if anyone even talks to each other. The resident I had yesterday was good, but today it's a new one. I get some new nurse every 12 hours, a new doctor every day; I don't even know who is taking care of me. I feel like I am just a name on someone's list. They just don't give a shit. The other day I went outside to smoke for 2 hours and no one even noticed I was gone. How am I supposed to expect them to help me when I get one of my severe pain attacks?" [**Decision Point 3**] You inquire about other vulnerability factors, and George reports frequent headaches, frequent feelings of boredom and emptiness, and not having been able to sleep for more than 2 hours since admission 4 days ago.

Together, you and George make a behavioral plan to structure the rest of his day. You contact the hospital's volunteer services to have the library cart brought to the patient's room and recommend to the team that they request a visit from the chaplain to give George an opportunity to discuss his current suffering. You also ask George to specify some actions that he might take when he feels the urge to scream, and the two of you generate a list of those things; the patient recalls that taking cold showers and applying ice packs to his face have been very helpful in the past. Before you go, you leave George with the task to create an organizational chart of everyone on his care team and to elicit help from staff, if need be, to complete it. You explain the advice you have provided the medical team on the behavior management protocol (see Table 4–4) and also put it in his chart for his care team. Now that he is emotionally regulated, you use this opportunity to give him feedback about his behavior earlier today. [**Decision Point 4**]

After your meeting with George, you check in with his nurse to inform her of his behavioral plan, actions that George found helpful in the past for reducing distressing emotions, and the task he is working on. You also inquire about the possibility of consistently assigning the same nurse to him as often as feasible and limiting disruptions between 11 P.M. and 6 A.M. to promote better sleep hygiene. The nurse remains somewhat frustrated and says, "I don't have time for all of this. I have other patients with real issues to deal with." You remind the nurse of the extra time and energy that George is placing on the treatment team and gently suggest that by promoting a more predictable and structured environment, George is less likely to get agitated, saving time in the longer run. You also ask whether she would be willing to experiment for a short time with preemptively checking on him briefly once per hour to see if he becomes less demanding. She is skeptical but agrees to trial this approach.

Later that day, you call George's primary care doctor and spouse to obtain collateral information. With the history obtained, you feel more confident in a diagnosis of BPD and contemplate giving this diagnosis to George the following day. [**Decision Point 5**]

On the next morning's rounds, you visit George as a follow-up patient and find him to be extremely somnolent and difficult to rouse. While reviewing his medication list, you see that the primary team has started him on olanzapine 10 mg every night at bedtime and that he has received multiple doses of diazepam for anxiety on the evening shift. His other medications include his home regimen of lithium carbonate 900 mg every night at bedtime, valproate 1,000 mg twice a day, citalopram 40 mg daily, clonazepam 1 mg twice a day, and quetiapine 300 mg every night at bedtime. You check with the team to assess the indication for diazepam and olanzapine the night before and discover that the olanzapine was started after the team saw the diagnosis of BPD in your consultation note. The medical intern believed that BPD was similar to bipolar disorder and that the paranoia that George was exhibiting the night before was evidence for psychosis. You educate the team on the interpersonal nature of BPD, including sensitivity to abandonment that often leads patients to display erratic, aggressive, and sometimes psychotic behaviors. You clarify that although short courses of an antipsychotic may at times be warranted, the long-term metabolic effects of ongoing antipsychotic use are associated with poor health outcomes. You advise several medication changes in your daily recommendations. [**Decision Point 6**]

Over the next 2 days, George remains in better behavioral control and is more alert and cooperative with his team. For 3 nights in a row, he has the same nurse who volunteers to check in with him to review whether he has adhered to his daily plan on the condition that he does not leave the floor for an unauthorized smoke break. George's Crohn's symptoms are improving, and he has successfully been transitioned to oral pain medications. He is now expressing anxiety about discharge to his primary team and appears more sullen when you meet with him on rounds that day. He says, "This is the nicest anyone has ever treated me. This place saved my life. I am afraid I will get sick again when I leave the hospital and I have no one to help me. Sometimes I wish I would die from my Crohn's." You validate the sadness he is feeling because of losing his current support system and remind him that during the course of his hospitalization, you observed that his mood brightened several times when he felt more connected to other people. You educate him on the difference between nonsustainable support that is generated through crises and long-standing supports that can be achieved through pursuing one's values and joining a group. You recommend that he begin to attend a free support group that the hospital hosts for patients with inflammatory bowel disease as well as join other community groups to strengthen his social support network. He expresses his gratitude for your help and understanding but is not fully committed to following through with your advice. [**Decision Point 7**]

After your final meeting with George, you meet with the primary team to discuss final recommendations for discharge and to sign off on the case. You proactively report your safety assessment and advise them not to place him on a psychiatric hold should he express further passive suicidal thinking. You also recommend limiting the supply of medications prescribed at discharge and flag him as a high-risk patient who would benefit from pain management through a structured pain clinic. You also suggest that the team place in the discharge summary the recommendation to taper his clonazepam once he returns to his primary care doctor. Last, you ask that the diagnosis of BPD be recorded in the medical record.

Decision Points: Alternative Responses

Rate each response in terms of its level of helpfulness with a rating of 1 (will be helpful), 2 (possibly helpful, continuing reservations), or 3 (not helpful—or even harmful).

1. In response to the medical intern's comments, the consulting psychiatrist should respond in what manner?

   A. "I get it. Patients like this are a waste of everyone's time. He probably just wants to get intravenous pain medication."
   B. "This patient sounds exceptionally difficult to manage, and I can't imagine how overwhelming this must feel. If you can hold off for a few minutes, I can meet you on your floor to come up with a plan."
   C. "Hold off on discharging, and don't do anything drastic until I see the patient."
   D. "Have you considered giving him some lorazepam and haloperidol to calm him down? Try that first and then call back if you still need a consult."

2. How would you describe your role as a consultant to George?

   A. "The medical team asked me to come because you can't seem to control your behavior."
   B. "Everyone is really concerned about you and thought you might need some extra support."
   C. "I'm here to help you and your team make better sense of what's gone on the past couple of days, and I think I can be useful in improving that relationship."
   D. "I am here to evaluate whether we need to adjust your medications based on the recent symptoms that you've been experiencing."

3. How is one to understand George's thoughts about the medical and nursing staff?

    A. His response reflects a psychotic thought process, and he should be medicated accordingly.
    B. George is demonstrating splitting and regression.
    C. The interpersonal stress attributed to frequent turnover, staff burnout, and separation from the primary support system is experienced as profoundly threatening and encourages maladaptive methods of reestablishing connection and avoiding aloneness and despair.

4. What feedback might you give George about his behaviors on the medical unit?

    A. "You can't scream at everyone here who does not respond to your needs immediately. That is unacceptable."
    B. "Your screaming frightens the staff and other patients. Are you aware that this is how you are coming across? Is this how you'd like to be perceived?"
    C. "I think I can help you to get the team to listen to you better, but it is going to require that you take a much gentler approach than the one you took this morning."
    D. "It makes sense to me that you would act the way you did this morning given how alone and upset you feel."

5. What is the role of the psychiatric consultant in disclosing a diagnosis of BPD to a patient for whom there is reasonable evidence to suggest the diagnosis?

    A. The consultant should refrain from diagnosis and defer to the outpatient team.
    B. The consultant should review the DSM-5 criteria for BPD with the patient and, while doing so, elicit the patient's feedback about the degree to which he identifies with each trait.
    C. The consultant should join the patient in discussing the diagnosis the patient believes he has, in this case bipolar disorder, without challenging the patient's conception of his illness.
    D. It is not the psychiatric consultant's role (nor is it possible) to accurately reach a diagnosis while the patient is under the acute stress associated with medical or surgical hospitalization.

6. Which of the following medication changes are in accordance with the GPM model?

   A. Discontinue olanzapine and double the dose of quetiapine to avoid prescribing two antipsychotic medications.
   B. Confirm George's clonazepam prescription with his pharmacy and, after confirmation, increase the dosage to 1 mg three times a day.
   C. Encourage the primary team to discontinue the olanzapine and diazepam if possible and to refrain from further use of anxiolytics. Also, encourage them to change all opioid medications to long-acting formulations as a standing order.
   D. Ask the team to check lithium and valproate levels to see if they are therapeutic.
   E. Add buspirone 5 mg twice a day for anxiety and depressive symptoms and ask the team to discontinue olanzapine and diazepam.

7. If George continues to become more symptomatic as his medical discharge approaches, what could be helpful?

   A. Validate the difficulty of transitioning back to full independence.
   B. Offer reassurance that George can and has managed to live outside of the hospital for many years and will likely do well once he is discharged.
   C. Reassure George that his insights into his own fears and worries are a sign of progress and underscore the importance of how useful joining a group can be in reducing his symptoms.
   D. Offer voluntary psychiatric hospitalization for further containment and treatment planning.

Discussion Points: Discussion

Numbers within brackets indicate level of helpfulness ratings.

1. In response to the medical intern's comments, the consulting psychiatrist should respond in what manner?

   A. "I get it. Patients like this are a waste of everyone's time. He probably just wants to get intravenous pain medication." [3] (Responding in this manner, although potentially validating, will not promote a better treatment alliance between patient and primary team.)

B. "This patient sounds exceptionally difficult to manage, and I can't imagine how overwhelming this must feel. If you can hold off for a few minutes, I can meet you on your floor to come up with a plan." [1] (This response is both validating and containing and is likely to best promote alliance with the consultee. It also communicates your desire to be both understanding and helpful. The offer to be present during these tensions also establishes your stance as a mediator.)

C. "Hold off on discharging, and don't do anything drastic until I see the patient." [2] (Although the message may be indicated, the tone is problematically reactive and demanding. The consultant should aim to both validate the difficulty in treating this patient and provide recommendations to soothe reactivity from the team.)

D. "Have you considered giving him some lorazepam and haloperidol to calm him down? Try that first and then call back if you still need a consult." [3] (This response is both dismissive to the team's concerns and potentially harmful to the patient. It is unclear from the information given to what extent the patient could be verbally de-escalated with a validating response, which can be achieved for most patients with BPD. This response is also likely to aggravate interactions with the patient if he is given a chemical restraint without a clear indication.)

2. How would you describe your role as a consultant to George?

A. "The medical team asked me to come because you can't seem to control your behavior." [3] (This response is not ideal because it communicates that the team is deficient in their skills. It also is problematic to endorse a goal of controlling the patient's behaviors. Rather, it is best to take an approach that demonstrates that you are advocating for both the patient and the team to reach specific goals—rather than vie in a power struggle—from the onset.)

B. "Everyone is really concerned about you and thought you might need some extra support." [2] (Although this clearly outlines the effect that the patient is having on the primary team, it does not invite the patient to accept more accountability or to problem solve. It also sets a less specific framework from which the psychiatric consultant can serve in the liaison between the medical service and the patient.)

C. "I'm here to help you and your team make better sense of what's gone on the past couple of days, and I think I can be useful in improving that relationship." [1] (This response begins with a simple and attainable focus that equally aligns with the medical team and the patient.)

D. "I am here to evaluate whether we need to adjust your medications based on the recent symptoms that you've been experiencing." [3] (Medications will likely have limited utility in the consultation recommendations for George.)

3. How is one to understand George's thoughts about the medical and nursing staff?

A. His response reflects a psychotic thought process, and he should be medicated accordingly. [3] (The rotation of hospital personnel is to be expected, but given the interpersonal hypersensitivity of patients with BPD, teams can expect more malevolent or paranoid interpretations of the team members' motives. These reactions do not demonstrate frank psychosis but rather distortions in perception under stress.)

B. George is demonstrating splitting and regression. [2] (Although this might be true, this framework may promote a pejorative view of George and not clarify a pathway to management.)

C. The interpersonal stress attributed to frequent turnover, staff burnout, and separation from the primary support system is experienced as profoundly threatening and encourages maladaptive methods of reestablishing connection and avoiding aloneness and despair. [1] (This way of understanding what George is saying allows for a descriptive outline of stressful factors that aggravated his BPD symptoms of intense anger and devaluation.)

4. What feedback might you give George about his behaviors on the medical unit?

A. "You can't scream at everyone here who does not respond to your needs immediately. That is unacceptable." [3] (Although this might be true, it insufficiently explains the problem George creates for his caregivers in their effort to provide optimal medical support. Being more specific about why the behavior is problematic from a position of promoting the patient's goals will strengthen his alliance with the consultant and his likelihood of getting on board with directives).

B. "Your screaming frightens the staff and other patients. Are you aware that this is how you are coming across? Is this how you'd like to be perceived?" [2] (This more descriptive approach, when delivered patiently, allows him to think about the effects of his behaviors on others. The response could be improved by connecting the effects of George's tendency to frighten others on the care he receives.)

C. "I think I can help you to get the team to listen to you better, but it is going to require that you take a much gentler approach than the one you took this morning." [1] (This approach will align with the patient's goals and feel more relatable as well as less blaming.)

D. "It makes sense to me that you would act the way you did this morning given how alone and upset you feel." [1] (This statement validates the patient's experience and allows you to instruct him on your interpretation that his anger or threatened state stems from feeling alone. This is the core formulation of BPD symptoms in GPM.)

5. What is the role of the psychiatric consultant in disclosing a diagnosis of BPD to a patient for whom there is reasonable evidence to suggest the diagnosis?

A. The consultant should refrain from diagnosis and defer to the outpatient team. [3] (The C-L psychiatrist can use the immediate context and interactions from the hospital setting to instruct George on the relevance of the diagnosis, which has been a key issue in interfering with the delivery of his medical care.)

B. The consultant should review the DSM-5 criteria for BPD with the patient and, while doing so, elicit the patient's feedback about the degree to which he or she identifies with each trait. [1] (This approach will often lead to an increased acceptance of the definitive diagnosis once it is given, while also gathering more clinical information to inform the prognosis and treatment approach. If the patient endorses the presence of even one trait of BPD while reviewing the criteria, research shows that this increases risk for hospitalization, depression, and suicidality [Zimmerman et al. 2012].)

C. The consultant should join the patient in discussing the diagnosis the patient believes he has, in this case bipolar disorder, without challenging the patient's conception of his illness. [3] (The consultant should not reinforce a misdiagnosis if his or her judgment aligns with a more accurate one. If a medical professional allowed patients to continue to believe they had conditions for which they did not actually meet criteria, this would be considered malpractice. Instead, accurate diagnosis promotes proper medical and self-care.)

D. It is not the psychiatric consultant's role (nor is it possible) to accurately reach a diagnosis while the patient is under the acute stress associated with medical or surgical hospitalization. [3] (Research shows that diagnostic disclosure and psychoeducation can improve symptoms of BPD [Zanarini et al. 2018]. Consultants can organize patient care by adding proper diagnosis to the record with resources such as the behavior management protocol [see Table 4–4].)

6. Which of the following medication changes are in accordance with the GPM model?

A. Discontinue olanzapine and double the dose of quetiapine to avoid prescribing two antipsychotic medications. [2] (The C-L psychiatrist should evaluate first whether or not a medication is helping the patient and taper those that are not. GPM would encourage the idea of reducing or simplifying the medication regimen.)

B. Confirm George's clonazepam prescription with his pharmacy and, after confirmation, increase the dosage to 1 mg three times a day. [3] (Benzodiazepines in particular are not proven effective in the treatment of BPD and can have disinhibiting effects that worsen rather than improve the situation.)

C. Encourage the primary team to discontinue the olanzapine and diazepam if possible and to refrain from further use of anxiolytics. Also, encourage them to change all opioid medications to long-acting formulations as a standing order. [1] (Simplifying medication plans by eliminating medications that have no indication for a patient's problem list, in addition to simplifying the medication administration schedule, can help patients use medications more predictably rather than reactively.)

D. Ask the team to check lithium and valproate levels to see if they are therapeutic. [2] (Although this is standard of care for the management of these medications, the optimal course of action is to reduce medications. A careful review of why these agents were started and what benefits they have is indicated prior to titration of dosing.)

E. Add buspirone 5 mg twice a day for anxiety and depressive symptoms and ask the team to discontinue olanzapine and diazepam. [2] (Discontinuing diazepam is a good idea because George is already taking clonazepam without clear indication. George is not complaining of depression and anxiety. He is distressed, not depressed.)

7. If George continues to become more symptomatic as his medical discharge approaches, what could be helpful?

A. Validate the difficulty of transitioning back to full independence. [1] (Transitions are difficult for patients with BPD, who will be anxious to know who will be helpful and understanding outside a caretaking system like the hospital. Naming this frames a problem you can work with him to troubleshoot.)

B. Offer reassurance that George can and has managed to live outside of the hospital for many years and will likely do well once he is discharged. [3] (As much as this might be true, this response invalidates the patient's fears of being on his own after a crisis in which he felt vulnerable and uncared for in a way that caused his BPD symptoms to flare up. Noting it will be difficult for the patient, while communicating your reassurance that he can manage, is a more balanced approach.)

C. Reassure George that his insights into his own fears and worries are a sign of progress and underscore the importance of how useful joining a group can be in reducing his symptoms. [1] (Impress upon patients that reflective insights about their fears can be communicated verbally in a way that brokers support. This is the goal: to increase verbal communication and decrease behavioral communication to get needs met. By appreciating George's efforts, the consultant can help build his confidence in the face of his fears.)

   D. Offer voluntary psychiatric hospitalization for further containment and treatment planning. [3] (Reactive hospitalization to prevent distress would only reinforce George's fears that he cannot manage. For him to build better coping skills and a life more worth living for him, he will need to have the opportunity to manage better on his own, between Crohn's flare-ups, to build his self-esteem and sense of security.)

Conclusion

Clinicians in C-L psychiatry can help medical and surgical colleagues understand that acute and chronic medical issues are more prevalent in patients with BPD than in the general population. General hospital teams may not have received proper formal education or guidance on the management of BPD in any setting. Patients with BPD are often identified as difficult or noncompliant, rather than as psychiatrically symptomatic, and experience stigma for both BPD and their concomitant medical diagnoses. C-L psychiatrists can use GPM principles to organize their consultation with their medical and surgical colleagues. GPM prepares C-L psychiatrists to confront misdiagnosis as well as educate their consultees on how to understand and accurately communicate with patients with BPD in managing their care. Like other referrals originating from busy and pressured medical and surgical hospital units, those involving patients with BPD require that the consultant speak to the team seeking the consult to clarify concerns, expectations, and observations before formulating a plan of interventions. The C-L psychiatrist's interventions include alliance building, advocacy, and education for both patient and consulting team regarding emotional reactivity and suboptimal medical decision making. The Behavior Management Protocol (see Table 4–4) is provided as a guide for managing reactivity and framing expectations about the organization of the patient's care as well as the staff's availability. With these interventions, the C-L psychiatrist can help colleagues in the general hospital transition from a reactive to a proactive position. These efforts help colleagues understand the interpersonal hypersensitivity model of BPD, which in turn allows them to objectively understand interpersonal interactions as symptoms of BPD rather than as outcomes of an inept or uncaring team or the fault of a "bad" patient. By clarifying a more productive and predictable way of understanding the patient with BPD in the general medical hospital, the C-L psychiatrist can also help the treatment team reduce unnecessary or harmful medication regimens aimed to control the behavior of the patient with BPD. Ultimately, restoring the medical and surgical team's ability to provide good care is the goal of the GPM C-L psychiatrist. Hopefully, this understanding can also reduce stigma and inconsistent care of patients with BPD, which is likely what both the professionals and the patients desire.

References

Al-Huthail YR: Accuracy of referring psychiatric diagnosis. Int J Health Sci (Qassim) 2(1):35–38, 2008 21475469

Bastien CH, Guimond S, St-Jean G, Lemelin S: Signs of insomnia in borderline personality disorder individuals. J Clin Sleep Med 4(5):462–470 2008 18853705

Bennett WR, Joesch JM, Mazur M, Roy-Byrne P: Characteristics of HIV-positive patients treated in a psychiatric emergency department. Psychiatr Serv 60(3):398–401, 2009 19252056

Breckenridge J, Clark JD: Patient characteristics associated with opioid versus nonsteroidal anti-inflammatory drug management of chronic low back pain. J Pain 4(6):344–350, 2003 14622692

Dilts SLJr, Mann N, Dilts JG: Accuracy of referring psychiatric diagnosis on a consultation-liaison service. Psychosomatics 44(5):407–411, 2003 12954915

Dixon-Gordon KL, Whalen DJ, Layden BK, et al: A systematic review of personality disorders and health outcomes. Can Psychol 56(2):168–190, 2015 26456998

Eren N, Şahin S: An evaluation of the difficulties and attitudes mental health professionals experience with people with personality disorders. J Psychiatr Ment Health Nurs 23(1):22–36, 2016 26272790

Fok MLY, Hayes RD, Chang CK, et al: Life expectancy at birth and all-cause mortality among people with personality disorder. J Psychosom Res 73(2):104–107, 2012 22789412

Frankenburg FR, Zanarini MC: Personality disorders and medical comorbidity. Curr Opin Psychiatry 19(4)428–431, 2006 16721176

Groves JE: Management of the borderline patient on a medical or surgical ward: the psychiatric consultant's role. Int J Psychiatry Med 6(3):337–348, 1975 1230444

Groves JE: Taking care of the hateful patient. N Engl J Med 298(16):883–887, 1978 634331

Gunderson JG, Links PS: Handbook of Good Psychiatric Management for Borderline Personality Disorder. Washington, DC, American Psychiatric Publishing, 2014

Hjorthøj C, Stürup AE, McGrath JJ, et al: Years of potential life lost and life expectancy in schizophrenia: a systematic review and meta-analysis. Lancet Psychiatry 4(4):295–301, 2017 28237639

Kahl KG, Greggersen W, Schweiger U, et al: Prevalence of the metabolic syndrome in patients with borderline personality disorder: results from a cross-sectional study. Eur Arch Psychiatry Clin Neurosci 263(3):205–213, 2013 22777277

Knesper DJ: My favorite tips for engaging the difficult patient on consultation-liaison psychiatry services. Psychiatr Clin North Am 30(2):245–252, 2007 17643841

Kontos N, Freudenreich O, Querques J, et al: The consultation psychiatrist as effective physician. Gen Hosp Psychiatry 25(1):20–23, 2003 12583923

Powers AD, Oltmanns TF: Borderline personality pathology and chronic health problems in later adulthood: the mediating role of obesity. Personal Disord 4(2):152–159, 2013 22686464

Ramchandani D, Lamdan RM, O'Dowd MA, et al: What, why, and how of consultation-liaison psychiatry. An analysis of the consultation process in the 1990s at five urban teaching hospitals. Psychosomatics 38(4):349–355, 1997 9217405

Riddle M, Meeks T, Alvarez C, et al: When personality is the problem: managing patients with difficult personalities on the acute care unit. J Hosp Med 11(12):873–878, 2016 27610608

Roepke S, Ziegenhorn A, Kronsbein J, et al: Incidence of polycystic ovaries and androgen serum levels in women with borderline personality disorder. J Psychiatr Res 44(13):847–852, 2010 20149393

Rothrock J, Lopez I, Zweilfer R, Andress-Rothrock D, et al: Borderline personality disorder and migraine. Headache 47(1):22–26, 2007 17355490

Sansone RA, Wiederman MW, Monteith D: Obesity, borderline personality symptomatology, and body image among women in a psychiatric outpatient setting. Int J Eat Disord 29(1):76–79, 2001 11135337

Semiz UB, Basoglu C, Ebrinc S, Cetin M: Nightmare disorder, dream anxiety, and subjective sleep quality in patients with borderline personality disorder. Psychiatry Clin Neurosci 62(1):48–55, 2008 18289141

Zanarini MC, Conkey LC, Temes CM, et al: Randomized controlled trial of web-based psychoeducation for women with borderline personality disorder. J Clin Psychiatry 79(3), 2018 28703950

Zimmerman M, Chelminski I, Young D, et al: Does the presence of one feature of borderline personality disorder have clinical significance? Implications for dimensional ratings of personality disorders. J Clin Psychiatry 73(1):8–12, 2012 22054015

Chapter 5

Generalist Adult Outpatient Psychiatry Practice

Daniel G. Price, M.D.

The genesis of good psychiatric management (GPM) as treatment for borderline personality disorder (BPD) involved the marriage of two distinct treatment paradigms. Its core represents a distillation of John Gunderson's *Borderline Personality Disorder: A Clinical Guide* (Gunderson and Links 2008). In the book's first edition, an experienced specialist wrote about something close to individual treatment in a private practice setting. GPM was born when this specialist wisdom was manualized by Paul Links to create a treatment easily teachable to generalists in a clinic setting for use as a robust comparison arm in research about dialectical behavior therapy (DBT; Gunderson and Links 2014; McMain et al. 2009, 2012). GPM's further elaboration in the *Handbook of Good Psychiatric Management for Borderline Personality Disorder* (Gunderson and Links 2014) has resulted in treatment not only appropriate for the generalist clinician encountering patients with BPD in private practice but also ideally suited for structuring the approach of a busy community clinic where patients with BPD exceed the availability of specialized therapies. Following the stepped care model proposed by Lois Choi-Kain (Choi-Kain et al. 2016; see Appendix B, "Stepped Care Model"), GPM and its principles can serve as a framework for diagnosing and treating patients with BPD who present via a variety of conduits (e.g., referrals from the emergency department and primary care providers as well as inpatient and partial hospitalization levels of care) and in a panoply of "guises" (e.g., substance abuse, bipolar disorder, treatment-resistant depression or anxiety, posttraumatic stress disorder [PTSD], psychotic disorders, or long-term therapy impasse cases).

GPM's clinical principles can, in fact, serve as "clinic" principles. Those principles—emphasizing the importance of clearly making and communicating the diagnosis, hopeful and active expectation of change, pragmatism, collaboration, multimodality and the use of groups, rationally addressing comorbidity, deemphasizing medications, fostering accountability, and setting measurable goals—are ideally suited for the demands of a busy clinic that is expected to take all comers despite limited resources. These are also principles, as discussed in this chapter, that mesh nicely with individual treatment plans required for all patients by regulators of such clinics. In this chapter, I delineate how GPM's principles can act as a scaffold for a clinic pragmatically supporting the treatment of a population of patients with BPD, analogous to how it acts as a scaffold for a clinician providing pragmatic support for the treatment of an individual patient with BPD.

Patients With Borderline Personality Disorder in the Outpatient Clinic: The Challenge

The prevalence of BPD in outpatient clinics is daunting. Approximately 10% of patients in psychiatric outpatient clinics have BPD (Zimmerman et al. 2010). These patients are disproportionately high utilizers of inpatient care (Comtois and Carmel 2016). Many of the patients who have BPD in such clinics have not been diagnosed or, if the diagnosis has been made, are either unaware of or not receiving treatment for the disorder.

Such underdiagnosis and undertreatment at outpatient clinics appear to stem from a host of causes. Given the traditional stigma of BPD, many patients *and clinicians* have resisted the use of the diagnosis. Additionally, frequent comorbidity can either obscure the diagnosis or lead to misplaced emphasis on the treatment of one or more other diagnoses to the exclusion of addressing BPD (Paris and Black 2015). Treatment choice may be determined by the treatments most widely available at the particular clinic. When faced with difficult patients and limited evidence-based care, available treaters choose the easiest option at their disposal (Paris 2015). Abraham Maslow's (1966, p. 15) so-called law of the instrument—"it is tempting, if the only tool you have is a hammer, to treat everything as if it were a nail"—might be recast as follows: "When all you have is 20-minute medication visits and Seeking Safety groups, everything looks like bipolar disorder or PTSD." Even when robust BPD treatment is available within a clinic (usually DBT in U.S. clinics), the scarcity of this resource frequently leads to the underdiagnosis and underemphasis of BPD treatment in the wider clinic. Clinicians often act as though they think, "Better to diagnose the depression I feel able to treat than the BPD that I don't and the DBT team can't accommodate." A recent study found that at some point during their career, as a result of either concerns about stigma or diagnostic uncertainty, 57% of clinicians had failed to disclose the diagnosis of BPD and 37% had failed to document it (Sisti et al. 2016). Of course, some clinicians in outpatient private practice can and do choose not to treat BPD at all; they can accurately diagnose BPD but choose to refer to others who "do DBT" or in some cases refer to other clinicians without informing patients of their diagnosis. Given the immediate benefits of discussing the diagnosis, the respect for a patient's autonomy that such a discussion shows, and the longer-term benefits that receiving an accurate diagnosis has on driving effective treatment, not disclosing the diagnosis may be unethical (Howe 2013). Even disclosing the diagnosis but referring "to DBT specialists" is of questionable value when these specialty services are in such limited supply.

Of course, in many mental health clinics (including where I work), treaters could not refer their patients with BPD elsewhere even if they would personally prefer to do so. Community-based clinics or health system–based clinics often have a mandate to care for all comers, sometimes regardless of patients' ability to pay. Community mental health clinics often serve patients who cannot afford treatment elsewhere, and therefore treatment for their BPD will be provided in the clinic *or nowhere.* The rise of accountable care organizations (ACOs) will likely amplify the problem. This care delivery model—encouraged by the Affordable Care Act—puts integrated health care and mental health care systems in charge of (and financially responsible for) all of a patient's health and mental health needs. If patients with BPD in an ACO are going to get a diagnosis and receive outpatient treatment for the diagnosis, it will happen within the ACO. If patients do not get diagnosed or treated for their BPD, their emergency department visits and hospitalizations will, nevertheless, be paid for by the system (ACO) itself. Although specialized treatments have been shown to be effective, they are generally in short supply nationally and in the clinic setting (Richter et al. 2016). Outpatient clinics in such a setting will need to devise a plan for diagnosing and treating BPD patients that proves to be more cost-effective than ignoring them, treating them as though they have something else, referring them out, or referring them to the overbooked DBT service.

Treatment Planning With GPM Principles

Outpatient mental health clinics must serve a lot of masters and please a lot of regulators. State agencies, the Centers for Medicare and Medicaid Services, and The Joint Commission (formerly Joint Commission on Accreditation of Healthcare Organizations) all require use of individual treatment plans for psychiatric patients with periodic updates (typically every 3 months). These plans are meant to ensure basic standards of care, transparent treatment, collaboration between treater and treated, achievable goals, and expectations for change. When positive change is not occurring, mandatory treatment planning can push patient and clinician to reconsider the treatment.

Most clinics have developed flexible treatment plan templates for major depressive disorder, generalized anxiety disorder, psychotic disorders, and other mental illnesses. We are now in the era of electronic medical records, virtual templates that are easily adaptable. These templates present a multicolumn menu of choices for naming targeted symptoms or problems related to the diagnosis, goals related to these symptoms or problems, and potential interventions. According to most regulatory agencies, the goals themselves are meant to be SMART (specific, measurable, achievable, relevant, and timely).

Fortunately, GPM's pragmatic, collaborative approach, in which positive change is expected, is almost tailor-made for elaborating individualized treatment plans. To start with, GPM's recommendations about how to prioritize comorbidities can be reified in a treatment plan template. For instance, if a patient has opioid use disorder along with BPD, the treatment plan could specify that the goals for the first 3 months are focused on the opioid use disorder as the targeted problem. The SMART goal for this might read, "The patient will have clean random drug screens for 3 consecutive months," and the intervention might be "referral to and treatment in a dual-diagnosis intensive outpatient program (DDIOP) with buprenorphine-assisted treatment." At 3 months, when the team and patient collaboratively evaluate this problem-goal-intervention triad, if the goal has been met, they can identify another problem-goal-intervention triad. In this example, if the patient's urine drug screens remain negative in an intensive outpatient program, it may make sense to focus on problems more directly related to her BPD—for example, hopelessness about BPD symptoms (see Table 5–1). A goal may be for the patient to have an understanding of the diagnosis, prognosis, and treatment options for her BPD, and an intervention could be framed in terms of psychoeducation (e.g., attendance at a BPD psychoeducation group).

A patient's fear of abandonment could likewise be explicitly addressed in a treatment plan. Here, GPM's predictions about the development of alliance (from a contractual alliance beginning in the first 3 weeks to 3 months to a relational alliance, which may take 6 months to a year) can be used to generate realistic measurable goals in a stepwise fashion. Thus, in the first month, the item "patient will report understanding of the frame—his or her role and role of the therapist—and establish treatment goals" could provide an achievable goal. Once this has been achieved, the more ambitious "patient will report experiencing therapist as caring, genuine, and understanding" can be identified as the new goal. Later, the item "patient will recognize difficult observations by therapist as being well intended," can serve as a more advanced milestone for measuring diminishing "fear of abandonment" in the patient. During this time, "collaborative, pragmatic, individual case management sessions" can be identified on the treatment plan as the main clinician intervention in service of these goals. Formal treatment plans can likewise mesh well with GPM's philosophy on medication usage. If a patient asks about trying a particular medication, the treatment plan review can present a concrete opportunity to establish what *problem* the medication (i.e., intervention) will be addressing and how (and in what time frame) the patient will help you determine whether the medicine is helping (i.e., SMART goal).

Used in this way, a formal treatment plan can be an effective way to reify GPM principles. The patient and treater are forced to collaborate, expect and document change, agree on achievable goals, and be clear about what interventions will be employed to achieve these goals. Importantly, such a treatment plan can also coordinate the elements of an overall GPM-informed treatment of BPD that an outpatient mental health clinic can provide. These elements in all good psychiatric treatments will include appropriate diagnosis, rational prioritizing of treatment of comor-

TABLE 5–1. Template of individualized treatment plan reflecting good psychiatric management (GPM) recommendations for the treatment of borderline personality disorder (BPD)

Problem: BPD

Target date	Short-term goals (SMART goals)
1 week	Patient will report understanding of diagnosis.
2 weeks	Patient will complete a safety plan with treater.
3 weeks	Patient will report understanding of the frame—his or her role and role of the therapist—and establish treatment goals (*contractual alliance*).
	Patient will regularly attend treatment.
	Patient will report decrease in subjective distress.
3 months	Patient will identify and use three adaptive coping skills to manage stress.
6 months	Patient will have decrease in dangerous behaviors, including self-harm, rages, and impulsive substance use.
	Patient will recognize significance of adverse interpersonal events, such as rejection or separations.
	Patient will report experiencing therapist as caring, genuine, and understanding (*relational alliance*).
9 months	Patient's Borderline Symptom List score will be reduced by half from baseline.
1 year	Patient will recognize difficult observations by therapist as being well intended (*working alliance*).
	Patient will have returned to meaningful work/school.

TABLE 5–1. Template of individualized treatment plan reflecting good psychiatric management (GPM) recommendations for the treatment of borderline personality disorder (BPD) *(continued)*

		Problem: BPD			
Treatment interventions					
Diagnosis	General	Family involvement	Individual therapy	Group therapy referral	
Discuss diagnosis with patient	Psychoeducation group therapy (8 weeks)	Family psychoeducation group	GPM treatment with ___	Self-assessment group	
Prioritize BPD as primary unless patient presents with	Completion of safety planning process	Review "Family Guidelines"[a]	DBT with ___	Self-help group (AA, etc.) Interpersonal group with	
Active substance dependence	Collaborative, pragmatic, individual case management sessions	"Family Connections"[b] multifamily group	MBT with ___		
Active anorexia nervosa	Referral to vocational services	Conjoint session with family		DBT skills group	
Active mania	Chain analysis as needed			MBT group	
Complex posttraumatic stress disorder	Patient-created autobiography				

Note. AA=Alcoholics Anonymous; DBT=dialectical behavior therapy; MBT=mentalization-based treatment; SMART=specific, measurable, achievable, relevant, and timely.

[a]See www.borderlinepersonalitydisorder.org/family-connections/family-guidelines/.
[b]See www.borderlinepersonalitydisorder.org/family-connections/.

bidities, expectations of positive functional change, and targeted use of medications, groups, and vocational services.

GPM Versus Specialized Borderline Personality Disorder Treatment in the General Adult Outpatient Setting

One may reasonably ask this question: If effective evidence-based treatments (EBTs) have been developed, why would an outpatient clinic bother to use a generalist treatment? If DBT were economical and DBT clinicians were plentiful, it might be rational for all patients with BPD to be treated with DBT. Unfortunately, DBT remains expensive monetarily and in terms of resource utilization. DBT in its standard format requires 1 hour weekly of individual therapy, around 1.5–2.5 hours weekly of skills group, availability of 24/7 coaching, and a 2-hour weekly DBT team consultation (Linehan et al. 2015). The therapists providing all of this treatment require hours of formal training and pretraining homework. Moreover, the cost of training currently stands at multiple hundreds of dollars per clinician for basic training and thousands for level-3 certification. It is likely for this reason that although 40,000 clinicians have attended a DBT workshop or training through the primary training institute for DBT (Behavioral Tech 2018), as of December 2018, there were only 240 DBT-Linehan Board of Certification–certified clinicians listed (see http://dbt-lbc.org/index.php?page=101163). Given the standard conservative estimate that approximately 2% of the population has BPD—and therefore, around 6 million people in the United States—it would require 600,000 clinicians capable of treating 10 patients with BPD at a time (a tall order for any clinician).

The numbers are only slightly more sanguine for other EBTs. Mentalization-based treatment (MBT) has also been shown in a number of studies to treat BPD effectively, but it too is both labor and training intensive. In addition to attendant supervision time, MBT generally requires 1 hour of individual therapy and 1.25 hours of group therapy weekly for each patient (Bateman and Fonagy 2016). Training requirements for MBT are less than for DBT but, nevertheless, require a 3-day course at a minimum. Although MBT is more widely distributed in Europe, fewer than 1,000 fully trained MBT therapists are estimated to exist in the United States, and only a few U.S. clinics are capable of providing anything like high-fidelity MBT care (Anna Freud National Centre for Children and Families 2018).

Transference-focused psychotherapy (TFP) also has built a significant evidence base. Generally eschewing groups, TFP is intended to be conducted as twice-a-week psychotherapy for at least a few years (Yeomans et al. 2015). Three days of training are also required for TFP, with a stated prerequisite of previous work as a psychodynamic therapist, along with 1 year of video-assisted group supervision—itself costing more than $1,000 a year. As a result of both the length of training and the prerequisite therapy experience, the number of TFP therapists will likely remain limited.

Although in an ideal world, specialist EBTs might represent the treatments of choice for BPD, they are usually not available as options for the reasons discussed. Even when EBTs are available at a particular clinic, they are rarely sufficient to treat all patients with BPD. In our clinic, where we have a DBT service, an MBT service, and a TFP clinician, our capacity for treating patients with BPD with these treatments is roughly 30 patients at a time. Given that the shortest recommended time for these specialist treatments is 1 year, 30 would be the total number of patients we could treat per year for BPD. Our clinic saw 2,664 unique outpatients last year (Masland et al. 2018). For all the reasons noted here, BPD is severely underdiagnosed in our clinic, but if we accept that 10% of all outpatients have BPD, as Zimmerman et al. (2010) suggest, we expect that our clinic in fact would have more than 250 patients with BPD. Most patients with BPD in our clinic, like most patients with BPD in the United States, simply cannot receive specialty EBTs (Zanarini 2008). In response to this chronic resource shortage, GPM's clinical principles can inform principles for a clinic and population health. Flexibility, eclecticism, and pragmatism encourage the use of a system of care not married to one type of treatment, especially one that is not feasible.

Fortunately, patients with BPD do not require intensive treatments to get better. In fact, the Collaborative Longitudinal Personality Disorders Study, which followed 175 patients with BPD naturalistically and longitudinally, found that more than 85% of patients with BPD remitted over 10 years, and the vast majority did not relapse once remitted (Gunderson et al. 2011). Few if any of these patients received intensive EBT (Gunderson et al. 2011), but the eclectic treatments they received were probably "good enough" (Zanarini 2008). Although there is some evidence about which comorbidities should be treated first (see next section), it remains unclear which characteristics of patients with BPD predict who will need intensive specialty treatments. Thus, a clinic charged with treating a population efficiently can benefit from offering the less intensive GPM first and reserving more intensive treatments for those patients for whom this usually "good enough" treatment was unsuccessful. The stepped care model outlined by Choi-Kain et al. (2016; see Appendix B) provides such a pragmatic and flexible approach. Readers can review Chapters 13, 14, and 15 in this volume for greater detail about integrating GPM with DBT, MBT, and TFP, respectively. In contrast to the modular approach of Livesley et al. (2016) proposing an eclectic use of many EBTs *within* one treatment or an attempt to distill the common principles of such treatments, Choi-Kain et al. (2016) proposed that GPM could serve as the initial treatment for mild, moderate, and even severe cases of BPD. For many, this practice may prove successful in inducing remission and have the advantage of "redistributing the bulk of BPD care to the generalist mental health professional" (Choi-Kain et al. 2016, p. 353).

GPM's expectation of change, its pragmatic espousal of frequently assessing whether treatment is useful, and its belief that treatment should be changed if it is ineffective can direct how the clinic approaches treatment structure. These practical GPM elements can be instantiated not only in the clinic's structure but also, as noted in the previous section, in the individualized treatment plan for the patient. If and only if patients are not improving as expected should a patient be offered more intensive specialist EBT treatment. In our clinic, patients with mild or moderate BPD symptoms are offered GPM first. Moreover, we only accept referrals to our EBT from outside the clinic for patients who have already received GPM and for whom the treatment failed. As with GPM treatment itself, this stepped care system works by emphasizing psychoeducation first. That is, GPM training can be offered to mental health workers in the clinic and the broader health care system, preparing them to diagnose, treat, and case manage the majority of BPD cases within the system. Our initial single-day training led to improved attitudes about BPD among mental health care clinicians from diverse disciplines, consistent with the findings of Keuroghlian et al. (2016). These changes persisted over a 6-month follow-up period (Masland et al. 2018), and we are utilizing this to broaden the reach of our stepped care model and effective BPD treatment within our system.

Comorbidity Management

One of the reasons why underrecognition and undertreatment are so common for patients with BPD is that comorbidity is the rule and pure BPD is the exception (Zanarini et al. 1998). Comorbidity is so common that some have argued that it should be a criterion for the diagnosis of BPD (Sansone and Sansone 2008). Given the complex comorbidity patterns found in patients with BPD (Table 5–2), deciding how treatment should proceed can be difficult. GPM argues that acknowledging the limited but growing data can guide treatment and its sequencing, and a clinic should build this sequencing into its treatment plans (see Table 5–1). As GPM sug-

TABLE 5–2. **Managing comorbidities in the treatment of borderline personality disorder (BPD)**

Comorbid condition	Subtype	BPD primary	How comorbidity should be approached
Anxiety disorders		Yes	Treat BPD, and anxiety disorder will likely resolve.[a]
Major depression		Yes	Treat BPD, and major depression will likely resolve.[b]
Bipolar disorder	Bipolar disorder I	No	If patient is manic, patient will be unable to benefit from BPD treatment; otherwise, treat both simultaneously.[c]
	Bipolar disorder II	Yes	Bipolar disorder II will stabilize as BPD stabilizes and can benefit from similar interventions.[c]
Substance use disorders	Dependence	No	Require sobriety/abstinence for a period of months prior to BPD treatment; proceed with diagnosis and psychoeducation but expect patient to work on sobriety first.[d]
	Abuse	Yes	If it will not interfere with therapy, treat substance abuse and BPD concurrently; remission of a substance use disorder is strong predictor of improvement in BPD.[d]
Eating disorders	Anorexia nervosa[e]	No	BPD treatment is not feasible if anorexia nervosa is active.[e]
	Bulimia nervosa;[f] eating disorder not otherwise specified	Yes	Treat BPD if physical health is stable.[f]

TABLE 5–2.   **Managing comorbidities in the treatment of borderline personality disorder (BPD)** *(continued)*

Comorbid condition	Subtype	BPD primary	How comorbidity should be approached
Posttraumatic stress disorder (PTSD)	Complex PTSD	No	Inability to trust therapist prevents establishment of alliance; treat complex PTSD before BPD.[a]
	Adult onset	Yes	If patient is able to participate in BPD treatment, treat BPD.[a]
Other personality disorders	Antisocial personality disorder	Unknown	Be cautious and determine whether treatment is being pursued for secondary gain.[c]
	Narcissistic personality disorder (NPD)	Yes	Treat BPD; NPD makes treating BPD more difficult, but NPD will improve if BPD does[c]; good psychiatric management for NPD can be adapted when BPD stabilizes (see Chapter 12, "Implementation of Good Psychiatric Management for Narcissistic Personality Disorder").

[a]Keuroghlian et al. 2015.
[b]Zanarini et al. 1998, 2004.
[c]Gunderson et al. 2014.
[d]Walter et al. 2009; Yen et al. 2004; Zanarini et al. 2011.
[e]Zanarini et al. 2010.
[f]Grilo et al. 2003; Zanarini et al. 2010.

gests, optimizing treatment requires determining either that 1) a comorbid condition precludes participating in BPD treatment or 2) the comorbid condition is likely to remit when BPD does. Depression and most anxiety disorders, including PTSD, fall into the "likely to remit" category, and thus a clinic should require that patients with these diagnoses comorbid with BPD receive treatment for BPD first. Not doing so sets these patients up to fail and results in poor use of clinic resources. Regarding the first determination, a clinician should consider whether a condition prevents a patient from maintaining motivation or participating in the active learning that GPM and all effective BPD treatments require. Certainly psychosis, ongoing mania, and the frequent intoxication found in substance use disorders fall into this category. The inability to trust anyone, including a clinician, engendered by *complex* PTSD also appears to preclude the stable use of any BPD treatment. Patients who are chronically physically ill or who lack motivation to change, as in active anorexia nervosa, or patients who are seeking treatment only for secondary gain (e.g., those with antisocial personality disorder) are unlikely to benefit from BPD treatment.

A clinic can and should be designed to make determinations regarding comorbidities and require patients with BPD to have definitive treatments for these comorbidities within their clinic or be referred elsewhere. For example, before being offered GPM or other BPD-specific treatment, an active heroin user should be required to receive intensive outpatient treatment and/or opioid replacement treatment leading to remission; a manic patient should have his or her mood stabilized; and an anorexic patient should attain a healthy weight and remission of behaviors threatening stable weight, perhaps through a residential program. Setting these expectations clearly will not only serve the best interests of the patient but also optimize the use of resources in an otherwise stretched clinic.

Utilizing Groups Effectively

Outpatient clinic settings often offer a variety of groups that may be helpful and uniquely effective in treating patients with BPD. Requiring that groups be a part of a patient's treatment plan (see Table 5–1) can help both the patient and the clinic. Groups can certainly be a mechanism for achieving and maintaining remission of the comorbidities that preclude effective BPD treatment (see previous section). Suboxone groups, Alcoholics Anonymous (AA), and Narcotics Anonymous can be key not only to getting a patient with substance use disorders clean but also to keeping the patient clean during BPD treatment. Likewise, patients with anorexia can improve in and be maintained in eating disorder–specific groups. In addition to treating comorbidities, groups can be an economical and readily available "midwife" for delivering effective BPD care.

Younger patients with BPD often have lives filled with chaotic family, romantic, and work relationships, demonstrating the external consequences of their interpersonal hypersensitivity. The psychosocial impairment wrought by such chaos frequently leaves older patients with BPD unemployed, estranged from family, and bereft of romantic relationships as well as friendships. For such patients, groups may offer the only arena for interpersonal hypersensitivity to be brought to light in the here and now. In BPD treatments, group work becomes crucial. Thus, clinics should require patients with BPD to attend groups to have the opportunity to integrate the group-generated material into individual work.

Fortunately, nearly any type of structured group can be useful in this way. Most widely available are self-help groups such as AA, Narcotics Anonymous, or peer-led groups through the National Alliance on Mental Illness and other organizations; these groups are available even outside a clinic setting, are usually free of charge, are open to everyone, and offer support and education. Perhaps more importantly, a patient can use such groups to begin rebuilding a social network. Most mental health clinics offer a number of other group types that will benefit patients with BPD. Self-assessment groups are some of the most common groups found in mental health clinics and offer an opportunity for patients with BPD to obtain support and also to work on skills in listening and expressing difficult feelings with others. Groups teaching patients particular skills to improve social functioning are likewise commonly available. DBT groups are probably the most common example of skills-building groups. However, clinics increasingly offer groups on mindfulness and other so-called third-wave cognitive therapies (e.g., acceptance and commitment therapy; Hayes et al. 2016). Overall, evidence for these groups in treating BPD specifically is limited, but the groups' focus on stress reduction and effectiveness for anxiety and depression more broadly are likely to be accepted by patients and be helpful adjuncts in their care. Mindfulness, long offered as a part of DBT, is increasingly a part of clinic group offerings. Mindfulness training on its own, in the form of DBT-M, was found in one study to enhance the clinical outcome of general psychiatric management of patients with BPD (Feliu-Soler et al. 2014).

Mindfulness is only one of the many skills that DBT therapists consider lacking in patients with BPD. A more detailed discussion of how GPM can integrate with DBT specialty care can be found in Chapter 13, "Integration With Dialectical Behavior Therapy," but given that DBT skills groups are perhaps the most widely available skills-building groups in U.S. mental health centers, we look briefly at how these can be utilized by a GPM practitioner.

As Gunderson and Links (2014) pointed out, GPM's emphasis on developing increased awareness and tolerance of emotions contrasts somewhat with DBT's tactic of learning skills designed to distract from emotions. However, as long as an individual clinician can help a patient utilize these skills, DBT is not incompatible with GPM work. Indeed, DBT skills group work appears to be very helpful to patients with BPD in its own right. A study comparing patients receiving standard DBT (individual DBT+DBT skills+24-hour skills coaching availability) with patients receiving DBT-I (individual DBT therapy only) and with patients receiving DBT-S (DBT skills group+case management) found that DBT-S outperformed DBT-I and was as effective as standard DBT on most measures (Linehan et al. 2015). Ironically, this important finding does not seem to have been embraced by much of the DBT community, but it provides intriguing evidence that DBT skills groups could be effectively paired with GPM, with its emphasis on case management.

In addition to utilizing preexisting groups in the clinic setting, we have found that specific groups, tied closely to GPM's principles, can serve as efficient hubs to facilitate implementation of a stepped care model. GPM argues that psychoeducation is important in reducing stigma, improving hope, and setting expectations about treatment and prognosis for patients with BPD. Indeed, a number of studies are beginning to bear out that simple psychoeducation interventions can be an effective treatment in their own right (Zanarini et al. 2018). To ensure that every patient with BPD in our clinic receives basic information about the diagnosis, etiology, neurobiological underpinnings, and (hopeful) prognosis of BPD, and about the treatment options and expectations in our clinic, we have created an eight-session psychoeducation group (Table 5–3). Every patient who is newly identified as having or potentially having BPD is referred to this group as his or her initiation into BPD treatment.

Beyond its role in ensuring that each patient is appropriately educated about the disorder, the group serves a number of other functions. Our vocational rehabilitation specialist leads part of one session introducing the importance that GPM places on "building a life worth living." Simultaneously, this session serves as an initial evaluation and contact for our patients with this specialist; they can then begin the process of consulting with vocational services to find the job or educational program that will begin this "building."

Later sessions in the group review the treatment options available in the clinic for BPD (in our case, GPM, DBT, and MBT). Patients are able to meet key practitioners in these modalities, participate in exercises consistent with each treatment, and see which approach resonates with them. Their knowledge of the treatments and methods helps patients set their expectations more realistically and becomes very helpful in the final group session. During the last session (week 8), patients meet with one or both of the group leaders in brief sessions in which the leaders present a pre-

TABLE 5–3.   **Sample curriculum outline for borderline personality disorder (BPD) psychoeducation group**

Session	Theme		Content
1	Diagnosis	a.	Introductions
		b.	General information and syllabus review
		c.	How is BPD diagnosed (review of criteria)?
		d.	How is BPD different from bipolar disorder?
		e.	What causes BPD?
		f.	Introduction to interpersonal hypersensitivity model of BPD
2	Course and prognosis	a.	Recap and questions from previous week[a]
		b.	Common myths about BPD explored
		c.	Course and prognosis of BPD
		d.	Which symptoms resolve more quickly and which persist longer?
3	"Building a life"	a.	Importance of using treatment to "build a life"
		b.	Work before love
		c.	How to get help: introduction to clinic's vocational services team[b]
4	Medications and comorbidities	a.	What is known about the role of medications in treatment
		b.	Overview of medication classes and side effects
		c.	What medications are helpful or harmful?
		d.	Comorbidities: how do we know when BPD is the diagnosis that requires prioritized treatment?
		e.	Medical comorbidities: what are the relationships between BPD and chronic medical illness?
		f.	Poor health-related lifestyle choices and health care utilization

TABLE 5–3. **Sample curriculum outline for borderline personality disorder (BPD) psychoeducation group** *(continued)*

Session	Theme	Content
5	Introduction to good psychiatric management (GPM)	a. Reintroducing interpersonal hypersensitivity model of BPD
		b. Emphasis on GPM's pragmatism and expectation of change
		c. Improvement generally involves feelings → behaviors → relationships → functioning
		d. Discussion of alliance and its temporal progression
		e. Discussion of GPM's pragmatic use of groups
		f. Discussion of safety planning, chain analysis, and other basic GPM tools
6	Introduction to dialectical behavior therapy (DBT)	Review of DBT theory and structure of treatment by DBT-trained clinician
7	Introduction to mentalization-based treatment (MBT)	Review of MBT theory and structure of treatment by MBT-trained clinician
Treatment team meeting during which all group participants are discussed and tentative treatment recommendations are developed		
8	30-minute individual meetings with patients	a. Discussion of team's recommendations and patient's thoughts about treatment going forward
		b. Decision about which track patient will begin based on acuity, availability, and patient preference

[a]Each session begins with recap and questions from previous week.
[b]Number of sessions can be modified according to clinic offerings (e.g., introduction to DBT and to MBT sessions can be eliminated in clinics where such sessions are not offered or are currently at capacity; other sessions can be added for clinics offering other evidence-based treatments).

liminary formulation to each patient (based on what the leaders learned from the patient in groups) and participate in shared decision making about their ongoing treatment plan. In our stepped care model, *early mild* cases, defined by Choi-Kain et al. (2016) as having one episode of threshold BPD with self-harm but no suicidal behaviors, are generally referred to GPM care with case management, with a potential group referral (see Appendix B). Sustained moderate cases can be offered a choice between the less-resource-intense GPM with medication management and DBT skills group, or one of our specialty care programs (DBT or MBT). We believe that because the patients have been introduced to the tenets and expectations of each treatment type in the education group, both the patient and the group leaders can more accurately predict which treatment scheme will be most beneficial.

A structured psychoeducation group contributes to improved patient flow within the clinic, as well. A referral to the BPD program from within our larger clinic results in an immediate referral to the psychoeducation group (see Table 5–1). Thereby, we ensure that every patient gains a basic understanding of GPM principles and the disorder. Additionally, by having two such groups started in staggered fashion, a patient can go from identification as a candidate for BPD treatment to beginning treatment within 1 month. Moreover, consistent attendance at the 8-week group serves as a marker for patient readiness to address the problem presented by BPD. Patients with poor attendance can be asked to attend sessions they missed before being referred to an individual GPM treater or to a specialist program.

Beyond having clinical utility, groups can also serve as a vehicle for clinician training. Groups commonly have coleaders, allowing a more seasoned clinician to teach one or more junior ones the elements necessary to care for patients with BPD. In the case of the psychoeducation group described above, psychiatry residents are coleaders with senior faculty. By rotating them in the coleader role, all residents working in the clinic become knowledgeable about and confident in teaching basic facts about BPD, its etiology, and its hopeful prognosis. Furthermore, cofacilitating such a group is an ideal way for residents to begin working with outpatients with BPD before having primary responsibility for patients—as advocated in Unruh and Gunderson's (2016) model of *good enough* psychiatry residency training in BPD.

Patients with BPD can benefit from any number of groups commonly found in the clinic setting. In addition to being cost-effective, groups can add things that individual treatment does not, including a supportive community, a laboratory in which the problems of social living are made explicit, and the valuable perspective of others dealing with the same problems in different ways. Moreover, a psychoeducation group based on GPM principles can support a generalist and a stepped care model approach to treating BPD by providing an efficient way to take in, evaluate, educate, and ultimately develop a treatment plan for BPD referrals in the clinic setting. In a clinic that trains clinicians, groups can also provide an adaptable arena for on-the-job training. Thus, as already noted, groups should be built into the treatment plans of all patients receiving BPD treatment in a clinic setting.

Case Vignette

The following case description includes decision points, each of which has several alternative responses listed at the end of the case. The reader will rate each alternative response in terms of its level of helpfulness. Discussions of responses follow.

> Lance is an unmarried 37-year-old male chef with a previous diagnosis of "clinical depression"; he presents to your outpatient clinic's partial hospitalization program after a 1-week admission to your health system's inpatient hospital. Lance was admitted after having fallen off the wagon following 13 months of sobriety. After Lance lost yet another position as a chef, his girlfriend of almost 1 year, Carol, said she was leaving him. He had been living in a communal living situation with some friends he knew from his most recent rehab. When Carol told him she could not put up with his continual financial and employment woes any longer, Lance became distraught. His craving for alcohol "came on like a freight train," and he went on a "a major bender." Later, he would say that he left his apartment because he did not want to "mess up anyone else's sobriety." He checked into a hotel room so he could drink alone and "maybe just do a *Leaving Las Vegas* kind of thing." A few days later, when Carol and one of his roommates found him in his hotel room, he was intoxicated, living in squalor, and not eating, and clearly had recently vomited. When they tried to reason with him, he broke a bottle and threatened to cut his neck. The police were called, and when he attempted to avoid them, he fell in the stairwell of the hotel, breaking his wrist. He was brought to the medical emergency department and, after having his wrist set, was sent to the psychiatric hospital because of the persistent suicidal statements he made in the emergency department.
>
> The subsequent week-long inpatient psychiatric admission—his first ever—led to referral to the partial hospitalization program. During Lance's 2-week partial hospitalization program stay, a preliminary evaluation by your colleague leads to concerns that Lance may have a personality disorder; your colleague asks if you would take Lance as a patient. [**Decision Point 1**]
>
> You agree to a consultation but do not promise to take on Lance as a patient. On taking a history, you learn that Lance has felt unhappy and empty "ever since I can remember." He felt out of place in high school and struggled with chronic suicidal thoughts. He started drinking at age 15 to "fit in," liking the way it numbed him out, especially when things became stressful. He never liked his schoolwork but followed many of his classmates to the large

state university in his hometown to study business. Quickly, he felt business school was a mistake, boring and "soul sapping"; a friend in the hotel and restaurant management school convinced him to take an introductory class. Lance found that he loved the class, and when he got a weekend job as a prep cook in a fine restaurant, he felt he had found his place. He loved the energy, creativity, and even emotional expressiveness of the kitchen. Although he did not like being yelled at, he did like the fact that a chef could "explode" on others and people tolerated it, and Lance earned good money. He completed his degree in culinary arts and moved up the ranks in a number of top kitchens, but despite this success, his emptiness and suicidal thoughts continued. In addition, although his talents allowed him to score prime jobs, his angry outbursts led to arguments at work and with intimate partners that sometimes led to his throwing things and often to the end of his job or relationships. He never "drank every day," but he often binged on alcohol when angry or when he wanted to relieve stress, and his binges often exacerbated problems at work or with partners. He tries to remain true to his partners, but he often cheats when he starts to feel that his girlfriend is "just going to leave me anyway." Using AA, he has had many lengthy periods of sobriety, but these frequently end with benders when he feels threatened at work or in his relationship. In the past, Lance periodically sought treatment from various primary care doctors, who diagnosed him with depression and anxiety. They prescribed various selective serotonin reuptake inhibitors (SSRIs), but the medications had only limited success. You have only 15 minutes left in the session. How might you use this time with Lance? [**Decision Point 2**]

You end the session by letting Lance know that you think he has both BPD and a significant alcohol problem. Furthermore, you let him know that because his drinking is often self-destructive and impulsive in the setting of interpersonal stress (and thus is in part a symptom of his BPD), he will need to have consistent sobriety to benefit from BPD treatment. You recommend that he attend your clinic's DDIOP, and you will resume treatment with him for his BPD when he has completed DDIOP.

After your discussion, Lance agrees that BPD sounds "a lot like me." Indeed, he wonders if his drinking may just be "this borderline thing...maybe I don't need alcohol treatment at all." [**Decision Point 3**]

As he heads out the door, Lance remembers that clonazepam has been helpful to chill him out and asks if you would be willing to prescribe this. [**Decision Point 4**]

Lance does well in DDIOP combined with frequent AA meetings. He even gets a sponsor. When DDIOP refers him back to you at discharge, he balks, saying, "I'm doing great, I'm working the program, I'm doing the steps—and now that I'm sober I just need to get back to work and work things out with Carol, and I don't need that borderline treatment." The DDIOP team, recognizing that Lance is doing much better, calls you in for a provider meeting with Lance to discuss next steps. [**Decision Point 5**]

Lance does return to see you, feeling that he needs to learn more about BPD. On his first visit he says he has a friend who has bipolar disorder, and Lance has wondered if he has it too because his moods are all over the place and "go from zero to angry" many times a day when his friends, romantic partners, or coworkers "let me down." [**Decision Point 6**] You explain to him that bipolar disorder and BPD can be differentiated and that given the rapidity of his mood shifts, and the fact that they often move toward anger, and the absence of concomitant neurovegetative changes, his symptoms are more consistent with BPD than bipolar disorder. Moreover, you point out that in almost every case, his mood changes result from interpersonal difficulties, and in fact it is his interpersonal hypersensitivity that not only lies at the heart of his BPD but also appears to drive his binge drinking. This is not what he learned in AA, he notes, but he would like to know more, asking, "Could we meet three times a week, like DDIOP, so I can really get going on this?" You remain pragmatic and tell him that patients with BPD rarely require such intense treatment and that you should begin with discussing some modest goals for his treatment, including restarting meaningful work, remaining sober, and learning more about BPD. He agrees to attend AA and your clinic's BPD psychoeducation group. From the latter, he learns about the hopeful prognosis of BPD, about its origins in interpersonal hypersensitivity, and about what is and is not useful in its treatment. Through your steady presence, wise advice, and holding him accountable for his "slips" with modified chain analyses to examine how they happen, he begins to see how interpersonal hypersensitivity often leaves him with uncomfortable affects. These affects, he learns, lead him to seek comfort in others, and if this is not available, to seek comfort in alcohol. With time and through the less interpersonally intense world of work, he is able to anticipate these situations better and access safer ways of coping, including calling his sponsor, getting to a meeting, or making a healthier choice, such as exercise.

Decision Points: Alternative Responses

Rate each response in terms of its level of helpfulness with a rating of 1 (will be helpful), 2 (possibly helpful, continuing reservations), or 3 (not helpful—or even harmful).

1. When asked by your colleague if you would begin personality disorder therapy with Lance, you

   A. Decline, saying that you are not a DBT expert.
   B. Decline, saying that he must be sober 6 months before you are willing to meet with him.
   C. Agree, but only if Lance is willing to do intensive, twice-weekly therapy.
   D. Agree to do a consultation to determine what could be the best way to proceed with Lance's treatment.

2. After gathering this history, how would you use the final 15 minutes of your session?

A. Schedule another session to gather more history before jumping to conclusions.
B. Prescribe an SSRI for Lance.
C. Tell him his problem is that he is an alcoholic and he needs to go to rehab; you cannot help him.
D. Review the criteria for BPD with Lance and begin educating him about the prognosis and how you would like to proceed.
E. Tell him he has BPD and is unlikely to get better.
F. Tell him he has BPD and he needs DBT.

3. As you end the session, you

A. Agree with Lance that his drinking is likely just a symptom of his BPD, and it will definitely resolve when his BPD does.
B. Agree with Lance that his drinking seems to be driven in part by his BPD but that you believe not addressing his drinking would be a mistake.
C. Disagree with Lance, indicating that his drinking is his only real issue, and once he has taken care of it, his other symptoms are likely to vanish.
D. Recommend AA.
E. Recommend a residential rehab.

4. When asked if you would prescribe clonazepam, you tell Lance,

A. "No, because it is against clinic policy to prescribe clonazepam for those with substance abuse problems."
B. "Yes, because it has been helpful for you before."
C. "Yes, because you have been using alcohol to self-medicate, and clonazepam is a better medication."
D. "No, because I worry that it is likely to be disinhibiting for you and will make things worse."

5. You should tell the DDIOP team and Lance the following:

A. It is Lance's choice.
B. Lance agreed to return for BPD treatment, so he should keep his word.
C. Lance should return to treatment with you, and now that he is done with DDIOP, he need not continue AA.

D. Although AA and the 12 steps are important and helpful, Lance's self-destructive pattern of interpersonal stress leading to binge drinking continued even when he did AA in the past and likely requires treatment of his BPD to avoid problems in the future.

E. Work has always been a part of Lance's stress, so he should not return to work and should just focus on patching things up with Carol, while continuing both AA and BPD treatment.

6. In response to Lance's concerns about bipolar disorder, you say,

A. "People with BPD can't have bipolar disorder."
B. "There is no similarity in symptoms between BPD and bipolar disorder."
C. "There is no way to differentiate the two, so you should probably be taking bipolar medications just to be safe."
D. "The symptoms of BPD and bipolar disorder can seem similar, and for that matter patients can have both, but there are some ways we can differentiate the two."
E. "If you treat BPD, the bipolar disorder will go away."

Decision Points: Discussion

Numbers within brackets indicate level of helpfulness ratings.

1. When asked by your colleague if you would begin personality disorder therapy with Lance, you

A. Decline, saying that you are not a DBT expert. [3] (Being helpful to patients with BPD does not require that you be an expert or that patients require subspecialist care.)
B. Decline, saying that he must be sober 6 months before you are willing to meet with him. [2] (Although sobriety is important for a number of reasons to allow a patient to consistently attend and benefit from care, such a waiting period to discuss the diagnosis and possible treatment options for BPD may lead to a lost opportunity in Lance's situation.)
C. Agree, but only if Lance is willing to do intensive, twice-weekly therapy. [3] (Treatment should be based on whether it is helpful. Most patients do not need twice-weekly therapy, and beginning with this as a requirement is not only overkill but may result in a treatment that scares off Lance.)

D. Agree to do a consultation to determine what could be the best way to proceed with Lance's treatment. [1] (A consultation is a pragmatic action in this situation. It allows for an assessment of Lance's diagnosis; consideration of his willingness to engage in treatment; the initiation of psychoeducation, which we know to be important for a patient's recovery; and prioritization of co-morbidities for treatment.)

2. After gathering this history, how would you use the final 15 minutes of your session?

A. Schedule another session to gather more history before jumping to conclusions. [2] (It may be useful to schedule another session, but Lance and the referring team no doubt would like some advice on the direction the treatment should take. If this can be done, it should be in this session. If at the end of this session more history is needed, encourage Lance to write out his autobiography as homework and email it to you before the next session or bring it to you then.)
B. Prescribe an SSRI for Lance. [3] (You do not have a great reason to prescribe an SSRI at this stage. Prescribing a medication without any other plan may, in fact, give Lance the wrong impression about what you expect to be helpful.)
C. Tell him his problem is that he is an alcoholic and he needs to go to rehab; you cannot help him. [3] (Although Lance does have a problem with alcohol, it is not clear that he needs rehab per se. More importantly, you have good evidence thus far that his drinking may be severely affected by his personality style, and leaving him with the impression that he only requires rehab would not only be incorrect but also feed into his tendency of black-and-white thinking.)
D. Review the criteria for BPD with Lance and begin educating him about the prognosis and how you would like to proceed. [1] (Making the diagnosis of BPD is one of the keys to providing appropriate treatment. Reviewing the criteria for BPD is also a good way to establish collaboration as an important part of treatment. Discussing the *hopeful* prognosis of BPD is the beginning of expecting change for Lance and having him expect it as well.)
E. Tell him he has BPD and is unlikely to get better. [3] (As stated in the explanation for option D above, discussing the diagnosis

is a good thing, but we now know that the prognosis for BPD is good overall.)

F. Tell him he has BPD and he needs DBT. [2] (Although Lance seems to have BPD, a more collaborative discussion of the diagnosis is more likely to be effective at this point. As noted, although DBT has an evidence base as a treatment for BPD, it is not the only treatment that can be effective, and narrowing the option down to DBT may not be practical in your clinic, depending on its availability.)

3. As you end the session, you

A. Agree with Lance that his drinking is likely just a symptom of his BPD, and it will definitely resolve when his BPD does. [3] (Although his drinking may in large part be an impulsive, risky behavior related to interpersonal hypersensitivity and may improve with his BPD, we do not have evidence that it will definitely resolve, and giving him this impression may lead him to eschew substance use disorders treatment.)

B. Agree with Lance that his drinking seems to be driven in part by his BPD but that you believe not addressing his drinking would be a mistake. [1] (See discussion under response A above.)

C. Disagree with Lance, indicating that his drinking is his only real issue, and once he has taken care of it, his other symptoms are likely to vanish. [3] (This has not been true in the past for Lance and is not likely to be now.)

D. Recommend AA. [2] (This is appropriate, as far as it goes, but is a mistake if this is the only thing recommended.)

E. Recommend a residential rehab. [2] (Residential rehab *can* be a part of the treatment but runs the risk of separating Lance from the clinic and from his newfound interest in figuring out the relationship between his drinking and BPD. An intensive outpatient program, preferably in your clinic, may be a better first step.)

4. When asked if you would prescribe clonazepam, you tell Lance,

A. "No, because it is against clinic policy to prescribe clonazepam for those with substance abuse problems." [2] (If this is true at your clinic, it is worth telling the patient, but presenting hard-and-fast rules without more explanation is not likely a way to establish collaboration with the patient.)

B. "Yes, because it has been helpful for you before." [3] (According to Lance, clonazepam has been helpful before; however, despite having used it in the past, he is in your office with alcohol, relationship, and occupational difficulties. Saying that it has been helpful sends a message that may reinforce Lance's previous pattern of preferring something that temporarily improves his affective distress while not improving [and perhaps worsening] his functioning.)

C. "Yes, because you have been using alcohol to self-medicate, and clonazepam is a better medication." [3] (See discussion under response B above. Clonazepam's tendency to be disinhibiting and decrease mentalizing may feel good for Lance, but the medication is not likely to be a good choice for him in the long run.)

D. "No, because I worry that it is likely to be disinhibiting for you and will make things worse." [1] (It is for this reason, in addition to clonazepam's addiction potential, that it is best to avoid this medication with Lance.)

5. You should tell the DDIOP team and Lance the following:

A. It is Lance's choice. [2] (In the end this statement is true, but this simplistic response is not in Lance's best interest. It is not surprising that having had some success in intensive outpatient treatment, Lance wishes he were all better, but this attitude is unrealistic. Before meeting you, Lance and his treaters have not formulated why this has been the case for him. You have a chance to remind him.)

B. Lance agreed to return for BPD treatment, so he should keep his word. [2] (In some respects this response does emphasize the GPM principle of accountability, but embarking on a treatment for BPD because it is "one's duty" seems an unlikely formula for success.)

C. Lance should return to treatment with you, and now that he is done with DDIOP, he need not continue AA. [3] (Lance is likely to need all the help he can get. Groups like AA have a number of advantages, including being free, being available throughout the week, and providing a ready-made supportive environment.)

D. Although AA and the 12 steps are important and helpful, Lance's self-destructive pattern of interpersonal stress leading to binge drinking continued even when he did AA in the past and likely requires treatment of his BPD to avoid problems in the future. [1] (Exactly.)

E. Work has always been a part of Lance's stress, so he should not return to work and should just focus on patching things up with Carol, while continuing both AA and BPD treatment. [3] (Work, no doubt, added to Lance's stress, but it will be key to his recovery. Although patients with BPD commonly seek exclusive relationships in hopes of filling their emptiness and scaffolding their unstable self, their interpersonal hypersensitivity and fear of abandonment make such relationships difficult to sustain. Work, on the other hand, provides structure, sense of purpose, financial stability, and less intense interpersonal situations that can serve as a safer learning ground for patients with BPD. Thus, GPM emphasizes work before love.)

6. In response to Lance's concerns about bipolar disorder, you say,

A. "People with BPD can't have bipolar disorder." [3] (Approximately 10%–15% of patients with BPD have bipolar disorder and vice versa.)

B. "There is no similarity in symptoms between BPD and bipolar disorder." [3] (This is not true, and this response would probably be experienced as invalidating by Lance, who comes to you wondering whether his symptoms represent bipolar disorder.)

C. "There is no way to differentiate the two, so you should probably be taking bipolar medications just to be safe." [3] (BPD and bipolar disorder can be differentiated. Although mood stabilizers and antipsychotics can be helpful for certain aspects of BPD, they are not curative and have many potential downsides. Therefore, they are not baseline treatment for BPD "just to be safe.")

D. "The symptoms of BPD and bipolar disorder can seem similar, and for that matter patients can have both, but there are some ways we can differentiate the two." [1] (This is an answer that both validates Lance's question and begins psychoeducation about this topic. Although superficially and nominally similar, the symptoms of BPD and bipolar disorder can be differentiated; however, doing so often requires the collaboration of the patient and others. Enlisting Lance in this collaboration, even at the point of differentially diagnosing, can be useful in creating a working alliance.)

E. "If you treat BPD, the bipolar disorder will go away." [3] (Unfortunately, this is not the case. On the contrary, BPD and bipolar disorder, when they exist in the same person, generally have independent courses and each requires its own targeted treatment.)

Conclusion

GPM has been designed to provide individual clinicians with a generalist approach to treating BPD. Fortuitously, because of its explicit and pragmatic approach, GPM can also serve as a blueprint for a large mental health clinic's strategy for addressing BPD in its population. For too long, clinics have either tacitly avoided identifying patients as having BPD (often treating them ineffectively for other diagnoses) or treated all of those with BPD as requiring resource-intensive, specialized (generally DBT) treatment. Both mistakes leave clinics paralyzed by the prevalence of BPD in their community.

GPM's pragmatism can serve as an antidote to this paralysis. Armed with hopeful data demonstrating that patients with BPD can and do get better, GPM emphasizes appropriate diagnosis of BPD. Further data regarding BPD's interaction with other illnesses have led to GPM developing a rational strategy for handling comorbid disorders—a strategy that can be employed by a clinic to drive individual treatment planning. An emphasis on a case management approach with liberal use of psychoeducation and groups can likewise be leveraged economically in a clinic setting. Indeed, much of the important psychoeducation and determination of the type and intensity of treatment that an individual patient requires can be done efficiently in a group designed for this purpose. Such a group can support the stepped care model with GPM at its base and can allow a clinic to appropriately distribute finite resources and maximize the mental health of the population for which it cares.

References

Anna Freud National Centre for Children and Families: Mentalization-Based Treatment: Basic Training, 2018. Available at https://www.annafreud.org/training/training-and-conferences-overview/training-at-the-anna-freud-national-centre-for-children-and-families/mentalization-based-treatment-basic-training/. Accessed January 2, 2019.

Bateman A, Fonagy P: Mentalization-Based Treatment for Personality Disorders: A Practical Guide. Oxford, UK, Oxford University Press, 2016

Behavioral Tech: Our impact, 2018. Available at https://behavioraltech.org/about-us/our-impact/. Accessed January 2, 2019.

Choi-Kain LW, Albert EB, Gunderson JG: Evidence-based treatments for borderline personality disorder: implementation, integration, and stepped care. Harv Rev Psychiatry 24(5):342–356, 2016 27603742

Comtois KA, Carmel A: Borderline personality disorder and high utilization of inpatient psychiatric hospitalization: concordance between research and clinical diagnosis. J Behav Health Serv Res 43(2):272–280, 2016 24875431

Feliu-Soler A, Pascual JC, Borràs X, et al: Effects of dialectical behaviour therapy-mindfulness training on emotional reactivity in borderline personality disorder: preliminary results. Clin Psychol Psychother 21(4):363–370, 2014 23494767

Grilo CM, Sanislow CA, Skodol AE, et al: Do eating disorders co-occur with personality disorders? Comparison groups matter. Int J Eat Disord 33(2):155–164, 2003 12616581

Gunderson JG, Links PS: Borderline Personality Disorder: A Clinical Guide, 2nd Edition. Washington, DC, American Psychiatric Publishing, 2008

Gunderson JG, Links PS: Handbook of Good Psychiatric Management for Borderline Personality Disorder. Washington, DC, American Psychiatric Publishing, 2014

Gunderson JG, Stout RL, McGlashan TH, et al: Ten-year course of borderline personality disorder: psychopathology and function from the Collaborative Longitudinal Personality Disorders Study. Arch Gen Psychiatry 68(8):827–837, 2011 21464343

Gunderson JG, Stout RL, Shea MT, et al: Interactions of borderline personality disorder and mood disorders over 10 years. J Clin Psychiatry 75(8):829 834, 2014 25007118

Hayes SC, Strosahl KD, Wilson KG: Acceptance and Commitment Therapy: The Process and Practice of Mindful Change, 2nd Edition. New York, Guilford, 2016

Howe E: Five ethical and clinical challenges psychiatrists may face when treating patients with borderline personality disorder who are or may become suicidal. Innov Clin Neurosci 10(1):14–19, 2013 23440937

Keuroghlian AS, Gunderson JG, Pagano ME, et al: Interactions of borderline personality disorder and anxiety disorders over 10 years. J Clin Psychiatry 76(11):1529–1534, 2015 26114336

Keuroghlian AS, Palmer BA, Choi-Kain LW, et al: The effect of attending good psychiatric management (GPM) workshops on attitudes toward patients with borderline personality disorder. J Pers Disord 30(4):567–576, 2016 26111249

Linehan MM, Korslund KE, Harned MS, et al: Dialectical behavior therapy for high suicide risk in individuals with borderline personality disorder: a randomized clinical trial and component analysis. JAMA Psychiatry 72(5):475–482, 2015 25806661

Livesley JW, Dimaggio G, Clarkin JF: Integrated Treatment for Personality Disorder: A Modular Approach. New York, Guilford, 2016

Masland SR, Price D, MacDonald J, et al: Enduring effects of one-day training in good psychiatric management on clinician attitudes about borderline personality disorder. J Nerv Ment Dis 206 (11):865–869, 2018 30371640

Maslow AH: The Psychology of Science: A Reconnaissance. New York, Harper and Row, 1966, p 15

McMain SF, Links PS, Gnam WH, et al: A randomized trial of dialectical behavior therapy versus general psychiatric management for borderline personality disorder. Am J Psychiatry 166(12):1365–1374, 2009 19755574

McMain SF, Guimond T, Streiner DL, et al: Dialectical behavior therapy compared with general psychiatric management for borderline personality disorder: clinical outcomes and functioning over a 2-year follow-up.Am J Psychiatry 169(6):650–661 2012 22581157

Paris J: Why patients with severe personality disorders are overmedicated. J Clin Psychiatry 76(4):e521, 2015 25919846

Paris J, Black DW: Borderline personality disorder and bipolar disorder: what is the difference and why does it matter? J Nerv Ment Dis 203(1):3–7, 2015 25536097

Richter C, Steinacher B, zum Eschenhoff A, et al: Psychotherapy of borderline personality disorder: can the supply meet the demand? A German nationwide survey in DBT inpatient and day clinic treatment facilities. Community Ment Health J 52(2):212–215, 2016 26323785

Sansone RA, Sansone LA: Borderline personality disorder: are proliferative symptoms characteristic? Psychiatry (Edgmont) 5(8):18–21, 2008 19727271

Sisti D, Segal AG, Siegel AM, et al: Diagnosing, disclosing, and documenting borderline personality disorder: a survey of psychiatrists' practices. J Pers Disord 30(6):848–856, 2016 26623537

Unruh BT, Gunderson JG: "Good enough" psychiatric residency training in borderline personality disorder: challenges, choice points, and a model generalist curriculum. Harv Rev Psychiatry 24(5):367–377, 2016 27603744

Walter M, Gunderson JG, Zanarini MC, et al: New onsets of substance use disorders in borderline personality disorder over 7 years of follow-ups: findings from the Collaborative Longitudinal Personality Disorders Study. Addiction 104(1):97–103, 2009 19133893

Yen S, Shea MT, Sanislow CA, et al: Borderline personality disorder criteria associated with prospectively observed suicidal behavior. Am J Psychiatry 161(7):1296–1298, 2004 15229066

Yeomans FE, Clarkin JF, Kernberg OF: Transference-Focused Psychotherapy for Borderline Personality Disorder: A Clinical Guide. Washington, DC, American Psychiatric Publishing, 2015

Zanarini MC: Reasons for change in borderline personality disorder (and other axis II disorders). Psychiatr Clin North Am 31(3):505–515, viii, 2008 18638649

Zanarini MC, Frankenburg FR, Dubo ED, et al: Axis I comorbidity of borderline personality disorder. Am J Psychiatry 155(12):1733–1739, 1998 9842784

Zanarini MC, Frankenburg FR, Hennen J, et al: Axis I comorbidity in patients with borderline personality disorder: 6-year follow-up and prediction of time to remission. Am J Psychiatry 161(11):2108–2114, 2004 15514413

Zanarini MC, Reichman CA, Frankenburg FR, et al: The course of eating disorders in patients with borderline personality disorder: a 10-year follow-up study. Int J Eat Disord 43(3):226–232, 2010 19343799

Zanarini MC, Frankenburg FR, Weingeroff JL, et al: The course of substance use disorders in patients with borderline personality disorder and Axis II comparison subjects: a 10-year follow-up study. Addiction 106(2):342–348, 2011 21083831

Zanarini MC, Conkey LC, Temes CM, et al: Randomized controlled trial of web-based psychoeducation for women with borderline personality disorder. J Clin Psychiatry 79(3), 2018 28703950

Zimmerman M, Ruggero CJ, Chelminski I, et al: Psychiatric diagnoses in patients previously overdiagnosed with bipolar disorder. J Clin Psychiatry 71(1):26–31, 2010 19646366

Chapter 6

College Mental Health Services

Richard G. Hersh, M.D.
Ellen F. Finch, B.A.

Borderline personality disorder (BPD) has a likely onset of symptoms in late adolescence or early adulthood and has been well described (Chanen and McCutcheon 2013). Although individuals with BPD are markedly different from their peers in both social functioning and overall health by age 24 years (Moran et al. 2016), certain BPD symptoms may emerge much earlier and are considered early signs or precursors of mental illness (Chanen and Thompson 2014; Choi-Kain and Gunderson 2015). Investigation confirms that the BPD diagnosis can be reliably made in adolescents and that early intervention may be of benefit in this population (Chanen et al. 2008). Early diagnosis and initiation of treatment of BPD would follow currently well-established recommenda-tions for proactive perspectives on the treatment of mood and psychotic disorders in this age group (McGorry 2013). However, clinicians histori-cally have been resistant to making a diagnosis of BPD in adolescent and young adult patients.

BPD is particularly salient on college campuses. College is a period of development during which independence is navigated and dependency abandoned. This transition in itself causes tumult, stress, and therefore risk for the development of a mental illness, be it depression, anxiety, sub-stance misuse, eating disorder, or BPD. Statistics suggest that patients with BPD are likely to first present to mental health professionals for individual psychotherapy or pharmacotherapy at approximately age 18 years, or around the time many may be entering college (Hersh 2013; Zanarini et al. 2001). In recent years, college counseling center directors have reported significant increases in the demand for services at their sites (Benton et al. 2003; Kitzrow 2003). These directors have identified a growing number of students arriving on campus with histories of hospitalization or outpa-tient psychotherapy and medication trials (Mowbray et al. 2006). In ad-dition, students with unusually complex psychiatric presentations are more commonly seen, posing particular challenges to campus counseling staff (Gallagher 2015).

The academic psychiatry community has responded to the increased demand for general mental health services on the college campus. Indeed, a volume of *Academic Psychiatry*, as introduced by Balon et al. (2015), was devoted to examining this emerging phenomenon from multiple perspec-tives. Surveys attempting to clarify the nature of the increasing demands made on college counseling personnel have identified rising rates of stu-dent anxiety and depressive disorders, eating disorders, substance use dis-orders, and nonsuicidal self-injurious behavior, among other mental health issues (American College Health Association 2017).

The most comprehensive surveys of psychopathology in the college-age population, examining both the general campus population and clin-ical samples from reports of campus mental health personnel, highlight the significant rates of symptomatology either consistent with BPD (im-pulsivity, suicidality) or reflecting syndromes commonly co-occurring with BPD (mood, eating, or substance use disorders). Unfortunately, sur-veys aimed at assessing trends in psychopathology by soliciting informa-tion from both clinicians in the campus setting and students accessing treatment do not routinely include detailed information about personality disorders. Despite the limited inclusion of specific questioning related to personality disorder pathology in many surveys of college student mental health, Meaney et al. (2016) were able to review 43 college-based studies that reported estimates of clinically significant BPD symptoms, and they determined that the prevalence of BPD in college samples ranged from 0.5% to 32.1%; this wide range of estimates reflects methodological or study sample factors.

This absence of more specific and consistent data on students with BPD may reflect the broader pattern exhibited by many mental health clinicians in their reluctance to diagnose personality disorders during adolescence or young adult years. A review of the contents of the previously cited volume of *Academic Psychiatry* dedicated to the topic of college student mental health concerns is illustrative of this phenomenon. There are articles on preparing and training the college mental health workforce (Riba et al. 2015), developing a psychiatry training elective in college mental health (Kirsch et al. 2015), and teaching college students about mental health (Shatkin and Diamond 2015), among others in the issue; however, material about the assessment and treatment of students with BPD or BPD traits is not included. In an earlier volume of the same journal, Zisook et al. (2012) described an overarching approach to preventing suicide on college campuses that does not include assessment and treatment of students with personality disorder symptoms; they did reference dialectical behavior therapy (DBT) groups as a possible intervention, describing the target disorder for the intervention as students "with impulsivity" but not specifically BPD or BPD traits.

Current Options for Treating Borderline Personality Disorder in the Campus Setting

There has been a growing emphasis on the use of evidence-based treatment interventions in the college setting (Cooper et al. 2008). The drive for use of evidence-based treatments has included interventions for depressive, anxiety, substance use, and eating disorders (Baez 2005; Birky 2005; Lee 2005; Resnick 2005). The emerging emphasis on the integration of evidence-based treatments in the campus setting has been a critical element in the recent introduction of DBT (Linehan et al. 1991) programs in this setting. Chugani (2015) reviewed the literature on DBT in the college counseling center setting, outlining the current knowledge and implications for practice. This article stresses the widely recognized trends in mental health issues on college campuses (more students with "severe and complex mental health issues, including non suicidal self-injurious behavior [NSSI], crises requiring immediate intervention, eating disorders, psychiatric medication issues, and substance abuse" [p. 120]) and the need for increased evidence-based treatment resources in this context.

Randomized controlled trials have demonstrated efficacy of comprehensive DBT in college settings for students with BPD features. Pistorello et al. (2012) compared DBT with optimized treatment as usual for a group of students with suicidality at baseline, a history of at least one lifetime nonsuicidal self-injurious behavior or suicide attempt, and at least three BPD diagnostic criteria. They found that those students in the DBT treatment group had better outcomes than those in the treatment-as-usual group across a number of domains. At Sarah Lawrence College, a comprehensive DBT program was developed due in part to the significant financial and administrative burdens associated with the actions of students with prominent BPD traits, including recurrent hospitalizations, withdrawal from school, and general disruption to "the living and learning community" (Engle et al. 2013). The preliminary results indicate that the treatment led to a reduction in hospitalizations and student medical leaves from school while providing an effective intervention for the target symptoms of BPD.

Importantly, comprehensive DBT entails for the patient weekly individual treatment and skills group participation, and for the clinician a weekly group supervision. In addition, the patient has access to the therapist between sessions through phone coaching. This resource-intensive structure precludes comprehensive DBT from being a viable option for most resource-constrained college counseling centers. At Sarah Lawrence College, for example, the option of comprehensive DBT treatment in the college counseling center was eventually altered because of cost concerns, although DBT skills groups remain an option for students (D. Nunziato, personal communication, December 2018). Chugani and Landes (2016) studied the trends in and barriers to implementation of DBT programs in campus settings. This electronic survey of college counseling center employees indicated that there were consistent barriers, including demands for productivity for the campus clinicians and a lack of individual therapists for the specific interventions for treating students with BPD. Implementation possibilities as suggested by the authors going forward included community outreach, "virtual" treatment teams, and additional strategic adaptation of the DBT model. Additional studies have examined pared-down versions of DBT as a possible treatment for BPD in college settings.

Meaney-Tavares and Hasking (2013) described a pilot study of a short-term, modified group DBT intervention that resulted in a reduction of depression and BPD traits and an increase in adaptive coping skills, problem solving, and constructive self-talk but no decrease in anxiety. In a small pilot study, Chugani et al. (2013) found that a short-term DBT skills training class developed for a student population with Cluster B personality disorder pathology led to improvement in increasing skills use and decreasing maladaptive coping skills, with a trend for improvement in difficulty regulating emotions. Another pilot study of short-term DBT skills groups for undergraduates with "significant emotional dysregulation" demonstrated that students had significant gains across measures of emotion regulation, affect, skills use, and functioning, without notable benefits observed from the addition of mindfulness skills (Rizvi and Steffel 2014).

These studies indicate that lower-intensity treatments may be efficacious with college-age populations, and given the prevalence of BPD in college settings, a feasible treatment is critically needed. Good psychiatric management (GPM) is a less intensive, less expensive intervention that can be adapted by college counseling centers working to treat students with BPD.

GPM in the College Setting

Central to the mission of GPM for BPD is a public health goal of providing consistent, informed treatment by generalists (Gunderson and Links 2014). The development and dissemination of efficacious interventions for the generalist may be responsible for the improving prognosis for BPD documented in recent years. The developers of GPM have stressed the need for solutions to two widely described phenomena related to the treatment of BPD: 1) limited access to appropriate, evidence-based care and 2) uneven care that risks worsening the course and/or prognosis of the disorder. Certainly, these two concerns may well affect treatment of the college student population. GPM is not designed as a replacement for one of the evidence-based psychotherapies for BPD, including DBT, transference-focused psychotherapy (Clarkin et al. 2007), schema-focused therapy (Giesen-Bloo et al. 2006), mentalization-based treatment (Bateman and Fonagy 1999), or Systems Training for Emotional Predictability and Problem Solving (Blum et al. 2008). GPM is accessible to clinicians of varied educational backgrounds without requiring extensive training and in some cases may serve as a prelude to treatment with one of the more extended evidence-based psychotherapies just listed.

Competence in providing GPM and adherence for practitioners rest on familiarity with the GPM handbook, its clinical examples, and its videos (Gunderson and Links 2014). It is important to stress that GPM was not intended for, and its practice should not be restricted to, practitioners with psychiatric training. Links et al. (2015) outlined the ways in which GPM can and should be used by clinicians of varied training, and they stressed that the pharmacotherapy component of GPM can easily be provided by prescribers in a split treatment model. In fact, GPM is designed to be practiced by psychologists, social workers, and other mental health clinicians, reflecting the relative limits in the number of psychiatrists available (as is often the case with campus psychological services) and the likely demands for access, given rates of BPD in the community, including in the college setting.

In this section, we present six principles of GPM adapted for the college mental health setting: diagnostic disclosure, psychoeducation, case management, focus on goals, multimodality, and flexible duration and intensity. These principles are widely applicable, commonsensical, and likely to integrate well with the approach of most clinicians in a college setting.

Diagnostic Disclosure

A first step toward helping the student with BPD symptoms is making and sharing the diagnosis of BPD. This can be done by reviewing the DSM-5 criteria for the disorder (American Psychiatric Association 2013) with the patient and collaboratively establishing the diagnosis and using the diagnostic disclosure script outlined in Figure 2-1 as a supplemental resource that can frame a patient's understanding of the diagnosis within a coherent narrative. Because of stigma associated with BPD among health care providers (Chanen and McCutcheon 2013), many clinicians fear that disclosing the diagnosis of BPD will upset the patient. They may therefore defer to mood, anxiety, eating, or substance use disorders as defined by DSM-5 (American Psychiatric Association 2013). This practice means that many students' BPD is undiagnosed; in fact, a recent review found that the true prevalence of personality disorders was 40 times higher than the diagnosed prevalence (Conway et al. 2017).

Promptly disclosing the BPD diagnosis informs the direction of care and allows open communication between clinician and student. The BPD diagnosis is the foundation of GPM, and withholding a diagnosis of BPD can increase the risk of iatrogenic harm (e.g., polypharmacy) and block the patient from receiving appropriate treatment (Chanen and McCutcheon 2013). It is important to note that in the multiple studies cited earlier in this chapter that used some or all elements of DBT, frank discussion about the BPD diagnosis was not necessarily expected during interventions. This distinguishes a number of these interventions from standard

DBT, which requires discussion of the diagnosis in the early stages of treatment, as is also the case with GPM.

GPM recommends that the clinician walk through the DSM-5 criteria for BPD (American Psychiatric Association 2013) with the student item by item, asking if each criterion fits the student's experience. The student will likely feel relief to know that his or her struggles are explained by a medical diagnosis and that there are other people who have the same problems. Once the diagnosis is collaboratively established, the clinician can move to the next critical element of GPM: psychoeducation.

Psychoeducation

GPM clinicians will routinely inform patients, families, and others involved of the BPD diagnosis and provide education about genetics, prognosis, comorbidities, and various treatment options. In the campus setting, this process of discussion of diagnosis can be complicated in certain cases by limitations on family involvement. In addition, GPM clinicians may need to provide information for resident advisors, deans, or others during the course of treatment. Although information available to students online or in counseling center waiting room reading material has traditionally had little, if any, information about BPD, some sites such as the ULifeline website (www.ulifeline.org) and Britain's YoungMinds mental health charity (www.youngminds.org.uk) now include pertinent and accessible psychoeducation material for the college-age population.

A central tenet of educating the student about a BPD diagnosis is explaining the model of interpersonal hypersensitivity as a central organizing concept. To this end, the therapist will explore symptoms as they emerge in the course of treatment as manifestations of interpersonal hypersensitivity, as might be the case with ruptured friendships or breakups. The GPM therapist will also explore interpersonal hypersensitivity as it emerges in the transference. It is crucial to have the shared framework of interpersonal hypersensitivity to help make sense of what is happening within the treatment and in the student's life outside of it.

Case Management

The GPM approach will stress the clinician's focus on what is happening in the student's life outside of treatment. GPM will not proceed along the lines of some other extended exploratory psychotherapies, with an exclusive emphasis on the patient's psychology or "what is happening in the room" and only limited attention to "nuts and bolts" concerns. Instead, the GPM clinician will attend to the patient's academic performance, involvement with activities, friendships, and engagement in student life as priorities. The GPM clinician will not shy away from providing case management to help the student deal with important logistical issues that are affecting his or her functioning.

Focus on Goals

GPM prioritizes the student's functioning in major spheres of activity and conceptualizes these goals (academic engagement, vocational involvement, relationships) as central to the treatment. In GPM, a focus on functioning is primary, with an assumption that a diminution in maladaptive behaviors associated with the BPD diagnosis will follow accordingly. Academic and vocational goals are always prioritized above romantic relationships; in other words, the focus is on work before love.

Multimodality

GPM supports and encourages the involvement of more than one clinician in any particular case. GPM does not prioritize the clinician-patient dyad, as occurred during the period when psychoanalytic theory dominated the treatment of personality disorder pathology. GPM welcomes the split treatment involving primary therapist and prescriber as well as the involvement of adjunctive treaters. In the college setting, treatment options might include campus-based self-help groups (e.g., 12-step groups, Weight Watchers, mindfulness groups). GPM would also be open to family therapy or couples therapy, if indicated.

Flexible Duration and Intensity

GPM emphasizes flexibility in the duration and intensity of treatment, in contrast to other evidence-based treatments for BPD that prescribe a specific model for treatment and usually specify frequency of meetings and duration of treatment at the outset. The GPM practitioner takes a different approach, tailoring the treatment to the individual patient's needs without dictating a particular treatment frame at the outset. In the campus setting, the GPM clinician's flexibility will allow for accommodation of the student's varying vacation schedule. (In this respect, GPM's flexibility is akin to the changes made in a "classical" DBT treatment in a number of the previously mentioned studies to fit students' academic schedules.) This flexible approach is especially important for college counseling centers that limit the number of sessions a student is allotted per semester.

Summary

The six elements discussed in this section provide the structural framework that scaffolds the GPM clinician's approach in treating a student with BPD. Additionally, GPM is characterized by a basic psychotherapeutic approach that helps guide the clinician. GPM clinicians are active but not reactive. They do not wait for the student to bring up an important issue. Instead, they actively and thoughtfully ask questions and bring up topics important to the student's functioning. The clinician should hold the student accountable for taking an active role in his or her treatment and working to get better. Change is expected, because BPD's longitudinal course is one of improvement, and the clinician should be acutely aware of any stagnation in the treatment and work with the student to address why the treatment is not working. The focus during appointments is consistently on life outside of treatment, and the clinician should routinely draw focus back to the student's functioning in the real world, as opposed to in the therapy room. Throughout all of this, the GPM clinician remains flexible and pragmatic. GPM prioritizes what is working above any set structure, and the clinician should feel comfortable making changes to adapt treatment to the many external factors that influence a college student's day-to-day life. This active, externally focused, and flexible therapeutic approach is illustrated in the case vignette.

Case Vignette

The following case description includes decision points, each of which has several alternative responses listed at the end of the case. The reader will rate each alternative response in terms of its level of helpfulness. Discussions of responses follow.

> Jane is an 18-year-old college freshman living away from home for the first time. Jane's high school years were notable for periods of binge-purge activity in the context of a tumultuous relationship with her high school boyfriend. During her high school years, Jane twice overdosed with over-the-counter medications, both times when she became convinced her boyfriend wanted to break off their relationship. Jane was seen in a hospital emergency department after both overdoses; after the second suicidal act, she was referred to a local clinic, where she was given a diagnosis of depression and prescribed an antidepressant medication that she took

only sporadically. Now in her first semester at college, Jane binge drinks three or four times per week. One weekend she learns through a friend that her boyfriend may be dating another girl back home. Jane becomes inconsolable, and cuts her wrists superficially with a dull kitchen knife. She tells her resident advisor that she is thinking about cutting her wrists again with a sharper knife and is then taken to the college counseling center during walk-in hours. As the on-call college counseling center social worker, you sit with Jane to review her history and conduct an evaluation. [**Decision Point 1**]

Toward the end of your first session, you follow standard GPM procedure by discussing with Jane your conjecture about a BPD diagnosis. Jane expresses a mixture of concern and relief on hearing the diagnosis. She agrees to include her parents via a phone call in your meeting so that she might share with them basic information about BPD's course, prognosis, genetics, and treatments.

You and Jane agree to a weekly meeting, with the proviso that you will frequently review Jane's goals and the effectiveness of the treatment as it unfolds. Jane's focus at the beginning of her treatment is on her desire to "win back" her boyfriend and somehow outdo the girl he is now dating. Jane begins by using extreme descriptions of her former boyfriend and his new girlfriend. [**Decision Point 2**]

Over the course of the first month of treatment, you work to understand the details of Jane's important relationships. At one point, you forget the name of her former boyfriend, and Jane erupts in anger. She yells, "I bet you're thinking more about that guy with the beard who you see every week before you see me. I'm guessing he's more important to you than I am." [**Decision Point 3**]

At your next appointment, you learn that Jane is significantly behind in her schoolwork and may fail two of her classes. She pleads with you to write a note to the dean excusing her from some requirements, because she "was really sick with BPD, and you know how hard the semester was." [**Decision Point 4**]

Following your advice, Jane decides to stay on campus during the weekends in an effort to engage in activities, focus on her schoolwork, and make new friends. She fails one class but passes her other three. She continues to cut and binge drink, but she is starting to feel more comfortable at college. After 6 months of treatment, during Jane's second semester of college, her preoccupation with her former boyfriend wanes. Jane brings this up during a session, remarking, "I haven't thought of him in weeks. I think my BPD is gone. I think this can probably be our last session." [**Decision Point 5**]

After discussion, Jane agrees to continue in treatment, and she completes her freshman year a few months later. You work together to find a treater for her to see while back home for the summer, and you encourage Jane to return to the summer job she held during high school. Jane is still struggling with her interpersonal relationships and occasionally binge drinks, but she is markedly less reactive and she passed all of her spring semester classes. You schedule an appointment for when she returns to campus in the fall.

Decision Points: Alternative Responses

Rate each response in terms of its level of helpfulness with a rating of 1 (will be helpful), 2 (possibly helpful, continuing reservations), or 3 (not helpful—or even harmful).

1. When learning about Jane's pattern of overdoses and threats to cut, you

   A. Immediately call to have Jane hospitalized—you can't risk another overdose.
   B. Determine that Jane will require intensive individual psychotherapy and may want to take a leave of absence from college.
   C. Ignore her cutting patterns and suicidality; they are a communication and not the cause of Jane's issues.
   D. Express concern about how Jane's impulsive, self-harming behavior may be undermining her adjustment to college and use these behaviors as examples as you explain your diagnosis of BPD.

2. When Jane suggests she might post an incriminating message about her former boyfriend on her social media account to drive away his new girlfriend, you

   A. Avoid addressing this comment and refocus the conversation on her plan to complete her academic work that weekend.
   B. Nod at Jane's suggestion and ask her to report back what happens at your next session.
   C. Directly outline the risks and potential consequences of Jane's plan. Ask Jane to wait another week and think carefully before posting the message. Then redirect the conversation to a group project for class that is challenging.
   D. Decide to involve Jane's ex-boyfriend in the therapy and set up a phone call with him.

3. When Jane screams at you about your other patient, you

   A. Profusely apologize for your error and ask how you can make it up to Jane. You explain that your other patient is not more important than Jane, and that you actually meet with Jane more than any other student.
   B. Recognize and apologize for your memory lapse and then question why Jane was so quick to yell at you about another patient.

C. Immediately end the session and ask Jane to leave. Her scream-ing is not acceptable behavior and should not be tolerated in a professional environment.

D. Determine that this explosive reaction is a sign that the treat-ment is not working and refer Jane to another therapist.

4. When Jane requests that you write a note to the dean to excuse her from some requirements, you

A. Contact the dean to reduce Jane's requirements. You agree that Jane was too sick to do work earlier in the semester and worry that failing classes will be a major barrier to her achieving her academic goals.

B. Explain to Jane that you are worried that intervening will be treating her as though she is incapable of taking responsibility for her actions. Instead of calling the dean, you work with Jane to come up with a plan to improve her academic standing over the rest of the semester and help her find tutors for the classes she is failing.

C. You sternly explain to Jane that asking you to call the dean is just a way for her to escape her self-made problems and that you are disappointed she would ask for such a thing.

D. Encourage Jane to have her parents call the dean. You do not see a medical reason for excusing her from academic commitments, but the dean may respond to family involvement.

5. When Jane proposes terminating treatment, you

A. Agree that Jane has improved a lot, and if she does not think that treatment is necessary, then you support her. You tell her that your door is always open if she wants to come back.

B. Acknowledge that Jane has made lots of improvements, but you still question whether her BPD is gone and whether ending treatment is a good idea. You bring up recent interpersonal problems she was having with her sorority sisters as an example of how her BPD symptoms may still be the cause of her prob-lems and suggest that the two of you keep meeting, at least until the end of the year.

C. Tell Jane that she is wrong and that her BPD is still very active. Explain that terminating a treatment that is working while Jane is still struggling with anger and cutting, not to mention her continued substance abuse problem, is a terrible idea.

D. Tell Jane that if she thinks her BPD is all better when it clearly is not, then this treatment is not working. Terminate the treatment and refer her to another treater.

Decision Points: Discussion

Numbers within brackets indicate level of helpfulness ratings.

1. When learning about Jane's pattern of overdoses and threats to cut, you

   A. Immediately call to have Jane hospitalized—you can't risk another overdose. [3] (A level-headed assessment of risk indicates that Jane's overdoses were minor (i.e., involving nonlethal amounts of over-the-counter medications) and interpersonally driven and that her risk of suicide is actually quite low. Jumping to hospitalization will remove Jane from the stressors she would do well to face and manage better and therefore may detract from a major opportunity in the treatment.)

   B. Determine that Jane will require intensive individual psychotherapy and may want to take a leave of absence from college. [3] (Although Jane's symptoms are serious, leaving college will provide only a temporary solution to relieve stress and not teach her how to understand her reactivity and cope more effectively in the long run. Her treatment needs to focus on stably functioning at college, and a less intensive, generalist treatment should be attempted before she takes a leave of absence.)

   C. Ignore her cutting patterns and suicidality; they are a communication and not the cause of Jane's issues. [2] (Jane's cutting and suicidality represent communication and should be addressed as such. However, they should not be entirely ignored and, instead, need to be understood within the model of interpersonal hypersensitivity and treated as a symptom of her BPD.)

   D. Express concern about how Jane's impulsive, self-harming behavior may be undermining her adjustment to college and use these behaviors as examples as you explain your diagnosis of BPD. [1] (This approach maintains the focus of functioning at college without ignoring the self-harm and suicidality altogether. It helps create a joint understanding around Jane's symptoms within the framework of BPD and interpersonal hypersensitivity.)

2. When Jane suggests she might post an incriminating message about her former boyfriend on her social media account to drive away his new girlfriend, you

   A. Avoid addressing this comment and refocus the conversation on her plan to complete her academic work that weekend. [2] (It is important to maintain a focus on Jane's academic functioning, and redirecting the conversation to this may be helpful. However, a plan to exact revenge via social media could backlash in serious ways, and the pragmatic GPM therapist would not ignore the potential ramifications of her plans.)
   B. Nod at Jane's suggestion and ask her to report back what happens at your next session. [3] (The GPM therapist is not passive but rather proactive at considering both interpersonal interchanges and consequences of behavior. It would not be pragmatic to allow Jane to proceed with such a harmful plan without thinking through the consequences.)
   C. Directly outline the risks and potential consequences of Jane's plan. Ask Jane to wait another week and think carefully before posting the message. Then redirect the conversation to a group project for class that is challenging. [1] (This approach both logically addresses Jane's problematic plan and refocuses the session onto one of Jane's goals, which is to successfully navigate the group project.)
   D. Decide to involve Jane's ex-boyfriend in the therapy and set up a phone call with him. [3] (Although GPM is multimodal and encourages involvement of family and/or significant others, involving Jane's ex-boyfriend would actively reactivate her interpersonal problems, which are not likely solved by one phone call with the ex-boyfriend. Jane would do better to achieve her goals at college rather than involve an ex-boyfriend who is the root of her current issues and past suicide attempts.)

3. When Jane screams at you about your other patient, you

   A. Profusely apologize for your error and ask how you can make it up to Jane. You explain that your other patient is not more important than Jane and that you actually meet with Jane more than any other student. [3] (Although your apology acknowledges the real elements of your relationship with Jane, this defensive reaction steers the conversation away from Jane's angry outburst, which is a symptom she should be working to address, and is unprofessional. Additionally, discussing appointments with another student is a violation of the Health Insurance Portability and Accountability Act [HIPAA].)

B. Recognize and apologize for your memory lapse and then question why Jane was so quick to yell at you about another patient. [1] (By apologizing, you acknowledge that your and Jane's relationship is real and that you are capable of error. Through not lingering on your error and instead moving the discussion to Jane's outburst, you reframe the incident as a discussion of how her BPD symptoms influence her relationships, such as yours and hers.)

C. Immediately end the session and ask Jane to leave. Her screaming is not acceptable behavior and should not be tolerated in a professional environment. [2] (This reaction appropriately holds Jane accountable for unacceptable behavior, and it is important for her to learn the consequences of her actions. However, angry outbursts are a symptom of BPD and should be understood as such. Automatically giving up the option to discuss what happened by ending the session is a missed opportunity, and as a GPM therapist you expect angry outbursts and are equipped to handle them.)

D. Determine that this explosive reaction is a sign that the treatment is not working, and refer Jane to another therapist. [3] (Although the GPM therapist does recognize sustained, problematic behavior as a sign that treatment is not working, Jane has only been in treatment with you for a month. Jumping to the conclusion that one angry outburst is cause for termination is too drastic. She is in treatment with you for help with these exact symptoms.)

4. When Jane requests that you write a note to the dean to excuse her from some requirements, you

A. Contact the dean to reduce Jane's requirements. You agree that Jane was too sick to do work earlier in the semester and worry that failing classes will be a major barrier to her achieving her academic goals. [3] (Although on the surface this may seem like a helpful thing to do, you are demonstrating to Jane that you do not think she is capable of completing her work and are allowing her to avoid the consequences of her actions.)

B. Explain to Jane that you are worried that intervening will be treating her as though she is incapable of taking responsibility for her actions. Instead of calling the dean, you work with Jane to come up with a plan to improve her academic standing over the rest of the semester and help her find tutors for the classes she is failing. [1] (By not lowering the bar for Jane, you hold her accountable for her behavior and demonstrate that you believe in her ability to be a successful student. At the same time, you recognize that Jane is struggling academically and use case management to help her get the academic assistance she needs.)

C. You sternly explain to Jane that asking you to call the dean is just a way for her to escape her self-made problems and that you are disappointed she would ask for such a thing. [2] (Holding Jane accountable for her academic standing is important, and the GPM therapist should do so. However, chastising Jane for her request does not leave room for collaborating on a solution and may discourage Jane from bringing up problems that she is having in the future.)

D. Encourage Jane to have her parents call the dean. You do not see a medical reason for excusing her from academic commitments, but the dean may respond to family involvement. [3] (This approach does not hold Jane accountable and encourages her to recruit others in order to dodge consequences. Although GPM encourages family involvement when appropriate, it does not promote using parents to solve problems that are of Jane's own making.)

5. When Jane proposes terminating treatment, you

A. Agree that Jane has improved a lot, and if she does not think that treatment is necessary, then you support her. You tell her that your door is always open if she wants to come back. [2] (It is important to acknowledge Jane's improvement, and GPM supports terminating treatment when it is no longer helpful. However, accepting Jane's explanation that not thinking about her ex-boyfriend means her BPD is gone is not pragmatic.)

B. Acknowledge that Jane has made lots of improvements, but you still question whether her BPD is gone and whether ending treatment is a good idea. You bring up recent interpersonal problems she was having with her sorority sisters as an example of how her BPD symptoms may still be the cause of her problems and suggest that the two of you keep meeting, at least until the end of the year. [1] (This is a thoughtful response that both validates Jane's excitement over her gains and draws into question her conclusion about terminating treatment. Through using examples from her current social environment, you help Jane to see how treatment could still be helpful without making her feel as though she has not improved after all.)

C. Tell Jane that she is wrong and that her BPD is still very active. Explain that terminating a treatment that is working while Jane is still struggling with anger and cutting, not to mention her continued substance abuse problem, is a terrible idea. [2] (Your statement is factually correct, and it is important to help Jane see another perspective on her decision to terminate. However, not validating Jane's excitement over her gains and noncollaboratively shutting down her idea is not a thoughtful approach and will likely drive Jane away.)

D. Tell Jane that if she thinks her BPD is all better when it clearly is not, then this treatment is not working. Terminate the treatment and refer her to another treater. [3] (Prematurely terminating a treatment that is helping Jane improve is harmful. GPM supports terminating treatments that are not working, but Jane had made significant gains. GPM calls for a more measured response.)

Conclusion

Working with students with BPD or BPD traits is an unavoidable reality for clinicians in today's college campus setting. Research indicates that more students than in the past are presenting to the university setting with complex presentations suggestive of primary or co-occurring personality disorder diagnoses. College and university officials are increasingly focused on symptoms often seen in students with BPD (suicidality, nonsuicidal self-injurious behavior, eating disorders, substance use disorders, or mood disorders). Some of these students may have primary personality disorder diagnoses or may have personality disorder traits or diagnoses co-occurring with other disorders, which would likely complicate response to standard treatment interventions.

The focus on treating students with BPD or BPD traits thus far has been on using DBT in the college campus setting. There have been attempts to use "classical" DBT with all four key components: weekly individual and skills group sessions for the patient, phone coaching for the patient, and weekly peer consultation for the clinician, as well as abridged versions of

DBT with changes either in the duration and intensity of the treatment or use of the DBT skills component only. Researchers have identified, among other impediments, ongoing difficulties in introducing DBT to the campus setting because of cost, lack of training available, and productivity expectations for college counseling center clinicians.

Because GPM is designed as an intervention to be used by clinicians of varied training, including "entry-level" clinicians, training in GPM may help college and university psychological services provide evidence-based treatment for students with BPD without incurring excessive expenses or requiring wholesale changes in the way care is delivered. GPM is premised on the idea that most clinicians with some elementary training can be "good enough" treaters for patients with BPD. Although some patients may require one of the more intensive evidence-based treatments, important prospective studies support the idea that most patients will get better relatively quickly even without treatment (Gunderson et al. 2011; Zanarini et al. 2006). GPM allows clinicians to supply a short-term, intermittent, nonintensive treatment, and it should confer even to novices a sense of self-confidence in their ability to treat patients with BPD.

References

American College Health Association: American College Health Association National College Health Assessment Fall 2016 Reference Group Data Report. Hanover, MD, American College Health Association, 2017. Available at: https://www.acha.org/documents/ncha/NCHA-II_FALL_2016_REFERENCE_GROUP_DATA_REPORT.pdf. Accessed July 23, 2018.

American Psychiatric Association: Diagnostic and Statistical Manual of Mental Disorders, 4th Edition, Text Revision. Washington, DC, American Psychiatric Association, 2000

American Psychiatric Association: Diagnostic and Statistical Manual of Mental Disorders, 5th Edition. Arlington, VA, American Psychiatric Association, 2013

Baez T: Evidence-based practice for anxiety disorders in college mental health, in Evidence-Based Psychotherapy Practice in College Mental Health. Edited by Cooper SE. New York, Haworth, 2005, pp 33–49

Balon R, Beresin EV, Coverdale JH, et al: College mental health: a vulnerable population in an environment with systemic deficiencies. Acad Psychiatry 39(5):495–497, 2015 26327172

Bateman A, Fonagy P: Effectiveness of partial hospitalization in the treatment of borderline personality disorder: a randomized controlled trial. Am J Psychiatry 156(10):1563–1569, 1999 10518167

Benton SA, Robertson JM, Tseng W, et al: Changes in counseling center client problems across 13 years. Prof Psychol Res Pr 34(1):66–72, 2003

Birky II: Evidence-based and empirically supported college counseling center treatment of alcohol and related issues, in Evidence-Based Psychotherapy Practice in College Mental Health. Edited by Cooper SE. New York, Haworth, 2005, pp 7–23

Blum N, St John D, Pfohl B, et al: Systems Training for Emotional Predictability and Problem Solving (STEPPS) for outpatients with borderline personality disorder: a randomized controlled trial and 1-year follow-up. Am J Psychiatry 165(4):468–478, 2008 18281407

Chanen AM, McCutcheon L: Prevention and early intervention for borderline personality disorder: current status and recent evidence. Br J Psychiatry Suppl 202 (s54):s24–s29, 2013 23288497

Chanen AM, Thompson K: Preventive strategies for borderline personality disorder in adolescents. Curr Treat Options Psychiatry 1(4):358–368, 2014

Chanen AM, Jackson HJ, McCutcheon LK, et al: Early intervention for adolescents with borderline personality disorder using cognitive analytic therapy: randomised controlled trial. Br J Psychiatry 193(6):477–484, 2008 19043151

Choi-Kain LW, Gunderson JG: Borderline Personality and Mood Disorders: Comorbidity and Controversy. New York, Springer, 2015

Chugani CD: Dialectical behavioral therapy in college counseling centers: current literature and implications for practice. J College Stud Psychother 29(2):120–131, 2015

Chugani CD, Landes SJ: Dialectical behavior therapy in college counseling centers: current trends and barriers to implementation. Journal of College Student Psychotherapy 30(3):176–186, 2016

Chugani CD, Ghali MN, Brunner J: Effectiveness of short term dialectical behavior therapy skills training in college students with Cluster B personality disorders. Journal of College Student Psychotherapy 27:323–336, 2013

Clarkin JF, Levy KN, Lenzenweger MF, et al: Evaluating three treatments for borderline personality disorder: a multiwave study. Am J Psychiatry 164(6):922–928, 2007 17541052

Conway CC, Tackett JL, Skodol AE: Are personality disorders assessed in young people? Am J Psychiatry 174(10):1000–1001, 2017 28965457

Cooper SE, Benton SA, Benton SL, et al: Evidence-based practice in psychology among college counseling center clinicians. Journal of College Student Psychotherapy 22(4):28–50, 2008

Engle E, Gadischkie S, Roy N, et al: Dialectical behavior therapy for a college population: applications at Sarah Lawrence College and beyond. Journal of College Student Psychotherapy 27(1):11–30, 2013

Gallagher RP: National Survey of College Counseling Centers 2014. Alexandria, VA, International Association of Counseling Services, 2015. Available at: http://d-scholarship.pitt.edu/28178/1/survey_2014.pdf. Accessed July 23, 2018.

Giesen-Bloo J, van Dyck R, Spinhoven P, et al: Outpatient psychotherapy for borderline personality disorder: randomized trial of schema-focused therapy vs transference-focused psychotherapy. Arch Gen Psychiatry 63(6):649–658, 2006 16754838

Gunderson JG, Links PS: Handbook of Good Psychiatric Management for Borderline Personality Disorder. Washington, DC, American Psychiatric Publishing, 2014

Gunderson JG, Stout RL, McGlashan TH, et al: Ten-year course of borderline personality disorder: psychopathology and function from the Collaborative Longitudinal Personality Disorders Study. Arch Gen Psychiatry 68(8):827–837, 2011 21464343

Hersh RG: Assessment and treatment of patients with borderline personality disorder in the college and university population. Journal of College Student Psychotherapy 27:304–322, 2013

Kirsch DJ, Domakonda M, Doerfler LA, et al: An elective in college mental health for training adult residents in young adult psychiatry. Acad Psychiatry 39(5):544–548, 2015 26105769

Kitzrow MA: The mental health needs of today's college students: challenges and recommendations. NASPA Journal 41(4):165–179, 2003

Lee CL: Evidence-based treatment of depression in the college population, in Evidence-Based Psychotherapy Practice in College Mental Health. Edited by Cooper SE. New York, Haworth, 2005, pp 23–33

Linehan MM, Armstrong HE, Suarez A, et al: Cognitive-behavioral treatment of chronically parasuicidal borderline patients. Arch Gen Psychiatry 48(12):1060–1064, 1991 1845222

Links PS, Ross J, Gunderson JG: Promoting good psychiatric management for patients with borderline personality disorder. J Clin Psychol 71(8):753–763, 2015 26197971

McGorry P: Prevention, innovation and implementation science in mental health: the next wave of reform. Br J Psychiatry Suppl 54(suppl 54):s3–s4, 2013 23288498

Meaney R, Hasking P, Reupert A: Prevalence of borderline personality disorder in university samples: systematic review, meta-analysis and meta-regression. PLoS One 11(5):e0155439, 2016 27171206

Meaney-Tavares R, Hasking P: Coping and regulating emotions: a pilot study of a modified dialectical behavior therapy group delivered in a college counseling service. J Am Coll Health 61(5):303–309, 2013 23768227

Moran P, Romaniuk H, Coffey C, et al: The influence of personality disorder on the future mental health and social adjustment of young adults: a population-based, longitudinal cohort study. Lancet Psychiatry 3(7):636–645, 2016 27342692

Mowbray CT, Megivern D, Mandiberg JM, et al: Campus mental health services: recommendations for change. Am J Orthopsychiatry 76(2):226–237, 2006 16719642

Pistorello J, Fruzzetti AE, Maclane C, et al: Dialectical behavior therapy (DBT) applied to college students: a randomized clinical trial. J Consult Clin Psychol 80(6):982–994, 2012 22730955

Resnick JL: Evidence-based practice for treatment of eating disorders, in Evidence-Based Psychotherapy Practice in College Mental Health. Edited by Cooper SE. New York, Haworth, 2005, pp 49–67

Riba M, Kirsch D, Martel A, et al: Preparing and training the college mental health workforce. Acad Psychiatry 39(5):498–502, 2015 26307363

Rizvi SL, Steffel LM: A pilot study of 2 brief forms of dialectical behavior therapy skills training for emotion dysregulation in college students. J Am Coll Health 62(6):434–439, 2014 24678824

Shatkin JP, Diamond U: Psychiatry's next generation: teaching college students about mental health. Acad Psychiatry 39(5):527–532, 2015 25743202

Zanarini MC, Frankenburg FR, Khera GS, et al: Treatment histories of borderline inpatients. Compr Psychiatry 42(2):144–150, 2001 11244151

Zanarini MC, Frankenburg FR, Hennen J, et al: Prediction of the 10-year course of borderline personality disorder. Am J Psychiatry 163(5):827–832, 2006 16648323

Zisook S, Downs N, Moutier C, et al: College students and suicide risk: prevention and the role of academic psychiatry. Acad Psychiatry 36(1):1–6, 2012 22362428

PART II
Providers

Chapter 7

Social Workers

Robert P. Drozek, M.S.W., LICSW

In recent years, the profession of social work has increasingly embraced the use of evidence-based therapies (EBTs) to guide and inform everyday clinical practice (Barth et al. 2012; Bertram et al. 2015; Bledsoe-Mansori et al. 2013; Howard et al. 2003; McNeece and Thyer 2004; Rubin 2011; Rubin and Parrish 2007). The National Association of Social Workers (2017) explicitly advances this commitment in its code of ethics, affirming that "Social workers should critically examine and keep current with emerging knowledge relevant to social work and fully use evaluation and research evidence in their professional practice" (p. 27). This principle is particularly relevant in the treatment of clients with borderline personality disorder (BPD). Given the high public health costs associated with BPD (Grant et al. 2008; Zanarini et al. 2008), as well as negative clinician attitudes toward clients with BPD (Sansone and Sansone 2013), there is an urgent need for further exploration of EBTs for BPD in clinical social work practice.

Dialectical behavior therapy (DBT) has received the majority of the attention in the social work literature on BPD (Chapman et al. 2011; Koons

2008; Panos et al. 2013; Schulz and Rafferty 2008; Washburn et al. 2016). Although DBT offers social workers a comprehensive resource for treating patients with BPD, given the complexity and intensity of DBT training and implementation (Carmel et al. 2014; Choi-Kain et al. 2016; Swales 2010), DBT may not be ideally suited for the community-based settings in which social workers traditionally practice, where time and resources can be severely limited. Furthermore, in focusing primarily on cognitive and behavioral skills acquisition, DBT fails to provide social workers with a clear framework for *clinical case management*, a therapeutic approach that is widely seen as the heart of social work practice.

In this chapter, I explore the various clinical, theoretical, and systemic benefits of good psychiatric management (GPM) for social work practice. Drawn from the pioneering clinical conceptualizations of John Gunderson (Gunderson 2001; Gunderson and Links 2008, 2014), GPM is the only EBT for BPD that operates from an explicitly case management framework. Therefore, as I suggest here, GPM offers considerable promise for harmonious integration with the key tenets of clinical social work. I outline GPM's main principles, attempting to illustrate what it might look like to apply GPM in everyday social work practice. I close by offering a clinical illustration of these ideas.

An Outline of GPM for Social Work Practice

It is widely understood that clinical social workers practice in a wide range of settings, including "community mental health centers, hospitals, substance use treatment and recovery programs, schools, primary health care centers, child welfare agencies, aging services, employee assistance programs, and private practice settings" (National Association of Social Workers 2005). Even within these contexts, social workers provide a diverse range of often-overlapping services, including individual counseling, clinical case management, psychotherapy, crisis intervention, and client education (National Association of Social Workers 2006). Given the numerous roles that social workers occupy, it would be difficult to propose a single formula for the use of GPM in social work practice. Instead, I review what I take to be the key elements of GPM, outlined in Tables 7–1 and 7–2, which can hopefully be flexibly tailored to the social worker's specific role. In particular, I try to highlight what GPM has to offer for social workers who primarily provide *case management* to clients with BPD, as well as those who primarily provide *psychotherapy* to these clients.

TABLE 7–1. **Good psychiatric management in social work practice**

Focus/goals	Improved psychosocial functioning
	Increased agency and autonomy
	Vocational meaning, "work before love"
Frequency	Once weekly or as needed
	Tailor frequency to support client's functionality
Therapeutic stance	Supportiveness, activity, humility, authenticity
Preliminary interventions	Give borderline personality disorder diagnosis
	Provide psychoeducation regarding etiology, course, effective treatment
	Clarify roles and goals
Foundational techniques	"Empathize and contextualize"

TABLE 7–2. **Moment-to-moment good psychiatric management strategies**

Case management strategies	
Goal	"Getting a life"
Specific techniques	Coaching regarding "how to live in the world"
	Willing to give advice, sharing wisdom and personal experience
	Role playing
	Reinforcing strengths, successes
	Assisting with concrete tasks
	Advocacy; resource identification, acquisition
	Serving as a liaison/referrer to other treaters, including psychopharmacology
Psychotherapeutic strategies	
Goal	Adaptation to reality
Specific techniques	Problem solving: "think first"
	Raising doubts about dependency; highlighting limitations of clinician, others

Goals and Focus of GPM

The overarching clinical goal of GPM is what has been called *social rehabil-itation*—that is, helping clients toward improved functioning in their vo-cational and relational endeavors (Gunderson and Links 2014). Whereas other EBTs for BPD focus on altering *internal* processes (e.g., improved cognitive and behavioral skills in DBT, enhanced mentalizing in mentaliza-tion-based treatment [MBT], integration of object relations in transference-focused psychotherapy [TFP]), on the assumption that such alterations will naturally result in the client's improved adaptation to his or her environ-ment, GPM focuses on directly addressing "observable social impairment and social adjustment issues" (Gunderson and Links 2008, p. 72). Essen-tially, GPM assumes that if clients are able to obtain an improved sense of meaning and purpose in their environments, they will naturally start to ex-perience improvements in the various forms of instability endemic to BPD symptomatology (e.g., emotional dysregulation, poor mentalizing, identity diffusion, splitting). Practically speaking, social rehabilitation could involve helping clients to start school, obtain volunteer work, resume a vocational role, increase household responsibilities, or improve reliability in an exist-ing set of responsibilities.

GPM's social rehabilitation focus mirrors social work's core assumption that the appropriate focus of clinical practice is the *person in adaptive rela-tionship with his or her environment*. As the International Federation of So-cial Workers (2014) affirmed, "Social work's legitimacy and mandate lie in its intervention at the points where people interact with their environ-ment." By focusing on environmental as well as psychological functioning, GPM also supports social work's ethical commitment to social justice: "So-cial workers should advocate for living conditions conducive to the fulfill-ment of basic human needs and should promote social, economic, political, and cultural values and institutions that are compatible with the realization of social justice" (National Association of Social Workers 2017, p. 29).

> **Practice points**
>
> For social workers providing case management
>
> - GPM validates the traditional focus of case management services, namely, improving the person's psychosocial functioning (Kanter 2011). Rather than conceptualizing such services as "superficial" compared to psychological therapies, GPM recognizes that case management might offer the most expedient path to improved stability for clients with BPD.

> **Practice points** *(continued)*
>
> For social workers providing psychotherapy
>
> • GPM recommends that psychotherapists focus not simply on psychological or "transferential" goals when working with clients with BPD. Rather, when collaborating with a client to develop the goals of a treatment, or when evaluating clinical outcomes, social workers should be consistently considering this question: How can this treatment help the client to lead a more engaged, productive, and meaningful life in his or her environment and community?

Frequency and Duration of GPM

Although GPM has been empirically validated in a once-weekly, year-long format (McMain et al. 2009), GPM advocates a flexible implementation tailored to the needs of the client: "No specific length and intensity are prescribed; patients and therapist collaborate in judging whether a therapy is effective" (Gunderson and Links 2014, p. 7). By making treatment frequency and duration contingent on clients' continued psychosocial progress, GPM seeks to encourage clients' efforts toward agency and autonomy while directly challenging the idea, often prevalent regarding BPD, that continued caretaking is predicated on clients remaining perpetually in the "sick" or "damaged" role.

This model mirrors the case management approach in clinical social work, where clinicians are encouraged to "titrate support so as to maximize a client's capacity for self-directed behavior" (Walsh and Manuel 2015, p. 822). Within a case management model, the frequency and duration of clinical contact is often determined by practical considerations, namely, how much support is needed to help a client achieve his or her goal or to address the reason for the referral (e.g., housing, transportation, entitlements).

> **Practice points**
>
> For social workers providing case management
>
> • In addition to validating case managers' practice of tailoring treatment intensity to the client's level of functioning, GPM grants case managers greater latitude in treating clients with BPD, allowing increases in the frequency and duration of clinical contacts as needed as long as the client is experiencing continued progress in psychosocial functioning.

> **Practice points** *(continued)*
>
> For social workers providing psychotherapy
>
> - If the client appears to be making good use of psychotherapy sessions, the social worker can feel comfortable increasing the frequency of appointments up to twice weekly. On the other hand, if the client starts to request additional sessions in the context of increased difficulties (e.g., emotional dysregulation, interpersonal conflict, self-harm), the social worker should proceed with caution, saying something like the following:
>
>   "I think it is really understandable that you would like to meet more frequently, given all the difficulties you have been having. However, I feel wary of giving you 'more' of a treatment that clearly hasn't been working that well for you. Let's look a bit more at what has been going on with you lately, so that we can come to a good decision about how to proceed."

Therapeutic Stance of GPM

The phrase *therapeutic stance* refers not so much to the specific interventions employed in a treatment but rather to the clinician's overall *attitude* and *approach* in the treatment relationship. In GPM, the clinician's stance involves several key elements:

- *Supportiveness:* warmth, reliability, interest, and concern
- *Activity:* asking questions, directly responding to clients, avoiding long silences, structuring the focus and trajectory of sessions
- *Humility:* flexibility, collaboration, thoughtfulness, willingness to take responsibility for mistakes, never presuming authoritative access to "the truth" about clients' experiences
- *Authenticity:* cautious transparency about ideas and opinions, comfort sharing "wise advice" about how the world works, operating both as a professional and as a "real person" in the treatment situation

GPM's therapeutic stance converges with the traditional approach in clinical case management. Supportiveness is a basic tenet of case management, "characterized by its direct concern for the well-being of the individual" (Woods and Hollis 2000, p. 35). Because case managers work with clients to address specific forms of psychosocial impairment, they often employ an active, engaged, and practically oriented clinical stance (Frankel and Gelman 2016). Furthermore, given social work's emphasis on collaboration, nonauthoritarianism, and client-centered practice, professional humility serves as a central feature of the case manager's guiding principles (National Association of Social Workers 2013). Finally, likely due to the practically oriented focus of case management, social workers tend to embrace the authenticity and down-to-earth approach advocated by GPM: "The social worker starts off as a 'real' person concerned with external events and people in the client's life, and in the course of intervention brings harmony between those two worlds" (Walsh and Manuel 2015, p. 821).

Practice points

For social workers providing case management

- When working with clients with BPD, social work case managers can feel confident that their clinical approach (emphasizing supportiveness, active involvement, humility, and authenticity) has theoretical, practical, and empirical support.

For social workers providing psychotherapy

- Social workers who tend to employ a more passive, nondirective stance in psychotherapy (e.g., dynamic clinicians, client-centered therapists) should consider increasing their level of activity and focus when using GPM to treat clients with BPD. This high level of activity is not unique to GPM but rather is central to all of the EBTs for BPD, likely because clients with BPD can regress and destabilize with insufficient structure.

- Similarly, social workers who employ a more technically "neutral" stance (e.g., refusing to answer clients' direct questions, not sharing opinions or ideas, avoiding any form of advice giving) are encouraged to cautiously practice greater transparency, authenticity, and self-disclosure in working with clients with BPD. Given the negative cognitive biases associated with BPD (Arntz et al. 2011), this approach can mitigate clients' tendency to read "neutrality" as negativity, thus improving the stability of the therapeutic alliance.

> **Practice points** *(continued)*
>
> For social workers providing psychotherapy *(continued)*
>
> • Social workers who employ models that assume a greater degree of clinician authority (e.g., first-wave cognitive and behavioral therapies, classical psychoanalytic theories) are encouraged to incorporate a greater sense of uncertainty and flexibility into their clinical stance. Such a posture decreases the chance of power struggles with clients with BPD, offsets clients' tendencies toward "polarized black-or-white thinking," and models a more balanced approach to interpersonal relationships (Gunderson and Links 2014, p. 15).

Preliminary Interventions

According to GPM principles, after becoming aware that a client likely meets three or more of the diagnostic criteria for BPD, the clinician should review and discuss the BPD diagnosis with the client. This recommendation can generate significant anxiety for social workers who do not already specialize in treating BPD. The social worker might worry that the client will react negatively to the diagnosis, that giving the diagnosis is not really necessary, or even that the very idea of a personality disorder contradicts the strengths-based perspective of social work practice. As stated by Corcoran and Walsh (2016), "Social workers should be concerned about using these diagnoses because they appear to describe the *total person* rather than particular aspects of the person, and they are often used in pejorative terms" (p. 452).

Although concerns such as these are well intentioned, they fail to appreciate many of the therapeutic benefits of explicitly discussing the BPD diagnosis with clients, benefits that often cannot be achieved by other means. In actual practice, most clients with BPD respond quite positively to receiving the diagnosis, because it explains and validates the challenges with which they have been struggling for most of their lives. According to Gunderson and Links (2008), "It is reassuring [for clients] to know they are not alone with their disorder and that a body of knowledge is available about this disorder and its treatment" (p. 81). Furthermore, clients have the right to know about their diagnosis, and providing clients with BPD-specific treatment *without* informing them contradicts the fundamental social work principle of informed consent (National Association of Social Workers 2017). Finally, disclosing the BPD diagnosis is entirely consistent with social work's strengths-based approach. In the definitive statement on the strengths perspective in social work, Saleebey (2013) advised, "Defining the problem situation or experience is an important first step in the helping process because it guides how the helping process will proceed (p. 191). Similarly, GPM assumes that "diagnosis giving" can actually be an *empowering* process for clients, helping them to mobilize their natural strengths to anticipate and address their emotional vulnerabilities in their interpersonal relationships and relational contexts.

Although clinicians can employ a variety of techniques to discuss the BPD diagnosis, I use an approach that I have found particularly helpful with my clients and that I see as consistent with the collaborative, client-centered philosophy of social work practice (Hepworth et al. 2017). When I feel confident that a particular client meets diagnostic criteria for BPD, and once I know the person well enough to provide examples from the client's history to illustrate these criteria, I usually say something like the following:

> As we've gotten to know each other better, I have been thinking that many of your symptoms are consistent with a specific diagnosis, which happens to be particularly amenable to treatment. Would you be open to discussing this a bit together?

If the client is interested in hearing more, I provide the client with a written list of the full diagnostic criteria for BPD, framed in colloquial, jargon-free language (e.g., the Zanarini Rating Scale for Borderline Personality Disorder [Zanarini et al. 2003]). We then proceed to review the criteria together.

> The diagnosis itself primarily involves problems with *instability*: instability in emotions, self-esteem, relationships, and behaviors. So the first issue is that the person often makes desperate attempts to avoid being abandoned, or even *feeling* abandoned by other people. Does that resonate with you at all?

If the client answers affirmatively, I invite the client to share examples from his or her own experience, explicitly validating these reflections if they seem applicable: "I guess you're right. It does sound like you've struggled with that a lot." If the person ever rejects a symptom that I see as relevant, I usually draw on my understanding of the client thus far.

> So it sounds like you don't feel that you really try to avoid rejection or abandonment by others. What about what you were telling me the other day about your boyfriend? You mentioned that you often feel quite anx-

ious that he's going to judge you or stop liking you, so you try to have sex with him a lot to make sure that those things don't happen. Could this ever be an attempt to avoid abandonment by him?

If the client continues to reject the criterion, I do not push the matter, instead moving on to consider other relevant symptoms. There is no profit to getting into a power struggle with clients about such matters. After reviewing all of the criteria with the client, I explain that these are all symptoms of BPD. By deemphasizing labels and privileging clients' own descriptions of their experiences, we decrease the chance of arousing clients' negative associations connected with the idea of having a "personality disorder." Instead, clients tend to feel understood and even validated, leaving the discussion with a sense of curiosity about the diagnosis and an eagerness to learn more about treatment.

After discussing the diagnosis, the clinician turns to the strategy of *psychoeducation*, which serves a central role in GPM. In GPM, psychoeducation involves providing the client with essential information about the BPD diagnosis, including heritability, biopsychosocial etiology, course, interpersonal dimensions, and responsiveness to treatment. Providing clients with this information can help them to cultivate a *balanced optimism* about their diagnosis—that is, they become increasingly aware of their basic vulnerabilities, which better positions them to make realistic plans for treatment and building a life while also developing a sense of hope about the high probability for improvement and success.

At first glance, because the term *education* can imply a power differential between instructor and trainee, it might appear that *psychoeducation* contradicts social work's emphasis on collaboration and empowerment. However, in addition to furthering social work's mandate to provide evidence-based care (Walsh 2008), psychoeducation embodies a strengths-based model of practice: "The patient/client and/or family are considered partners with the provider in treatment, on the premise that the more knowledgeable the care recipients and informal caregivers are, the more positive health-related outcomes will be for all" (Lukens and McFarlane 2006, p. 291–292).

Finally, at some point in the early stages of treatment, the clinician works with the client to clarify what GPM calls "roles and goals." *Roles* refers to the social worker and client's explicit, collaborative expectations about "the frame" of the treatment relationship, such as appointment schedule, fees, cancellation policy, intersession availability, and the social worker's interaction with other parties relevant to the treatment (e.g., psychiatrist, family supports). *Goals* refers primarily to the client's time-limited, discrete, measurable, and obtainable aims (e.g., decreasing suicidal behavior, asking for help when in crisis, implementing communication skills with a partner, finding volunteer work).

Practice points

- Although the strategies described here are an essential part of the early phases of GPM, social workers should feel free to return to them as needed throughout the course of treatment—for example, by continuing to contextualize a person's difficulties in terms of the BPD diagnosis or by invoking a client's goals in order to stimulate shared reflection about the progress of the treatment.

- For many social workers, there is often a temptation to quickly jump to *solutions* (e.g., recommending resources in case management, employing cognitive restructuring in psychotherapy) in response to a client's difficulties. When applying GPM to social work practice, social workers are advised to temporarily resist this "righting reflex" in the early phases of treatment (Hohman 2012) and to remember that diagnosis giving, psychoeducation, and clarification of goals and focus of GPM *are effective clinical interventions in and of themselves* that play an essential role in the effective treatment of clients with BPD.

Foundational Techniques: "Empathize and Contextualize"

In any given session of GPM, the clinician frequently employs two primary techniques: *validation* and *contextualization of affect*. GPM defines *validation* as "affirming the reality of patients' perceptions or the justification for their feelings" (Gunderson and Links 2008, p. 68). GPM's validation, also understood as "support" or "empathetic recognition," implies not simply accurately describing clients' experiences (e.g., "It sounds like that comment really hurt your feelings") but affirming that it is *reasonable* and *understandable* that clients would experience the world in this way, given their history and experiences (e.g., "That *was* really hurtful; I think anyone in your shoes would have been upset by that"). Given the vulnerabilities to self-criticism and interpersonal hypersensitivity of clients with BPD (Gunderson and Lyons-Ruth 2008), this approach serves as a necessary condition for productive therapeutic work with these clients.

A second foundational technique in GPM is *contextualization of affect*. Many clients with BPD tend to experience their emotional and behavioral challenges (e.g., depression, self-loathing, suicidal thinking and gestures) in markedly decontextualized terms (e.g., "I'm just depressed—that's the way I've always been," "There wasn't really a trigger for cutting my wrists— the idea just came into my head, so I did it"). These decontextualized experiences can contribute to the feelings of confusion, powerlessness, and hopelessness that are so common for clients with BPD.

GPM observes that the emotional dysregulation in BPD is usually triggered by some form of stress in interpersonal relationships, often involving feelings of rejection, abandonment, or aloneness. In GPM, when clients present with difficulties with emotional dysregulation or impulsivity, clinicians actively inquire about the thoughts, emotions, and situations that preceded these challenges, with an emphasis on how they were feeling about themselves and others before, during, and after the event. This tactic overlaps significantly with DBT's use of chain analysis (Linehan 1993) as well as MBT's technique of mentalizing functional analysis (Bateman and Fonagy 2016). As Gunderson and Links (2014) pointed out, "This review is essential for understanding (increasing self-awareness, accepting the impact of others), developing a sense of agency, and preventing recurrences" (p. 42).

Practice points

- Social workers have long recognized the central role of empathetic validation in everyday clinical practice (Hamilton 1951; Turner 1978; Woods and Hollis 2000). In addition to providing justification for this approach with clients with BPD, GPM offers further guidance on the practical application of empathetic validation, recommending that social workers regularly employ this technique to accommodate the fundamental emotional/interpersonal vulnerabilities of patients with BPD and especially underscoring the importance of using this approach when clients are in states of emotional and behavioral dysregulation.

- As noted earlier in the section "Goals and Focus of GPM," social work embraces the person-in-environment model of human experience, which "highlights the importance of understanding an individual and individual behavior in light of the environmental contexts in which that person lives and acts" (Kondrat 2008, p. 348). By advocating the contextualization of affect with clients with BPD, GPM validates the theoretical and clinical approach already employed by most social workers in everyday clinical practice.

> **Practice points** *(continued)*
>
> • When clients with BPD present in states of emotional distress, GPM recommends that, rather than responding with some "change-oriented" intervention (e.g., advice giving, problem solving), social workers should slow down the entire process—first validating clients' experiences and then working with them to contextualize these experiences in terms of recent scenarios of abandonment, aloneness, and rejection in interpersonal relationships. Once clients feel sufficiently safe and aware of the relational meaning of their experiences, they will be better equipped to productively utilize the change-oriented strategies that are an essential component of GPM.

Moment-to-Moment Strategies

Compared with the other EBTs for BPD, GPM spends little time specifying "on-model" and "off-model" interventions, instead advocating a clinical approach that is "inherently flexible, pragmatic, and adapted to each patient" (Gunderson and Links 2014, p. 3). GPM's case management strategies involve a hands-on, practical, "roll-up-your-sleeves" approach to working with clients, one that has substantial overlap with the social work approach to case management practice (Frankel and Gelman 2016). GPM's specific case management interventions include coaching; giving advice; role-playing; reinforcing strengths and successes; assisting clients with concrete tasks (e.g., building a resume, completing an application for housing or other benefits); serving as a liaison and "point person" between the client and important parties in the client's life (e.g., family members, other clinicians, agency contacts); providing education and advocacy regarding available resources; and, when appropriate, making referrals for additional clinical care (e.g., psychopharmacologist, day treatment programs, family therapy) and resource-related support (e.g., housing, transportation, financial and nutritional assistance). All of these interventions further GPM's main aim: helping clients to "get a life," to directly improve their functioning in the real world.

Above all, GPM's psychotherapeutic strategies focus on encouraging clients' *adaptation to reality*: "The goals of treatment are to help BPD patients learn to tolerate such stressors better and to accept limitations in themselves and in others" (Gunderson and Links 2014, p. 77). Along these lines, GPM strongly supports the use of *problem solving*—that is, helping clients to consider cognitive and behavioral strategies to address their challenges with emotional, behavioral, and interpersonal instability. Problem solving can be employed preemptively, such as when clients anticipate a triggering situation and reflect on how they might respond should it arise (e.g., by practicing positive self-talk, or by pressing "pause" on the situation and taking some time to cool down). Social workers can also practice problem solving retroactively, for example, by considering clients' emotional and behavioral response to a challenging scenario and encouraging them to reflect on more adaptive responses that they might have employed in the moment (e.g., following strategies listed on a safety plan, practicing healthy assertiveness rather than criticizing). Over time, clients come to internalize these strategies, resulting in an enhanced ability to "think first" before acting: "Learning to think about the relation of cause and effect, regarding both feelings and interpersonal relationships, introduces delays of impulse discharge or avoidance behaviors" (Gunderson and Links 2008, p. 299).

GPM's second major therapeutic strategy is that of *exploring limitations in interpersonal relationships*. Consistent with Kernberg's (1975) seminal formulations, GPM recognizes the tendencies toward extreme idealization and devaluation that characterize the interpersonal experiences of clients with BPD. As these dynamics unfold in the course of a GPM treatment, the clinician is instructed to 1) empathetically validate the client's longings for these idealized models of relatedness and 2) act as a "representative of reality" by gently questioning the feasibility of these longings. This approach can take a range of shapes: the social worker can help clients to recognize and accommodate their own limitations in relationships (e.g., by providing psychoeducation about the genetic vulnerabilities involved in BPD); highlight the potential impracticality of some of their hopes and demands for other people (e.g., by commenting that it is perhaps unrealistic that they expect that other people automatically know their needs and wants without their communicating them); and explicitly acknowledge his or her own limitations as a clinician, for example, by reminding clients about the external boundaries of the social worker's role, acknowledging that the social worker is "not omniscient, clairvoyant, or omnipotent" (Gunderson and Links 2014, p. 41), and "expressing skepticism about the patient's level of dependency on the relationship" (Choi-Kain et al. 2016, p. 352). The hope is that clients, over time, will come to internalize these ideas and to feel increasingly connected and "cared for" in their relationships, even in the face of the unavoidable limitations in themselves and others (Gunderson and Links 2014).

Practice points

- When practicing GPM, social workers should consider using techniques that lie outside of their traditional clinical repertoires. For example, social work case managers can work with clients to practice problem-solving strategies and to explore the limitations in Self and Other. Social work psychotherapists can expand their clinical approach by not simply employing internally focused strategies (e.g., skills training, interpretation, bolstering mentalizing) but also by utilizing the range of case management strategies listed in Table 7–2 to directly improve clients' functioning in the "real world."

- In general, GPM offers minimal guidance about "which intervention to use when." After employing the basic interventions already reviewed (e.g., diagnosis giving, psychoeducation, "empathizing and contextualizing"), clinicians are encouraged to use "common sense" in deciding what to do next: What problems appear most pressing for the client at this particular moment? What interventions have the potential to be the most helpful for him or her, based on previous experiences with the client? Clinicians are encouraged to be flexible and pragmatic in their choices, discontinuing an approach if it appears ineffective and comfortably trying out new strategies if so inspired.

Case Vignette

The following case description includes decision points, each of which has several alternative responses listed at the end of the case. The reader will rate each alternative response in terms of its level of helpfulness. Discussions of responses follow.

> You are employed as a clinical social worker in an urban community mental health clinic. Monica is a 33-year-old single white woman referred to you by a psychiatrist in your clinic for "counseling and case management." At Monica's psychiatry appointment today, she informed her prescriber, alternating between sobbing and extreme rage, that she was getting kicked out of her Section 8 apartment by "those asshole slumlords." She insisted that she was going to "end up homeless again" and would have to return to sex work to support herself. Before you meet Monica, while reviewing her chart, you notice that the psychiatrist has diagnosed her with major depressive disorder, posttraumatic stress disorder, and BPD.

In your first several sessions with Monica, you obtain a full psychosocial history. Monica describes a history of early developmental abuse and neglect, reporting that she grew up in poverty with a single mother who herself was highly volatile and would frequently "smack me around to keep me in line." Monica shared a long history of chaotic, intense relationships with older, controlling men: "These guys always start out great, but once they realize that I'm not just a doormat, they can't deal with me anymore." Given Monica's historical diagnosis of BPD, you ask her a range of questions to assess for the diagnosis. Monica confirms long-standing difficulties with impulsivity (e.g., in sex and spending), feelings of self-hatred and emptiness, and self-injury by cutting, often in response to arguments with her boyfriends. She also reports difficulties with alcohol, from which she has now been abstinent for the past 3 years, with intermittent attendance at Alcoholics Anonymous (AA) meetings. You learn that she has recently been getting into "knock-down, drag-out fights" with her boyfriend, Harry, as well as heated arguments with the management staff in her apartment building when they have attempted to discuss these fights with her. Management has informed her that if these conflicts continue, she will be at risk for eviction. You start to feel quite confident that she meets the diagnostic threshold for the diagnosis of BPD. [**Decision Point 1**]

You decide to directly discuss the BPD diagnosis with Monica, reviewing the diagnostic criteria, considering examples from Monica's own experience, and providing psychoeducation about its heritability, course, and responsiveness to treatment. To your surprise, she responds quite well to this discussion, admitting that other treaters have mentioned that she had BPD before, but no one had explained it in this level of detail. She says, "I've always known that I had really bad anger problems and that I get a little messed up in relationships, but I didn't know it was so involved." She shares that although she does not want to let Harry and the apartment managers "off the hook," she definitely would like to work on her anger issues with you, because she does not want to lose her apartment. You discuss together your mutual expectations for the treatment (e.g., appointment schedule, clinic policies, fees), and you agree to meet on a weekly basis to work on these issues.

Monica storms into the following session in a state of extreme agitation, yelling, "Those bastards!" She explains that she had gotten into another argument that morning with the assistant manager of her apartment building. "They don't care about me. They don't care about the other tenants. It's all about the money for them." [**Decision Point 2**]

You choose to ask Monica more about her interaction with the assistant manager that morning. She explains that she had gone to the management office to pay her rent, and the manager made her wait for 15 minutes before providing her with a receipt for her payment. You ask Monica what she was thinking and feeling as she waited. She replied, "I was just getting more and more angry. Who does he think he is, to make me wait like that? If I didn't have a Section 8 voucher, do you think he would have made me wait? That bastard—he does not know who he is dealing with." You observe that it sounds like Monica was feeling judged and rejected by the assistant manager, and Monica agrees with this, sharing about the shame that she feels about having a Section 8 voucher and her worries that people look down on her for this. At this point, Monica appears to have calmed down. She starts to tell you about how she has been spending her days—alone in her apartment, watching television and researching "housing discrimination" on the Internet while waiting for her boyfriend to get home. As the day goes on, she starts to feel more and more angry and upset, but she always experiences significant relief when her boyfriend comes over around dinnertime, like now her day can finally begin. [**Decision Point 3**]

You collaborate with Monica to identify a range of triggers that could signify her impending agitation and rage (e.g., feelings of insecurity and restlessness, thoughts about the unfairness of her housing situation), as well as coping skills that could be helpful to her in her future interactions with management staff (e.g., counting to 10 before responding to staff's comments, checking Facebook on her phone). You work to write these all up in the form of a crisis plan, and provide her with a paper copy. You also verbalize your concerns about her lack of daytime structure, to which she is somewhat receptive: "I don't want to go overboard here, but I could start going back to that noontime AA meeting I used to attend. I've been meaning to go back there anyway, because it's been a while."

Over the next several months, Monica begins to experience notable improvements. On her own, she starts reading through her crisis plan prior to all of her interactions with apartment building staff. Her arguments with them largely subside, and she reports an improved ability to "stop" herself before speaking, even when she is feeling judged. She also starts attending the AA meeting several days per week. She rekindles some friendships with other members there, even assuming a service position of making coffee. She tells you, "It makes me feel good to be giving back, even a little bit, the way that everybody helped me when I first started coming around."

About 3 months after starting to work together, Monica arrives for her appointment upbeat and beaming. "I've got some great news," she says. "Harry is moving in with me!" You are caught off guard by this. Monica's housing situation has just started to stabilize, and this decision could directly interfere with all the progress she has made. In addition to increasing the potential for conflicts between them, this could place Monica's Section 8 voucher at risk because Harry is not listed on her HUD-50058 form. You share these concerns with Monica, and she explodes at you: "I can't believe you! This is the first time that I've been happy about something in so, so long. Your job is to *support* me, not to bring me down." [**Decision Point 4**]

You share with Monica that you can understand why she would feel so upset with you, given how pessimistic you were and how excited she was about this new plan. Your reaction seems to catch Monica off guard, and she says, "I'm glad that you can see this about yourself." You continue, "Well, don't let me off the hook too quickly. Even though I could have gone a bit easier on you, I can't agree that it's my job to just support every decision you make. What if I think you're making a bad decision? Aren't I allowed to share that with you and still be helpful to you if we happen to be on different pages?" Monica admits that she cannot really argue with you on this point. This opens up a helpful discussion about how you and Monica can work together productively even if you disagree with each other and even if she potentially feels judged or criticized by you. Over time, you and Monica begin to explore the relevance of these themes in her other interpersonal relationships, such as with Harry and the apartment building management.

Decision Points: Alternative Responses

Rate each response in terms of its level of helpfulness with a rating of 1 (will be helpful), 2 (possibly helpful, continuing reservations), or 3 (not helpful—or even harmful).

1. Now that you understand Monica's situation more fully, you consider taking the following courses of action:

    A. Open a discussion about Monica's possible BPD diagnosis, sharing information about the diagnosis, etiology, course, and effective treatment.

    B. Recommend to Monica that the two of you call the apartment building management together, so that you can try to broker a solution to prevent Monica from getting evicted. You feel that although discussing the BPD diagnosis might be useful at some point, this housing situation should take priority.

    C. Ask Monica if she would like to learn additional communication skills for managing these conflicts with Harry and the management staff. If she is able to practice greater interpersonal effectiveness in these relationships, then the BPD diagnosis could become a nonissue.

2. After empathizing with Monica's feelings of anger, you consider employing the following approaches:

    A. Inform Monica that she likely felt rejected or criticized by the assistant manager in this interaction, and provide psychoeducation about GPM's model of interpersonal hypersensitivity in BPD.

    B. Invite Monica to try role-playing this scenario with you in session to consider strategies that she might employ in the future to decrease the chance of conflict with the management staff.

    C. Ask Monica to tell you more about what happened in this interaction with the assistant manager.

3. In light of Monica's recent difficulties, you consider the following interventions:

   A. Share your concerns about Monica's lack of daytime structure, asking if she would be interested in discussing ways that she could spend her time that might help her obtain a greater sense of purpose and meaning in her life.
   B. Invite Monica to share more about her relationship with her mother when she was younger. Without a deeper understanding of the developmental antecedents of her difficulties with interpersonal hypersensitivity, it will be difficult for Monica to make progress on these matters.
   C. Work with Monica to identify the early "warning signs" of her conflicts with management staff and to consider strategies for emotional regulation and effective communication in these moments.

4. Recognizing that this is a pivotal moment in the treatment, you consider responding in the following ways:

   A. Consistent with GPM's emphasis on humility, you apologize for saying what you said and agree that you should support Monica's own goals rather than your agenda for her life.
   B. Remark that Monica's response reminds you of her interpersonal pattern with the apartment building staff: when she feels criticized, she is likely to become angry and critical of others.
   C. Empathize with Monica's frustration with you and attempt to gently challenge her unrealistic expectations of you.

Decision Points: Discussion

Numbers within brackets indicate level of helpfulness ratings.

1. You consider taking the following courses of action:

   A. Open a discussion about Monica's possible BPD diagnosis, sharing information about the diagnosis, etiology, course, and effective treatment. [1] (Given your confidence that Monica meets diagnostic criteria for BPD, both options B and C risk creating a superficial and avoidant dynamic in the treatment to which clients with BPD are exquisitely sensitive and which can subtly undermine the therapeutic process. Furthermore, commencing with option A increases the possible efficacy of options B and C; if Monica is more fully informed about the essential nature of her challenges, she will likely be more receptive to traditional psychotherapeutic and case management interventions that specifically address her vulnerabilities toward emotional and interpersonal sensitivity.)

B. Recommend to Monica that the two of you call the apartment building management together, so that you can try to broker a solution to prevent Monica from getting evicted. You feel that although discussing the BPD diagnosis might be useful at some point, this housing situation should take priority. [2] (Although there could be substantial value in attempting options B and C at some point in Monica's treatment, GPM would recommend postponing these interventions until you have frankly discussed her potential diagnosis and its impact on her daily life [option A], especially because Monica is not in any immediate danger of being evicted.)

C. Ask Monica if she would like to learn additional communication skills for managing these conflicts with Harry and the management staff. If she is able to practice greater interpersonal effectiveness in these relationships, then the BPD diagnosis could become a nonissue. [2] (See option B discussion.)

2. After empathizing with Monica's feelings of anger, you consider employing the following approaches:

A. Inform Monica that she likely felt rejected or criticized by the assistant manager in this interaction, and provide psychoeducation about GPM's model of interpersonal hypersensitivity in BPD. [2] (Suggesting underlying issues behind her actions risks undermining GPM's emphasis on clinical humility because it privileges the social worker's own authority and knowledge without sufficient emphasis on understanding and validating Monica's experiences.)

B. Invite Monica to try role-playing this scenario with you in session to consider strategies that she might employ in the future to decrease the chance of conflict with the management staff. [2] (This option feels a bit premature, because it will be difficult for Monica to effectively utilize role-playing techniques [or any other behavioral strategy, for that matter] if she does not yet possess a sufficient sense of self-awareness and agency in this situation.)

C. Ask Monica to tell you more about what happened in this inter-action with the assistant manager. [1] (Consistent with GPM's recommendation to "empathize and contextualize," GPM would recommend that you ask for further details about the interper-sonal interaction that led to Monica's current state of emotional dysregulation. Although Monica is clearly assuming that manage-ment does not care about her, it is not yet evident *what happened* in this interaction that led her to arrive at this conclusion.)

3. You consider the following interventions:

A. Share your concerns about Monica's lack of daytime structure, asking if she would be interested in discussing ways that she could spend her time that might help her obtain a greater sense of purpose and meaning in her life. [1] (GPM would favor inter-ventions that directly address Monica's most pressing difficulties with psychosocial functioning, in this case her risk of homeless-ness related to interpersonal conflicts. Because you have already worked to "empathize and contextualize" Monica's conflict with the assistant manager, GPM allows for considerable latitude in selecting further clinical interventions with Monica. As noted in GPM's "Moment-to-Moment Strategies" (discussed in the previ-ous section), options A and C would both be viable choices at this point. In GPM, the social worker would assume that some positive, meaningful structure could act as a buffer for Monica's vulnerabilities toward interpersonal sensitivity.)

B. Invite Monica to share more about her relationship with her mother when she was younger. Without a deeper understanding of the developmental antecedents of her difficulties with inter-personal hypersensitivity, it will be difficult for Monica to make progress on these matters. [3] (In GPM, the social worker would not assume that Monica needs to acquire historical insight in or-der to improve her impulse control. The here-and-now focus is prioritized.)

C. Work with Monica to identify the early "warning signs" of her conflicts with management staff and to consider strategies for emotional regulation and effective communication in these mo-ments. [1] (See option A discussion. Problem-solving interventions might help Monica improve her impulse control, thereby decreasing conflict with management staff.)

4. After expressing concerns about Monica's "great news," you consider responding in the following ways:

   A. Consistent with GPM's emphasis on humility, you apologize for saying what you said and agree that you should support Monica's own goals rather than your agenda for her life. [2] (Although option A embodies GPM's principles of validation and humility, it is perhaps *too* supportive, missing the clinical opportunity to challenge Monica's idealizing tendencies.)

   B. Remark that Monica's response reminds you of her interpersonal pattern with the apartment building staff: when she feels criticized, she is likely to become angry and critical of others. [3] (Option B contradicts GPM's emphasis on empathetic validation; it runs the risk of making Monica feel blamed for her feelings while problematically shifting the focus off her relationship *with you*, which is the current, emotionally charged arena for interpersonal learning.)

   C. Empathize with Monica's frustration with you and attempt to gently challenge her unrealistic expectations of you. [1] (Given Monica's intense emotionality in this moment, GPM principles would recommend that, first and foremost, you respond by empathizing with Monica's distress, in the hope that this validating intervention would enable her to reflect further on the feasibility of her expectations of you. This approach could help to strengthen Monica's ability to accept the limitations of other people, which, in turn, would lead to improvements in Monica's long-standing challenges with interpersonal hypersensitivity.)

Conclusion

In this chapter, I have attempted to illustrate the key principles of GPM, the application of these principles in social work practice, and the substantial areas of overlap between GPM and the fundamental tenets of social work. In closing, I would like to suggest that there are compelling reasons to consider GPM not simply as a *viable* treatment for BPD but as a primary, organizing framework for the care of BPD in clinical social work.

First, GPM offers significant resource-related advantages for social work practice. Compared with all of the other EBTs for BPD, GPM involves the least training time, the lowest training costs, and the fewest number of weekly clinical resource hours (Choi-Kain et al. 2016). This makes GPM ideally suited for the community-based settings in which many social workers traditionally practice, where time and resources are often in short supply.

Second, GPM's decreased intensity is highly consistent with social work's emphasis on client self-determination and autonomy (National Association of Social Workers 2017). Rather than automatically assume that all clients with BPD require highly intensive, dependency-inducing treatments, GPM holds that many clients can obtain substantial functional improvements from less-intensive support. This approach is justified by research suggesting that many clients with BPD experience symptom remission even without any treatment (Gunderson et al. 2011; Zanarini et al. 2010).

Third, GPM's generalist model is particularly well suited for the heterogeneous nature of the social work profession. Because all other EBTs for BPD are primarily psychotherapeutic, they are useful primarily for social workers providing psychotherapy. In contrast, GPM's generalist model—accessible, pragmatic, and framed primarily in terms of broad principles of care—is flexible enough to be tailored to the diverse roles that social workers occupy, including the substance abuse counselor working in a partial hospitalization program, the emergency department clinician (Hong 2016), the individual therapist in private practice, the clinical case manager working with veterans, and so on.

Furthermore, GPM's explicit focus on case management, a signature feature that distinguishes it from other EBTs for BPD, makes it uniquely hospitable to the social work profession. As discussed in this chapter, GPM involves a sensitive integration of psychotherapeutic and case management principles, situated within a case management framework. Given the foundational importance of case management in social work (National Association of Social Workers 2006), there is good reason to embrace an EBT for BPD that allows social workers to comfortably utilize the range of interventions central to the profession. In addition to serving as a first-line treatment for BPD, GPM could also serve as a "meta-frame" for the clinical care of BPD in social work. If a client could benefit from therapeutic interventions found in another EBT for BPD (e.g., mindfulness skills in DBT, MBT's model of mentalizing polarities), rather than completely adopt that model and abandon the client's case management needs, the social worker could simply add those interventions to supplement the "psychotherapeutic strategies" listed earlier in Table 7–2. In this way, social workers could feel free to tailor their psychotherapeutic interventions to address the unique needs of their clients without sacrificing the case management focus on strengthening client autonomy and improving psychosocial functioning.

Finally, more so than any of the psychotherapeutically oriented EBTs for BPD, GPM helps to fulfill social work's explicitly stated mandate to promote "continued development of the evidence base for social work case management" (National Association of Social Workers 2013, p. 8). Although many of the EBTs for BPD contain case management components (Bateman and Fonagy 2016; Linehan 1993), case management is rarely seen as a central therapeutic ingredient in the effectiveness of these models. However, the equivalent efficacy of GPM and DBT (McMain et al. 2009), as well as the comparable utility of "standard" DBT and DBT skills groups with case management (Linehan et al. 2015), raises this interesting question: To what extent does the these treatments' efficacy derive from the psychotherapeutic strategies that receive the most attention in the EBT literature versus the case management strategies often operating "behind the scenes" in these treatments. As Choi-Kain et al. (2016) argue, "Case management remains an understudied but important clinical approach that might do more to help BPD patients' functioning than any manualized psychotherapy alone" (p. 353). Given social work's status "as a leader within the field of case management" (National Association of Social Workers 2013, p. 8), this perspective opens up the door for the important role that social workers might play in the evidence-based clinical care of clients with BPD. GPM offers social workers an effective, accessible, and commonsense framework to organize and direct these efforts.

References

Arntz A, Weertman A, Salet S: Interpretation bias in cluster-C and borderline personality disorders. Behav Res Ther 49(8):472–481, 2011 21621746

Barth RP, Lee BR, Lindsey MA, et al: Evidence-based practice at a crossroads: the timely emergence of common elements and common factors. Res Soc Work Pract 22(1):108–119, 2012

Bateman A, Fonagy P: Mentalization-Based Treatment for Personality Disorders: A Practical Guide. New York, Oxford University Press, 2016

Bertram RM, Charnin LA, Kerns SE, et al: Evidence-based practices in North American MSW curricula. Res Soc Work Pract 25(6):737–748, 2015

Bledsoe-Mansori SE, Bellamy JL, et al: Agency-university partnerships for evidence-based practice: a national survey of schools of social work. Soc Work Res 37(1):179–193, 2013

Carmel A, Rose ML, Fruzzetti AE: Barriers and solutions to implementing dialectical behavior therapy in a public behavioral health system. Adm Policy Ment Health 41(5):608–614, 2014 23754686

Chapman AL, Turner BJ, Dixon-Gordon KL: To integrate or not to integrate dialectical behaviour therapy with other therapy approaches? Clin Soc Work J 39(2):170–179, 2011

Choi-Kain LW, Albert EB, Gunderson JG: Evidence-based treatments for borderline personality disorder: implementation, integration, and stepped care. Harv Rev Psychiatry 24(5):342–356, 2016 27603742

Corcoran J, Walsh J: Clinical Assessment and Diagnosis in Social Work Practice, 3rd Edition. New York, Oxford University Press, 2016

Frankel AJ, Gelman SR: Case Management: An Introduction to Concepts and Skills, 3rd Edition. New York, Oxford University Press, 2016

Grant BF, Chou SP, Goldstein RB, et al: Prevalence, correlates, disability, and comorbidity of DSM-IV borderline personality disorder: results from the Wave 2 National Epidemiologic Survey on Alcohol and Related Conditions. J Clin Psychiatry 69(4):533–545, 2008 18426259

Gunderson JG: Borderline Personality Disorder: A Clinical Guide. Washington, DC, American Psychiatric Publishing, 2001

Gunderson JG, Links PS: Borderline Personality Disorder: A Clinical Guide, 2nd Edition. Washington, DC, American Psychiatric Publishing, 2008

Gunderson JG, Links PS: Handbook of Good Psychiatric Management for Borderline Personality Disorder. Washington, DC, American Psychiatric Publishing, 2014

Gunderson JG, Lyons-Ruth K: BPD's interpersonal hypersensitivity phenotype: a gene-environment-developmental model. J Pers Disord 22(1):22–41, 2008 18312121

Gunderson JG, Stout RL, McGlashan TH, et al: Ten-year course of borderline personality disorder: psychopathology and function from the Collaborative Longitudinal Personality Disorders Study. Arch Gen Psychiatry 68(8):827–837, 2011 21464343

Hamilton G: Theory and Practice of Social Case Work, Revised Edition. New York, Columbia University Press, 1951

Hepworth DH, Rooney RH, Rooney GD, et al: Direct Social Work Practice: Theory and Skills. Boston, MA, Cengage Learning, 2017

Hohman M: Motivational Interviewing in Social Work Practice. New York, Guilford, 2012

Hong V: Borderline personality disorder in the emergency department: good psychiatric management. Harv Rev Psychiatry 24(5):357–366, 2016 27603743

Howard MO, McMillen CJ, Pollio DE: Teaching evidence-based practice: toward a new paradigm for social work education. Res Soc Work Pract 13(2):234–259, 2003

International Federation of Social Workers: Global Definition of Social Work. Rheinfelden, Switzerland, International Federation of Social Workers, July 2014. Available at: http://ifsw.org/get-involved/global-definition-of-social-work/. Accessed July 24, 2018.

Kanter J: Clinical case management, in Theory and Practice in Clinical Social Work, 2nd Edition. Edited by Brandell JR. Thousand Oaks, CA, Sage, 2011, pp 561–586

Kernberg OF: Borderline Conditions and Pathological Narcissism. New York, Jason Aronson, 1975

Kondrat ME: Person-in-environment, in Encyclopedia of Social Work, 20th Edition. Edited by Mizrahi T, Davis LE. New York, Oxford University Press, 2008, pp 348–354

Koons CR: Dialectical behavior therapy. Soc Work Ment Health 6(1–2):109–132, 2008

Linehan M: Cognitive-Behavioral Treatment of Borderline Personality Disorder. New York, Guilford, 1993

Linehan MM, Korslund KE, Harned MS, et al: Dialectical behavior therapy for high suicide risk in individuals with borderline personality disorder: a randomized clinical trial and component analysis. JAMA Psychiatry 72(5):475–482, 2015 25806661

Lukens EP, McFarlane WR: Psychoeducation as evidence-based practice: considerations for practice, research, and policy, in Foundations of Evidence-Based Social Work Practice. Edited by Edited by Roberts AR, Yeager KR. New York, Oxford University Press, 2006, pp 291–313

McMain SF, Links PS, Gnam WH, et al: A randomized trial of dialectical behavior therapy versus general psychiatric management for borderline personality disorder. Am J Psychiatry 166(12):1365–1374, 2009 19755574

McNeece CA, Thyer BA: Evidence-based practice and social work. J Evidence-Based Soc Work 1(1):7–25, 2004 28879812

National Association of Social Workers: NASW Standards for Clinical Social Work in Social Work Practice. Washington, DC, National Association of Social Workers, 2005

National Association of Social Workers: Assuring the Sufficiency of a Frontline Workforce: A National Study of Licensed Social Workers. Executive Summary. Washington, DC, National Association of Social Workers, 2006

National Association of Social Workers: Code of Ethics of the National Association of Social Workers. Washington, DC, National Association of Social Workers, 2017

National Association of Social Workers: NASW Standards for Social Work Case Management. Washington, DC, National Association of Social Workers, 2013

Panos PT, Jackson JW, Hasan O, et al: Meta-analysis and systematic review assessing the efficacy of dialectical behavior therapy (DBT). Res Soc Work Pract 24(2):213–223, 2013

Rubin A: Teaching EBP in social work: retrospective and prospective. Journal of Social Work 11(1):64–79, 2011

Rubin A, Parrish D: Views of evidence-based practice among faculty in master of social work programs: a national survey. Res Soc Work Pract 17(1):110–122, 2007

Saleebey D: The Strengths Perspective in Social Work Practice, 6th Edition. Boston, MA, Pearson, 2013

Sansone RA, Sansone LA: Responses of mental health clinicians to patients with borderline personality disorder. Innov Clin Neurosci 10(5–6):39–43, 2013 23882440

Schulz SC, Rafferty MP: Combined medication and dialectical behavior therapy for borderline personality disorder. Soc Work Ment Health 6(1–2):133–144, 2008

Swales MA: Implementing dialectical behaviour therapy: organizational pre-treatment. Cogn Behav Ther 3(4):145–157, 2010

Turner FJ: Psychosocial Therapy: A Social Work Perspective. New York, The Free Press, 1978

Walsh J: Psychoeducation, in Encyclopedia of Social Work, 20th Edition. Edited by Mizrahi T, Davis LE. New York, Oxford University Press, 2008, pp 453–456

Walsh J, Manuel J: Clinical case management, in Social Worker's Desk Reference, 3rd Edition. Edited by Corcoran K, Roberts AR. New York, Oxford University Press, 2015, pp 820–824

Washburn M, Rubin A, Zhou S: Benchmarks for outpatient dialectical behavioral therapy in adults with borderline personality disorder. Res Soc Work Pract 1–12, 2016, doi.org/10.1177/1049731516659363

Woods ME, Hollis F: Casework: A Psychosocial Therapy, 5th Edition. Boston, MA, McGraw-Hill, 2000

Zanarini MC, Vujanovic AA, Parachini EA, et al: Zanarini Rating Scale for Borderline Personality Disorder (ZAN-BPD): a continuous measure of DSM-IV borderline psychopathology. J Pers Disord 17(3):233–242, 2003 12839102

Zanarini MC, Frankenburg FR, Reich DB, et al: The 10-year course of physically self-destructive acts reported by borderline patients and Axis II comparison subjects. Acta Psychiatr Scand 117(3):177–184, 2008 18241308

Zanarini MC, Frankenburg FR, Reich DB, et al: Time to attainment of recovery from borderline personality disorder and stability of recovery: a 10-year prospective follow-up study. Am J Psychiatry 167(6):663–667, 2010 20395399

Chapter 8

Primary Care Providers

Karen A. Adler, M.D.

Ellen F. Finch, B.A.

Ana M. Rodriguez-Villa, M.D., M.B.A.

Lois W. Choi-Kain, M.D., M.Ed.

Primary care providers (PCPs) are likely to see at least one patient with borderline personality disorder (BPD) in every 16 visits on their daily schedule (Gross et al. 2002). Although patients with BPD do not typically come to primary care settings seeking long-term psychiatric care, they do present with general medical complaints to their PCP, just like any other patient. What distinguishes them is that their primary medical care is complicated by the interpersonal sensitivity and reactivity symptomatic of their personality disorder. The co-occurrence of BPD with medical problems makes for a formidable challenge for PCPs in their time-pressured care management. Nonadherence with usual treatment recommendations further complicates treatment of these patients. Often, neither the patient nor the PCP feels comfortable with the care provided or the interaction around it. Commonly, the patient feels his or her needs are not met, and the PCP finds that administering the standard care of good medical practice is difficult at best or futile at worst.

In practice, individuals with BPD interface with their PCP frequently for treatment of usual and sometimes preventable medical complaints. Problems related to BPD influence not only patients' interactions with their PCP but also their specific health issues and high utilization of health care (Ansell et al. 2007). Research demonstrates that patients with active BPD are more likely to suffer from obesity, diabetes mellitus, osteoarthritis, and urinary incontinence than are patients who have remitted from BPD (Keuroghlian et al. 2013). This increase is due in part to prolonged exposure to the side effects of medications, such as atypical antipsychotics, that are known to impact weight and metabolism. Patients with BPD are also found to have poorer health habits, which include higher rates of smoking and drinking alcohol, as well as less frequent exercise. Lastly, functional and pain disorders such as fibromyalgia, temporomandibular joint disorders, low back pain (Frankenburg and Zanarini 2004; Sansone and Sansone 2004), and migraine headaches (Sansone and Sansone 2004) are also more prevalent in patients with BPD than in those without.

Given these elevated rates of obesity and its related medical sequelae, poor self-care, and high rates of complex pain syndromes, patients with BPD are prone to feel that they need medications and subsequently use medications in more problematic ways. They are characterized by elevated rates of polypharmacy (Sansone and Sansone 2004), sustained use of prescribed opioid analgesics (Frankenburg et al. 2014), and daily use of sleep aids (Frankenburg and Zanarini 2004; Plante et al. 2009). Nearly one-third of patients with BPD acknowledge misusing medications that have been prescribed to them (Sansone and Sansone 2004). The high rates of prescription opioid use as well as the high prevalence of pain syndromes may relate to a general central nervous system hypersensitivity to physical and emotional pain as well as abnormalities in endogenous opiate neurotransmission in BPD (Frankenburg et al. 2014).

Alone, these health issues are easily identified and addressed by the clinician. However, the patient's concurrent interpersonal reactivity often overshadows his or her chief medical complaint. Inherent to BPD is sensitivity to caregiving and perceived neglect, best understood within the framework of interpersonal hypersensitivity (see Appendix C, "Interpersonal Coherence Model"). Interpersonal hypersensitivity is a core feature of BPD. It is activated in situations where there is an expectation of caregiving. The desire of the patient with BPD to feel fully cared for, understood, and "taken seriously" is often at odds with the focus on efficiency in current practice settings, where managed care dictates that PCPs manage symptoms conservatively, avoiding high-cost, invasive, and unnecessary procedures. Patients with BPD feel reassured by visible acts of care, which may lead PCPs to engage in unsustainable or excessive measures. These PCP responses often function to rescue patients with BPD from some sort of perceived threat around which they feel helpless. In medicine, reactionary responses to a patient's bids for urgent or extensive medical attention can result in recurrent high-cost interventions that do not ultimately resolve the patient's complaints and instead lead the patient in and out of the hospital and its services.

This trajectory of medical care and services will sound familiar to the PCP. PCPs can predict that patients with BPD will at times experience their health care encounters to be too brief or impersonal. When this happens, patients are likely to become reactive and may push boundaries or make demands that challenge practice standards. Common challenges include appeals to extend appointment times or attempts to contact the provider by phone or electronic means in between or in lieu of office visits (Sansone and Sansone 2004). Patients may cancel scheduled appointments and follow up with demands for urgent accommodation. Angry outbursts when demands are not met are common. Other ways in which patients engage the PCP outside the standard of a professional relationship include overly personal questions, hugs, gifts, or pleas for the PCP to manage all their health care needs rather than accepting appropriate referrals. The PCP will find that the BPD patient's confidence that he or she is being cared for and taken seriously fluctuates, and interactions with the PCP and the clinic staff may be characterized by oscillations between the poles of idealizing the primary care staff and deriding them for negligence or for not truly understanding the severity of his or her problems.

Considering these dynamics that are prototypical to the patient with BPD and his or her caregiver, it is not surprising that these patients' health care utilization patterns are distinct and inefficient. Of course, these tendencies further complicate the patient-provider relationship. Patients with BPD utilize more high-cost medical services, such as emergency department evaluations and expensive imaging studies (Keuroghlian et al. 2013). This pattern reflects two of the disorder's defining characteristics: high reactivity to stressors and poor tolerance of distress. It fuels the BPD patient's pursuit of "quick fixes" for problems.

Patients with BPD have difficulty sustaining effort toward longer-term goals. In a psychiatric setting, these goals may be sobriety, maintaining employment, or avoiding hospitalization. In a primary care setting, common goals are maintaining preventive care or making use of pain management strategies, such as physical therapy, that are lower risk but require sustained effort. It is common for patients with BPD to interpret a lack of immediate and tangible symptom reduction as evidence that a treatment plan is not working and subsequently abandon the long-term treatment plan. This dynamic between clinician and patient, as well as between legitimate medical needs and the BPD symptoms that cloud them, understandably confuses or frustrates PCPs. It is a dynamic that can be managed effectively and, when addressed, benefits both parties.

Given the frequency with which patients with BPD present in primary care settings and the difficulty that their symptoms pose, it is critical that PCPs be able to recognize BPD as part of the diagnostic picture. This capability will enable them to manage the way BPD symptoms influence the care interaction in the primary care setting. Good psychiatric management (GPM), an evidence-based (McMain et al. 2009), generalist approach to treating BPD, serves as an ideal foundation for developing guidelines for treating BPD in the primary care setting. Like much of modern evidence-based medicine, GPM is founded on up-to-date medical knowledge about the etiology, neurobiology, course, and treatment responsiveness of BPD. Because it can be adapted to psychiatric settings of brief or longitudinal nature, we believe it can also be adapted to the nonpsychiatric professional when distilled to consider the types of problems PCPs in particular face in providing care for patients with BPD.

This chapter outlines six GPM-based guidelines for providers to follow when working with BPD patients in a primary care setting. These strategies are not a focused treatment for BPD itself. If a patient with BPD desires more intensive care for psychiatric symptoms and hopes for psychological change—or if medically dangerous self-harm or suicidality does not attenuate—referral to psychiatric care is needed. Rather, the strategies outlined here help PCPs maintain standard practices while managing the unique challenges introduced by their patients with BPD.

GPM Tips for the Primary Care Provider

To help PCPs manage encounters with their patients with BPD, we discuss six guidelines adapted from GPM. Summarized in Table 8–1, these guide-

---

TABLE 8–1.   Good psychiatric management guidelines for primary care providers

---

1. Frame clinical problems with consideration of the borderline personality disorder diagnosis.
2. Validate the patient's subjective distress.
3. Tolerate anger empathetically but do not give in to demands.
4. Maintain standards of good care.
5. Prescribe conservatively.
6. Respond to self-harm or suicidal statements with concern and assessment of risk.

---

lines, which organize and structure the prototypical oscillations in the treatment relationship, instruct GPM-informed PCPs to 1) frame clinical problems with consideration of the borderline personality diagnosis; 2) validate the patient's subjective distress; 3) tolerate anger empathetically but do not give in to demands; 4) maintain standards of good care; 5) prescribe conservatively; and 6) respond to self-harm and suicidal statements with concern and assessment of risk.

Frame Clinical Problems With Consideration of the Borderline Personality Disorder Diagnosis

Many PCPs may fear that disclosing the diagnosis of BPD will upset the patient or disrupt the patient-doctor relationship. Even psychiatrists frequently defer the BPD diagnosis to focus on an issue that appears more feasible to treat by prescribing medications. Research demonstrates, however, that BPD in and of itself renders common psychiatric disorders such as depression more treatment resistant until the BPD is addressed (Skodol et al. 2011). Prompt diagnostic disclosure is the standard for good medical care in general. When PCPs suspect BPD, they should share their diagnostic impression with the patient, as they would if they suspected depression, anxiety disorder, substance use disorder, or any other medical problem. With diagnosis, the PCP informs the direction of care and promotes accurate communication with the patient. Diagnosis medicalizes the disorder for both patient and treater, highlighting the treatable nature of presenting symptoms as opposed to perpetuating their understanding as character flaws of the patient or failures of the treatment staff. For example, hostility and impulsivity are symptoms of BPD; when perceived as flaws in the patient's character, both patient and provider develop suspicion, sensitivity, and poor communication in their exchanges. Practitioners should expect that in the context of their diagnosis, a patient with BPD may be predictably hypersensitive toward any caregiver, including medical providers. Sharing the diagnosis of BPD and providing basic education about its symptoms can reduce impulsivity and interpersonal instability (Zanarini and Frankenburg 2008). Nondisclosure of the BPD diagnosis can increase the risk of iatrogenic harm (e.g., polypharmacy) and prevent the patient from receiving appropriate treatment (Chanen and McCutcheon 2013).

Owing to stigma around the disorder, some clinicians may find sharing the diagnosis of BPD challenging. We recommend that clinicians use DSM-5 (American Psychiatric Association 2013) to walk the patient through the criteria and explain the diagnosis (see Chapter 2, Figure 2–1; see also American Psychiatric Association 2014). Often, patients feel relief when they discover that their struggles are explained by a coherent diagnosis. It suggests that other people share these same problems, thereby normalizing them. The GPM model of interpersonal hypersensitivity (see Appendix C) also provides a framework around which the patient can develop insight into his or her often-problematic behavioral patterns. Armed with the knowledge of the BPD diagnosis and ways it can affect caregiver relationships, the PCP and patient can predict in a nonpejorative and clinical manner how this diagnosis may affect their relationship going forward.

Validate the Patient's Subjective Distress

Validation has become a buzzword in the mental health community. The core task of validation is understanding the patient's experience, no matter how pathological or symptomatic it is, especially regarding how it might make the patient feel. Then, the key is to communicate that it makes sense that the patient would think or act in specific ways related to the stress and emotions involved. This is distinct from communicating either agreement or disagreement. Importantly, validating an emotional response does not mean the provider is agreeing to change medical decision making or office policies to alleviate the patient's distress. In fact, validation can mitigate the need to take action to prove understanding of the patient's distress.

The PCP can acknowledge the patient's experience with a statement that shows an understanding of what the patient with BPD is trying to communicate (e.g., "It sounds like you are in a lot of pain" or "I can tell that this is something you want to have taken care of as soon as possible"). Validation allows the patient to feel comfortably connected once again, decreasing limbic system activation and allowing prefrontal cortex–driven decision making to reemerge. For this reason, it is helpful to validate the patient's emotions prior to using logic or justifications for policies and decisions. Until the emotional reaction has subsided, such communication cannot be processed and typically leads to further escalation by the patient in an attempt to have his or her perspective heard.

Tolerate Anger Empathetically but Do Not Give in to Demands

Although validation is important, it is equally important to neither condone nor reinforce behaviors considered inappropriate or unsafe in the office (e.g., screaming, throwing things, mistreating office staff, making demands outside standard of care). Practitioners following GPM should maintain a calm presence and outward nonreactivity during such events and explain that these behaviors make it difficult to provide patients with the help they seek. Given that patients with BPD have a low tolerance for emotional or physical distress, they may become pleading or even hostile if treatment recommendations do not appear to offer immediate relief of pain or distress. The PCP should hold the patient accountable for his or her actions and should not tolerate behaviors that would be unacceptable from any other patient.

Maintain Standards of Good Care

When the patient with BPD makes bids for more or different care than the standards offered, PCPs may be tempted to bend the rules and usual course of care. The most effective long-term care is provided when the PCP maintains the same standards of care for the patient with BPD as for any other patient. The following are guidelines to help maintain standards and limits:

1. *Set limits and observe them.* Share your own limits, standards, and policies in a way that takes ownership of them rather than implies that the patient is asking for something unreasonable. Acknowledging the difference in perspectives while calmly enforcing the standard policies and practices is generally both necessary and sufficient. Although it may solve the immediate problem to "bend the rules" and agree to a request that is outside the norm of your setting, doing so will likely perpetuate the patient's emotional outbursts and demands for special treatment.

2. *Schedule frequent visits that are brief and consistent.* Predictable visits help the patient with BPD feel cared for without compromising office policies and standards. Knowing that there is a set routine will help your patient accept limits you set on intersession contact and show that you are invested in their care.

3. *At each appointment, prioritize the most urgent medical issue.* Patients may have a constellation of symptoms and complaints that seem impossible to address at once. Help the patient to prioritize what is the greatest problem for him and address that issue as a team. This approach is not unique in a primary care setting but is of heightened importance for the patient with BPD who is prone to dysregulation and disorganization when confronted with a medical or psychological stressor.

4. *Set goals to accomplish between appointments.* At each appointment, work with the patient to set small, achievable tasks that he or she should accomplish before the next appointment (e.g., seeing a specialist for an injury). Hold the patient accountable for what he or she says he or she will do. This may include making lifestyle changes that the patient has struggled to make in the past because the patient finds the magnitude of these changes overwhelming, the ultimate reward too abstract, or the timeline too long. These goals should be small, measurable, and attainable within the time provided. Help the patient to track progress in a way that holds him or her accountable, and do not let your patient off the hook.

5. *Communicate proactively with other medical professionals.* When making referrals for patients with BPD, PCPs can proactively contact the specialist consultant to provide background information, answers to specific consultation questions, and directives. This is standard procedure for PCPs, but the time pressures of current-day medical practice make it difficult to do this for any patients, regardless of whether they have BPD. Although more work for the PCP in the short term, this communication aims to ensure that all the efforts by the PCP, patient, and specialist help the patient reach goals in the long term. This added effort by the GPM-informed PCP to proactively enact a systematic, organized, and responsive treatment plan can actually save time in the long term by avoiding reactive, haphazard, and overly complicated courses of treatment.

Prescribe Conservatively

Any medication should be prescribed cautiously, because no medication has been found to be uniformly or dramatically helpful for the treatment of BPD and none have been approved by the U.S. Food and Drug Administration for this purpose (American Psychiatric Association Practice Guidelines 2001; Ingenhoven 2015; Ingenhoven et al. 2010). Polypharmacy is common in patients with BPD and should be avoided because it increases the risk for side effects and promotes dependency. Importantly, benzodiazepines are generally contraindicated; they can worsen BPD symptoms and increase disinhibition.

Respond to Self-Harm or Suicidal Statements With Concern and Assessment of Risk

Consider self-harming behavior and suicidal statements to be predictable symptoms of BPD. Keep in mind that these symptoms are often a communication of distress, most likely as a result of interpersonal stressors (see Appendix C). The patient may be trying to demonstrate the magnitude of his or her distress, express dissatisfaction with care, or pressure the provider to grant requests. Respond to these communications by validating pain or distress, showing concern, evaluating risk and medical dangerousness (e.g., previous suicide attempts, lethality of plan, access to means), and referring the patient to a mental health provider or emergency care if needed.

Case Vignette

The following case description includes decision points, each of which has several alternative responses listed at the end of the case. The reader will rate each alternative response in terms of its level of helpfulness. Discussions of responses follow.

> Crystal is a 32-year-old single woman with a medical history of chronic, severe migraine headaches, frequent bronchial infections, and irritable bowel syndrome. Her health habits are notable for daily tobacco use; she smokes one or two packs per day. She also reports frequent anxiety and trouble sleeping due to her "stress level." She recently disclosed to you that when she is particularly "stressed" by arguments with her boyfriend or "being singled out and yelled at" by her supervisor at work, she will sometimes cut her arm superficially or binge on sugary foods in an effort to manage her feelings.
>
> During the initial visit, you spent significant time counseling Crystal about lifestyle modifications such as smoking cessation, relaxation training, and sleep hygiene. In addition, you provided referrals to a neurologist for her migraines and to wellness groups for stress management and smok-

ing cessation. She appeared earnest and attentive and thanked you for being so helpful and for taking her seriously.

At the follow-up visit, you learn that Crystal has not followed through with any lifestyle changes or referrals. [**Decision Point 1**] She is apologetic but cites problems outside of her control, implores you not to "get mad" or "drop her as a patient," and requests medications to help with pain, sleep, and anxiety. [**Decision Point 2**]

With your guidance, Crystal is able to identify that her top priority is improving her sleep because her poor sleep seems to lead to both migraines and worsened mood and anxiety. You give her a written handout with principles of sleep hygiene and help her identify three specific changes she will make before the next visit. Together, you identify and problem-solve barriers to those changes. She agrees to defer management of her migraine headaches to the neurologist. She is engaged and appears calm. Your scheduler knocks on the door to tell you that the next available appointment with neurology is in 8 weeks. Crystal suddenly becomes acutely distressed, tears come to her eyes, and she tells you, "I'm sorry but I can't do this. It's too much. I'm not going to be here in 8 weeks."[**Decision Point 3**]

You are able to empathetically reflect Crystal's feelings: "It sounds like it's going to be really hard for you to wait that long to get some help with your headaches." Crystal stops crying and speaks more calmly. You perform a brief risk assessment and are reassured that she is safe and can remain safe. Then you work on formulating a plan for how she might tolerate the wait time for the neurology appointment. [**Decision Point 4**]

By the end of the visit, Crystal agrees to follow the plan to modify her sleep hygiene and manage her head pain with over-the-counter analgesics as directed before returning to see you in 2–3 weeks for follow-up. She appears calm but somewhat disappointed. As you are walking out of the exam room, she asks you what she should do if she needs to see you before the next appointment. [**Decision Point 5**]

Decision Points: Alternative Responses

Rate each response in terms of its level of helpfulness with a rating of 1 (will be helpful), 2 (possibly helpful, continuing reservations), or 3 (not helpful—or even harmful).

1. In response to Crystal's disclosure that she did not follow up on lifestyle modifications and referrals, you should

   A. Validate how difficult it is to make changes while clearly stating that nothing will improve without significant effort on her part.
   B. Tell her you can see that giving her so many tasks was overwhelming and offer for you or your staff to set up appointments with specialists on her behalf.

C. Tell her that until she has attended the specialist appointments and put the lifestyle modifications into practice, there is nothing to be done and she should not come back to see you until she has completed these tasks.

D. Work with her to identify the problem that is bothering her the most (e.g., migraine headaches, insomnia, anxiety) and then work on a detailed plan of how to tackle that problem, setting clear, concrete, small goals for the next appointment.

2. In response to Crystal's request for multiple medications, you should

A. Agree to prescribe a short-term supply of tramadol for migraines, zolpidem for sleep, and lorazepam for anxiety.

B. Agree to prescribe medications but avoid narcotics and benzodiazepines (e.g., consider a triptan for migraines and hydroxyzine for sleep and anxiety).

C. Provide Crystal with education on the risks of using multiple potentially habit-forming medications given her BPD diagnosis.

D. Ask Crystal about her substance use history.

3. How should you interpret Crystal's sudden statement that she will not "be here" in 8 weeks?

A. She is suicidal and needs to be hospitalized.

B. She is not suicidal but is intentionally manipulating you to feel fear and sympathy so that you will prescribe narcotics for her.

C. She has poor distress tolerance, and she has become scared and dysregulated upon getting the information that she has to wait 2 months to have her migraines assessed and treated. You need to validate her distress and calm her emotions before conducting a risk assessment and formulating a plan.

D. She is not suicidal but is communicating that her pain is too severe to wait months for an appointment with a specialist. Therefore, you should reassess your willingness to manage her symptoms in the interim.

4. How do you proceed with the medical management of Crystal's headaches?

A. Extend the appointment so you can take a more complete headache history, confirm the migraine diagnosis, and determine whether it is appropriate to prescribe an abortive agent such as a triptan.

B. Normalize Crystal's feelings by sharing that most patients are frustrated by the long wait times to see specialists but also share that 8 weeks is a typical wait time.

C. Redirect Crystal to the goals you set up for the visit and the tasks to be worked on between visits. Ask her to schedule a follow-up appointment with you in 2–3 weeks, at which time you will focus on management of headaches.

D. Explain to Crystal how to use over-the-counter analgesics (e.g., acetaminophen and ibuprofen) to manage head pain until your follow-up appointment.

5. How do you respond to Crystal's question about needing access to care prior to the next scheduled appointment?

A. Tell her that she can call for a same-day appointment or use urgent care or the emergency department if anything happens that cannot wait until the next scheduled appointment.

B. Tell her that none of her complaints warrant such frequent care and she needs to be able to wait a few weeks between visits.

C. Instruct her to use the nurse call-in line or patient portal to communicate with you if she has concerns, and advise her that you or one of the nurses will let her know if she needs to come in sooner than planned.

Decision Points: Discussion

Numbers within brackets indicate level of helpfulness ratings.

1. In response to Crystal's disclosure that she did not follow up on lifestyle modifications and referrals, you should

A. Validate how difficult it is to make changes while clearly stating that nothing will improve without significant effort on her part. [1] (Using empathy at the start decreases defensiveness and allows for more effective interventions. It is very important not to let the patient off the hook, which reinforces helplessness and is not change oriented. A main tenet of GPM is to make patients aware of their responsibility in their own care and recovery.)

B. Tell her you can see that giving her so many tasks was overwhelming and offer for you or your staff to set up appointments with specialists on her behalf. [2] (It is likely true and worth acknowledging that the number of action items and referrals the patient was tasked with generated overwhelming anxiety. Offering to have staff schedule appointments on her behalf could be helpful and might be appropriate if this is standard practice in your office. If it is not in your practice's general standard of care and would constitute bending the rules or create an undue burden on your staff, this action is best avoided.)

C. Tell her that until she has attended the specialist appointments and put the lifestyle modifications into practice, there is nothing to be done and she should not come back to see you until she has completed these tasks. [3] (This is not helpful in creating a working alliance and will not motivate a patient with BPD to rise to the challenge, especially given the number and scope of assigned tasks. She will more likely drop out of your care and seek care in higher-cost venues [e.g., emergency department].)

D. Work with her to identify the problem that is bothering her the most (e.g., migraine headaches, insomnia, anxiety) and then work on a detailed plan of how to tackle that problem, setting clear, concrete, small goals for the next appointment. [1] (This is the recommended strategy for making visits with patients with BPD manageable for both you and the patient.)

2. In response to Crystal's request for multiple medications, you should

A. Agree to prescribe a short-term supply of tramadol for migraines, zolpidem for sleep, and lorazepam for anxiety. [3] (Patients with BPD are at high risk of prolonged use of narcotics and misuse of prescription medications. In addition, benzodiazepines are not recommended for patients with BPD because these medications can worsen disinhibition. Finally, treatment plans should not be made based on the level of distress or demand expressed by the patient with BPD. These responses by practitioners lead to escalation of demands and risk for poor outcomes and dangerous prescribing patterns.)

B. Agree to prescribe medications but avoid narcotics and benzodiazepines (e.g., consider a triptan for migraines and hydroxyzine for sleep and anxiety). [2] (This is a more conservative approach than option A and may be appropriate, but it still runs the risk of establishing a pattern in which the patient's distress is appeased by action, specifically prescriptions. It may ultimately lead to more pressure placed on you for a quick fix and diminish her efforts to change poor health habits.)

C. Provide Crystal with education on the risks of using multiple potentially habit-forming medications given her BPD diagnosis. [1] (This is an important piece of patient education that can be delivered in the context of her BPD-related symptoms.)

D. Ask Crystal about her substance use history. [2] (Substance use history is an important component of patient history and should not be avoided in patients with BPD. However, in this vignette, the timing of the question might produce an angry, defensive response that will not yield useful information. Her complaints can be adequately addressed with a continued focus on lifestyle modifications and/or conservative prescribing of noncontrolled substances.)

3. How should you interpret Crystal's sudden statement that she will not "be here" in 8 weeks?

A. She is suicidal and needs to be hospitalized. [3] (Reflexive hospitalization of patients with BPD who make vague suicidal statements should be avoided. It is typically unnecessary, interferes with the ability of the patient to engage in meaningful work and life activities, and is costly to the health care system.)

B. She is not suicidal but is intentionally manipulating you to feel fear and sympathy so that you will prescribe narcotics for her. [2] (Although this might be true and you certainly may feel manipulated and scared, most patients with BPD are not doing this intentionally. They are instead trying to convey their level of desperation regarding their poor ability to manage their own distress. Holding this attitude may lead the PCP to an unproductive level of irritation toward the patient with BPD and does not facilitate the goals of the PCP.)

C. She has poor distress tolerance, and she has become scared and dysregulated upon getting the information that she has to wait 2 months to have her migraines assessed and treated. You need to validate her distress and calm her emotions before conducting a risk assessment and formulating a plan. [1] (A key principle of GPM is to understand and validate the emotions associated with statements about suicide/safety; therefore, the PCP should conduct a risk assessment and formulate a plan based on level of medical risk. Note that this clinical response does not make any assumptions about Crystal's level of suicidality prior to following the steps outlined here.)

D. She is not suicidal but is communicating that her pain is too severe to wait months for an appointment with a specialist. Therefore, you should reassess your willingness to manage her symptoms in the interim. [3] (The first part of the statement may be true, and it is appropriate for you as the PCP to treat the headaches until neurology can assume management. However, you should not modify your treatment plan on the basis of the BPD patient's expression of subjective distress or threats of suicide. Over time, if the PCP modifies the treatment plan because of the patient's expressed distress or suicidal threats, this can reinforce the patient's expression of distress through suicidal statements.)

4. How do you proceed with the medical management of Crystal's headaches?

A. Extend the appointment so you can take a more complete headache history, confirm the migraine diagnosis, and determine whether it is appropriate to prescribe an abortive agent such as a triptan. [3] (Although you may need more time to gather history before prescribing an abortive agent, extending the current appointment is an instance of bending the rules for the patient with BPD based on subjective distress. It is better to schedule a follow-up appointment.)

B. Normalize Crystal's feelings by sharing that most patients are frustrated by the long wait times to see specialists but also share that 8 weeks is a typical wait time. [1] (Validate what is valid but do not bend reality for the patient. It is important to reorient the patient to what is standard care, directly communicating that what is being asked of her is a standard that patients are required to tolerate.)

C. Redirect Crystal to the goals you set up for the visit and the tasks to be worked on between visits. Ask her to schedule a follow-up appointment with you in 2–3 weeks, at which time you will focus on management of headaches. [1] (This response incorporates two key principles of GPM: first, brief, frequent, and consistent appointments with a small, concrete focus for each and, second, tasks for the patient to complete between appointments.)

D. Explain to Crystal how to use over-the-counter analgesics (e.g., acetaminophen and ibuprofen) to manage head pain until your follow-up appointment. [1] (It is appropriate to provide safe pain management to all patients, and there should be time left in the appointment to give the patient concise directions on the use of over-the-counter pain relievers.)

5. How do you respond to Crystal's question about needing access to care prior to the next scheduled appointment?

A. Tell her that she can call for a same-day appointment or use urgent care or the emergency department if anything happens that cannot wait until the next scheduled appointment. [3] (Although such a response may be appropriate with other patients, patients with BPD are at high risk for overusing high-cost medical care, such as urgent care sources and the emergency department, and should not be encouraged to do so unless medically necessary.)

B. Tell her that none of her complaints warrant such frequent care and she needs to be able to wait a few weeks between visits. [2] (This statement might be true and could be effective if delivered with humor or more empathy after knowing the patient for more than two visits. However, in this scenario, it is an unhelpful redirection and will cause the patient to feel angry, rejected, and not taken seriously.)

C. Instruct her to use the nurse call-in line or patient portal to communicate with you if she has concerns, and advise her that you or one of the nurses will let her know if she needs to come in sooner than planned. [1] (This is the preferred response, provided that you have the appropriate resources available. It provides the patient with an appropriate channel for communication of concerns but allows the care team to dictate the next encounter based on knowledge of the medical dangerousness of the symptoms reported rather than permitting the patient to determine the frequency and setting of care based on her level of fear or distress about her symptoms.)

Conclusion

The GPM principles adapted for primary care are not unlike those applied to other psychiatric disorders. They are basic tenets of *good general* psychiatric management. Perhaps they are fundamental to *good general* medical care. Stigma associated with BPD specifically and the dearth of practical training about BPD interfere with consistent, systematic, and optimal care of these patients. GPM principles are designed to help psychiatrists and PCPs alike achieve their usual goal of providing optimal care while also helping patients in the goal of receiving good medical care. Ultimately, providing care for patients with BPD remains challenging for psychiatrists and PCPs, but these basic guidelines can provide a road map in the face of predictable challenges.

References

American Psychiatric Association: Diagnostic and Statistical Manual of Mental Disorders, 5th Edition. Arlington, VA, American Psychiatric Association, 2013

American Psychiatric Association: Handbook of Good Psychiatric Management for Borderline Personality Disorder (video file). Arlington, VA, American Psychiatric Association, 2014. Available at: https://vimeo.com/84897040. Accessed June 15, 2018.

American Psychiatric Association Practice Guidelines: Practice guideline for the treatment of patients with borderline personality disorder. Am J Psychiatry 158 (10 suppl):1–52, 2001 11665545

Ansell EB, Sanislow CA, McGlashan TH, et al: Psychosocial impairment and treatment utilization by patients with borderline personality disorder, other personality disorders, mood and anxiety disorders, and a healthy comparison group. Compr Psychiatry 48(4):329–336, 2007 17560953

Chanen AM, McCutcheon L: Prevention and early intervention for borderline personality disorder: current status and recent evidence. Br J Psychiatry Suppl 202 (s54):s24–s29, 2013 23288497

Frankenburg FR, Zanarini MC: The association between borderline personality disorder and chronic medical illnesses, poor health-related lifestyle choices, and costly forms of health care utilization. J Clin Psychiatry 65(12):1660–1665, 2004 15641871

Frankenburg FR, Fitzmaurice GM, Zanarini MC: The use of prescription opioid medication by patients with borderline personality disorder and Axis II comparison subjects: a 10-year follow-up study. J Clin Psychiatry 75(4):357–361, 2014 24500123

Gross R, Olfson M, Gameroff M, et al: Borderline personality disorder in primary care. Arch Intern Med 162(1):53–60, 2002 11784220

Ingenhoven T: The place of trauma in the treatment of personality disorders. Eur J Psychotraumatol 6, 2015

Ingenhoven T, Lafay P, Rinne T, et al: Effectiveness of pharmacotherapy for severe personality disorders: meta-analyses of randomized controlled trials. J Clin Psychiatry 71(1):14–25, 2010 19778496

Keuroghlian AS, Frankenburg FR, Zanarini MC: The relationship of chronic medical illnesses, poor health-related lifestyle choices, and health care utilization to recovery status in borderline patients over a decade of prospective follow-up. J Psychiatr Res 47(10):1499–1506, 2013 23856083

McMain SF, Links PS, Gnam WH, et al: A randomized trial of dialectical behavior therapy versus general psychiatric management for borderline personality disorder. Am J Psychiatry 166(12):1365–1374, 2009 19755574

Plante DT, Zanarini MC, Frankenburg FR, et al: Sedative-hypnotic use in patients with borderline personality disorder and Axis II comparison subjects. J Pers Disord 23(6):563–571, 2009 20001175

Sansone RA, Sansone LA: Borderline personality: a primary care context. Psychiatry (Edgmont) 1(2):19–27, 2004 21197375

Skodol AE, Grilo CM, Keyes KM, et al: Relationship of personality disorders to the course of major depressive disorder in a nationally representative sample. Am J Psychiatry 168(3):257–264, 2011 21245088

Zanarini MC, Frankenburg FR: A preliminary, randomized trial of psychoeducation for women with borderline personality disorder. J Pers Disord 22(3):284–290, 2008 18540800

Chapter 9

Psychopharmacologists

Deanna Mercer, M.D., FRCPC
Paul S. Links, M.D., M.Sc., FRCPC

The challenges of prescribing medications for people who have borderline personality disorder (BPD) are best summed up by Dr. Kenneth Silk (2011, p. 312):

> It is…not clear when one should medicate (or not medicate) during a crisis and/or an upsurge in dyscontrolled behavior or affect…. [P]atients present with statements about increasing psychological pain (and perhaps suicidal ideation) accompanied by pleas that something must change immediately. These pleas and the obvious pain and distress that the patient is experiencing add further difficulty to the prescribing physician's decision as to whether to prescribe more of the same, to add something, to change prescriptions, to wait out the crisis, or to conjure up an unusual combination of medications that has not been tried before.

TABLE 9–1.   **Good psychiatric management principles for prescribing medications to patients with borderline personality disorder**

- •   Build an alliance
- •   Avoid a dichotomous stance
- •   Select appropriate medications
- •   Address comorbidity

For anyone who has prescribed medications to patients struggling with BPD, this passage will feel eerily familiar. The challenge of prescribing medications to an acutely distressed individual with BPD is compounded by the scarcity of research to provide guidance. Although research clearly supports the benefits of psychotherapy for BPD, the message that psychotherapy is the treatment of choice is not reassuring to an individual who is acutely suffering, cannot access psychotherapy, or has yet to see its expected benefits.

So how do we as psychopharmacologists respond? The research is clear on this point—we prescribe medications frequently, often in combination, even when patients are actively engaged in psychotherapy (Hörz et al. 2010; McMain et al. 2009). However, clinical guidelines of countries such as the United Kingdom (National Institute for Health and Clinical Excellence 2009) and Australia (National Health and Medical Research Council 2012), as well as systematic reviews such as the Cochrane Review (Stoffers et al. 2010), all emphasize that medications do not appear to be effective in reducing the overall severity of BPD, although they are indicated for treatment of co-occurring disorders.

Good psychiatric management (GPM) principles (Table 9–1) provide a map for us to negotiate the difficult task of prescribing medications in the face of intense client distress and limited knowledge of effectiveness of medications, while recognizing that we need to encourage participation in psychotherapy instead of reinforcing the notion that medications are the cure. GPM recommends focusing on building the therapeutic alliance first, recognizing that in the end this may be more therapeutic than the medications prescribed. Only then are medications prescribed in line with what is known about their use in the treatment of BPD.

Build an Alliance

The effort that we put into building a therapeutic alliance with our patients with BPD almost always pays off. When it does not, we can at the

---

TABLE 9–2.   Guidelines for alliance building

Provide psychoeducation.	Describe central role of interpersonal hypersensitivity.
	Clarify adjunctive role of medications.
	Discuss limitations of current knowledge.
Show concerned attention.	Appreciate subjective distress.
	Be available for queries between sessions.
	Respond to negative attitudes with curiosity and reassurance.
Emphasize need for collaboration.	Identify target symptoms for medications.
	Develop a system to monitor effects and potentially adverse side effects of medications.
Be active, not reactive.	If a patient requests medications even if not depressed, offer a selective serotonin reuptake inhibitor.
	If a patient does not want medications but is depressed, encourage their use but do not push.

---

very least say we have tried, and usually our patients will acknowledge our efforts. In the long run, the patient's relationship with the prescriber and the messages about the role of medications in BPD may be more therapeutic than the medication prescribed. The cornerstones of alliance building, as listed in Table 9–2, are psychoeducation, concerned attention, emphasizing the need for collaboration, and being active rather than reactive.

Provide Psychoeducation

Central to building the alliance is psychoeducation about interpersonal hypersensitivity as the core problem in BPD. Patients often report that they have been given other diagnoses and treatments that they did not feel accurately reflected their inner reality, but they were in so much distress that they felt their only option was to accept the treatment offered. The description of *interpersonal hypersensitivity*—intense emotional distress in the face of real and perceived relationship difficulties, including loneliness—captures the essence of the experience of BPD. When we take the time to communicate this understanding of their difficulties, our patients often feel relieved and grateful that someone understands.

Once they feel understood, patients are often more able and willing to accept the next two important messages of psychoeducation: that medications are adjunctive and empirical support for their use is limited.

Show Concerned Attention and Respond to Negative Attitudes With Curiosity and Reassurance

Once we recognize that a patient's problem is interpersonal hypersensitivity, we can then alter our ways of interacting with the patient to address this reality and improve the chances of establishing a strong therapeutic alliance. We begin to show concerned attention by responding with empathy to the patient's subjective reports of distress ("It has to be difficult to be experiencing so much suffering") and by providing practical help, such as offering to be available to answer medication-related questions that arise between appointments.

Through the lens of interpersonal hypersensitivity, negative attitudes toward clinicians ("You see me as a diagnosis," "You are ignoring what I am saying") and toward medication ("I don't want to take meds," "I think I just need to change my attitude and stop being so emotional") are transformed into opportunities to be curious about patients' experiences. When we respond with curiosity rather than rejection or impatience, we model an alternative way for patients to respond to their own and others' negative attitudes.

Emphasize Need for Collaboration

A key element of GPM is helping patients learn to "think first." This is particularly important when it comes to the use of medications. Medications have a small to at most moderate effect for BPD. In the face of an interpersonal event that causes a wave of severe distress, any benefit may be difficult to detect, and the person may discontinue a medication, believing it to be ineffective. Also, sometimes medications that are ineffective, or perhaps even harmful, are continued. Ask questions that help in developing clear goals for medication ("What are the symptoms that you are hoping medication will help with?") and a method to monitor the impact of the medication and potential side effects ("It will be important for us to know for sure whether this medication is helping you over the long term. Would you be willing to record your anger each day on a calendar, and then we can check together to see if this is doing what we hope?"). Thinking first also involves encouraging patients to read about the prescribed medications and to bring up any concerns.

Be Active, Not Reactive

GPM encourages us to be "active, not reactive." This means that we should be thoughtful and balanced in our approach to the prescription of medications. For example, we might still offer a selective serotonin reuptake inhibitor (SSRI) to a patient who is requesting medications but does not seem depressed. SSRIs may have a small benefit for impulsivity and questionable benefit for mood instability and anger (Mercer et al. 2009). They also have a favorable safety and side-effect profile. Offering an SSRI, highlighting the uncertain benefits, and requesting that the patient monitor the effect of the medication ("It will be important for you to monitor the effect of this medication") promote patient curiosity about his or her response to the medication and present an opportunity for the psychiatrist to reinforce the need for participation in psychotherapy ("Although I think this may have some benefit, I am more convinced about the potential benefit from your therapy, so it will be important for you to continue your therapy").

Being thoughtful and balanced in our approach can also be helpful with a patient at the opposite end of the spectrum who appears to be severely depressed but does not want medications. Where we feel medications might be helpful, providing gentle encouragement is indicated: "Given that medications have not seemed particularly helpful in the past, I understand your reluctance to try another medication. At the same time, I do think that medication has the potential to be helpful. If you were to consider trying this medication, it would be important for both of us to monitor the effect of the medication and any side effects."

Avoid a Dichotomous Stance

The balanced approach to medication management reflects the GPM principle of avoiding a dichotomous stance: avoiding the assertion that medications either will or will not be helpful. Instead, a thoughtful approach is advocated: "I am not certain if medications will work. They may be helpful. It is important that we monitor."

Select Appropriate Medications

GPM guidelines regarding selection of medications (Table 9–3) include assessment of relevant case factors, knowledge of what medications can and cannot accomplish, and avoidance of polypharmacy.

TABLE 9–3.   Guidelines for selecting medications

Assess relevant case factors	Consider patient motivation.
	Take into account symptom type and severity.
	Review current medications.
	Assess patient distress—acutely distressed patients need to learn self-soothing and may respond to new medications with a placebo effect.
Know what medications can and cannot accomplish	Know medications' potential helpfulness for decreasing aggression and anger.
	Recognize medications' limited benefit for depressive symptoms and self-harm
Avoid polypharmacy	Taper a medication if the patient fails to respond to it before beginning another.
	Cross-taper if the patient is in severe distress.

Assess Relevant Case Factors

Deciding which medication is best will depend on patient motivation, symptoms to be targeted (reviewed in later section "Pharmacological Management of Borderline Personality Disorder"), symptom severity, and the medications the patient is currently taking. As a general rule, if patient motivation for medications is low, or if there is concern about a patient's ability to take medications regularly, SSRI antidepressants or short-term atypical antipsychotics are safest, whereas the mood stabilizers and tricyclic antidepressants should be avoided. When symptoms are severe or are having a significant impact on function, mood stabilizers and atypical antipsychotics could provide benefit.

Know What Medications Can and Cannot Accomplish

Meta-analyses of medications (Binks et al. 2006; Duggan et al. 2008; Herpertz et al. 2007; Ingenhoven et al. 2010; Lieb et al. 2010; Mercer et al. 2009; Nosè et al. 2006; Vita et al. 2011) suggest that, in general, medications may be helpful for decreasing anger and aggression but have limited benefit for addressing depressive symptoms (although SSRIs and other antidepressants are indicated in the case of a major depressive episode) and self-harm.

Before a medication is prescribed for a patient in severe distress, it is important to communicate that although medications may provide some benefit, the most effective way for the patient to cope with acute distress is to learn self-soothing. Medications may help to some degree, but they are not a substitute for learning how to soothe oneself in the face of a crisis ("I know from what you have told me that you are having a very tough time. I think that this medication may help to some degree. It is important that you know that skills like self-soothing can be even more powerful than medications in helping you to survive difficult interpersonal events.").

Avoid Polypharmacy

Given that national guidelines (National Health and Medical Research Council 2012; National Institute for Health and Clinical Excellence 2009) highlight that current evidence does not support a role for medications in reducing overall severity of BPD, and the high rate of side effects from medications, GPM advocates clearly setting a framework for avoiding polypharmacy. Prior to prescribing, it is useful to establish a policy that if the patient is failing to respond to a medication, that medication will be tapered before another medication is introduced, unless the patient is in severe distress, in which case cross-tapering can occur.

Address Comorbidity

Addressing comorbidities requires discerning and informed prioritization of the comorbid disorder relative to BPD. See Table 9–4 for guidelines.

Pharmacological Management of Borderline Personality Disorder: Recent Developments

Patients with BPD will request and are often given prescriptions for multiple medications, even though the use of medication in the management of BPD is highly controversial. The National Institute for Health and Care Excellence (2015) in the United Kingdom stated that medications are "not to be used" in the management of BPD. These treatment guidelines are known to be stringent and directly contradict those of the American Psychiatric Association (2001), which recommends a symptom-targeted approach to the pharmacological management of patients with BPD. Even in psychosocial randomized controlled trials (RCTs) involving patients

TABLE 9–4.   Guidelines for addressing comorbidity

Action	Consideration	Examples of comorbidity
Prioritize comorbidity when	Comorbidity precludes involvement or active learning.	Mania, disordered substance use, anorexia
Prioritize borderline personality disorder (BPD) when	Comorbidity is unlikely to remit or more likely to recur unless BPD is in remission.[a]	Depression, anxiety, social phobia, remitted bipolar disorder (I, II), bulimia
Stabilize BPD before addressing comorbidity to	Increase patient's ability to tolerate medication for comorbidities (Keuroghlian et al. 2015).	Panic disorder, posttraumatic stress disorder, obsessive-compulsive disorder

[a]This does not preclude trials of medications appropriate for the other conditions.

with BPD that try to set up ideal conditions, patients were still exposed to two different medications on average over the course of treatment (McMain et al. 2009). In spite of the controversy and the need for further research, medication can play a role in the management of symptoms and improvement of functioning in patients with BPD.

In this section of the chapter, recent research evidence supporting the use of medication is reviewed and discussed by drug type. The review also makes mention of some novel approaches that require further research but may open new avenues for managing patients with BPD. The section concludes with a discussion of the limitations of the current research.

Medication Types

Antipsychotic Medication

Major meta-analytic studies and recent reviews from 2009 onward (Hancock-Johnson et al. 2017; Ingenhoven et al. 2010; Lieb et al. 2010; Mercer et al. 2009; Stoffers and Lieb 2015) suggest that antipsychotic medications have a small but statistically significant effect compared with placebo in managing certain symptoms in patients with BPD. Antipsychotic medications seem useful in lessening anger, impulsivity, aggression, and the cognitive perceptual disturbances found in patients with BPD. Many of the second- and third-generation antipsychotics have been used with patients with BPD; however, all of the studies used small samples and were of short duration. The one exception is the study by Zanarini et al. (2011), in which olanzapine was tested versus placebo in a large RCT involving 451 outpatients. In this 12-week study, olanzapine 5–10 mg/day was superior to placebo in lessening symptoms of BPD. During a 12-week open-label extension study, in which both the active and the placebo groups from the previous study were given a 12-week course of open-label olanzapine, placebo participants improved in a fashion similar to that of the active group (Zanarini et al. 2012). Although benefits were evident, the adverse effects of olanzapine were considerable, including somnolence, fatigue, and increased appetite and weight gain. In addition, the Cochrane Review mentioned at the beginning of this chapter (Stoffers et al. 2010) raised a potential concern with olanzapine, finding in two trials that olanzapine had a tendency toward increased suicidal ideation and self-mutilation when compared with placebo; however, two other trials found a decrease in suicidal ideation and one trial found no difference between olanzapine and placebo. This finding is inconsistent but presents a caution worth noting for further study.

Another major study compared quetiapine extended release (ER) 300 mg/day, quetiapine ER 150 mg/day, and placebo in an 8-week RCT involving 95 participants with BPD (Black et al. 2014). A large effect size was found for the low-dose quetiapine ER versus placebo on borderline symptoms (Cohen's $d = -0.79$). The comparison between moderate-dose quetiapine and placebo was not significant, and there were no significant differences between the quetiapine groups. On secondary outcomes, including verbal and physical aggression, both quetiapine doses were superior to placebo. However, side effects were common, particularly with the moderate-dose quetiapine ER. Side effects such as sedation predicted participants' discontinuation of the study. Because this study had fairly stringent exclusion criteria for comorbid disorders, further studies are clearly indicated to generalize the findings to the majority of patients with BPD who present with multiple comorbid disorders.

In summary, antipsychotic medication at low doses appears to have some utility for symptoms of BPD such as anger, impulsive aggression, and the cognitive perceptual features. Owing to risks of sedation and weight gain, as well as a possible increase in suicidal ideation, antipsychotic medications need to be monitored carefully and their risk-benefit ratio reassessed at 3–6 months.

Mood Stabilizers

Mood stabilizers such as lamotrigine had initially shown promise in the treatment of patients with BPD, with effectiveness in small studies for reducing anger, impulsivity, and perhaps also depression (Reich et al. 2009; Tritt et al. 2005). However, a large and well-designed RCT recently conducted by Crawford et al. (2018) failed to show superiority of lamotrigine to placebo, casting doubt on the effectiveness of this class of medications.

Omega-3 fatty acids (eicosapentaenoic acid [EPA] and docosahexaenoic acid [DHA]) have also been evaluated in two studies with patients with BPD and may have modest benefit on mood symptoms, aggression, and suicidality. The studies used doses of ethyl EPA plus DHA in the range of 1–2 g/day (Hallahan et al. 2007; Hancock-Johnson et al. 2017; Stoffers and Lieb 2015; Zanarini and Frankenburg 2003).

In summary, mood stabilizers can be very useful in patients with BPD, and there is reasonable evidence to support their use. Most of the trials have been of short duration. However, an investigation of the long-term effectiveness of lamotrigine in patients with BPD failed to demonstrate its superiority to placebo (Crawford et al. 2018; Gunderson and Choi-Kain 2018). Again, these medications have significant side effects, particularly for women in the childbearing years, and the risks versus benefits must be carefully evaluated.

Antidepressants

Meta-analytic and systematic reviews of pharmacological treatment in patients with BPD suggest that antidepressants have a limited role in the management of these patients (Hancock-Johnson et al. 2017; Ingenhoven et al. 2010; Lieb et al. 2010; Mercer et al. 2009; Nosè et al. 2006; Stoffers and Lieb 2015). However, some evidence suggests that anger, depression, and perhaps affective instability can be symptom targets when using these medications. For example, a pilot study of patients with BPD taking duloxetine suggested that impulsivity, anger, and affective instability improved (Bellino et al. 2010). However, there is no robust evidence supporting the efficacy of antidepressants in treating BPD as a whole. Most often, antidepressants are used to treat comorbid depression or anxiety disorders. The use of antidepressants for these comorbid disorders is justified, but the patient has to be realistic about the expected outcomes. For example, the longitudinal course of comorbid depression in patients with BPD is significantly improved if patients receive an evidence-based psychotherapy for BPD (Cristea et al. 2017).

Methylphenidate

Attention-deficit disorder is often found to be comorbid with BPD, raising the question of whether stimulants such as methylphenidate should be prescribed for patients with BPD. To the best of our knowledge, no RCT evidence examining the use of methylphenidate in patients with BPD has been completed at the time of this review. However, there are two studies that are of relevance to this question. A 12-week open-label prospective study of 14 adolescent females with BPD and attention-deficit/hyperactivity disorder (ADHD) examined the effect of prescribing methylphenidate up to 60 mg/day on several outcomes (Golubchik et al. 2008). The study excluded adolescents with psychosis or substance abuse diagnoses. The findings indicated that the ADHD and aggressive symptoms were improved, and, interestingly, three of the patients stopped self-harming after exposure to methylphenidate. There was no worsening of the borderline symptoms and no development of psychoses. The study requires replication but suggests that, for certain patients, aggressive and self-mutilating behavior may be helped by methylphenidate.

A second 4-week prospective naturalistic study compared BPD patients without ADHD to BPD patients with ADHD, some of whom were taking methylphenidate (Prada et al. 2015). All of these patients were going through an intensive dialectical behavior therapy (DBT) program throughout the course of the investigation. BPD patients with ADHD who were taking methylphenidate showed significant improvement compared to BPD patients with ADHD who were not taking methylphenidate on measures of motor impulsiveness, overall impulsiveness, ADHD severity, state anger, and depression severity. In addition, the study suggested that patients who had their ADHD symptoms treated with methylphenidate were more able to benefit from the DBT program, implying that methylphenidate may have a role in making BPD patients with ADHD better able to participate in psychosocial interventions. Such findings illustrate that studies of pharmacological interventions should not only focus on symptom improvement but also investigate other aspects of functioning.

These two small, short-term, open-label studies suggest that stimulants may play a role in the treatment of BPD comorbid with ADHD. Because these results are preliminary, we recommend that patients first be assessed for a history of substance dependence and that the diagnosis of ADHD be confirmed with collateral or school records. Long-acting preparations are preferred because they may reduce the risk of stimulant misuse. When stimulants are prescribed, benefits should be particularly apparent in terms of improvements in functioning, either in treatment programs or work settings; otherwise, given the potential for diversion and misuse, the medication should be discontinued.

Other Approaches

Opioid antagonists such as naltrexone have been tested in female patients with BPD and have shown nonsignificant effects on dissociative symptoms. Clonidine has been used to decrease inner tension and hyperarousal and may be useful in patients with BPD and comorbid posttraumatic stress disorder (PTSD; Hancock-Johnson et al. 2017; Stoffers and Lieb 2015); however, further studies are needed to clarify the role of these medications in patients with BPD and comorbid PTSD.

Because patients with BPD often struggle in interpersonal relationships, several medications have been advanced as possible approaches to improving prosocial behavior. Oxytocin in the general population has been shown to promote group trust and cooperation and improve social cognitive abilities such as emotional recognition (Amad et al. 2015). Therefore, oxytocin was felt to have possible benefits for improving deficits in mentalizing and the bias to negative-valenced social stimuli that are found in patients with BPD. At this point, no clinical trials of oxytocin in patients with BPD have been reported, and most of the studies that have been done have examined laboratory outcomes related to prosocial behavior (Amad et al. 2015). These studies show a mixture of results in patients with BPD, with some evidence that oxytocin can improve hypersensitivity to social threats but then contradictory findings that oxytocin may lessen trust and cooperative behaviors in certain social dilemmas. These mixed results may be explained by the social salience hypothesis (Shamay-Tsoory et al. 2009), which suggests that oxytocin may modulate the salience to both positive- and negative-valenced social emotions and therefore may lead to contradictory outcomes in certain contexts. Although interest remains in studying the role of oxytocin in patients with BPD, all of these findings come from laboratory studies, and this research has not controlled for various confounders such as gender differences, menstrual cycle effects, and medication interactions.

Research is underway to determine whether medication could modify the social pain experienced by patients with BPD in the face of actual or perceived social rejection. In an RCT, Yovell et al. (2016) investigated the efficacy of exogenous opioids in the reduction of separation distress and the risk of suicide in severely suicidal adult patients. This study tested buprenorphine up to 0.8 mg/day versus placebo in severely suicidal adult patients without current substance use to determine if the medication would reduce suicide ideation. These patients were not selected for having BPD, although more than half of the participants met criteria for the disorder. Over the course of the 4-week trial, buprenorphine led to significant reductions in suicidal ideation and suicide probability compared with placebo. The study also found a reduction in depressive symptoms; however, this reduction was smaller than the impacts on suicide risk. On the basis of these results, the mechanism of action was thought to be through reducing social pain associated with rejection and abandonment as opposed to impacting and reducing depressive symptoms. The study was limited by a high dropout rate, the short duration of follow-up, and the need to further study the safety of buprenorphine. However, this research indicates a unique line of inquiry to determine whether modifying social pain can reduce suicidal crisis in patients with BPD. Other medications that have been implicated in the attenuation of social pain include acetaminophen and marijuana (Deckman et al. 2014; Dewall et al. 2010).

There are several case reports concerning the use of transcranial magnetic stimulation (TMS) on patients with BPD. A few case reports, which focused on the dorsolateral prefrontal cortex, have suggested that TMS may have an impact on borderline symptoms such as anger and affective instability (Arbabi et al. 2013; Cailhol et al. 2014). Feffer et al. (2017) focused on the dorsomedial prefrontal cortex and documented improvement in depressive rather than borderline symptoms in three patients with BPD. TMS deserves further study in patients with BPD, particularly regarding its impact on mood and affective instability.

Limitations

Although there is some evidence supporting the value of medication over placebo for certain symptom targets in patients with BPD, this evidence has many limitations. Most studies considered here have largely female samples, making it difficult to generalize these findings to men with BPD. In addition, the sample sizes in the studies are small, trial durations are short, and the exclusion criteria are unrealistically stringent, excluding participants with Axis I comorbidities (DSM-IV-TR; American Psychiatric Association 2000), further challenging the generalizability of these findings. Furthermore, the quality of the studies is often questionable, with an ever-present risk of bias. Finally, because patients with BPD are often exposed to medication, there has been insufficient attention given to the side effects and reasons for withdrawal in previous pharmacological trials. Thus, more research on the psychopharmacological management of patients with BPD is advised.

Case Vignette

The following case description includes decision points, each of which has several alternative responses listed at the end of the case. The reader will rate each alternative response in terms of its level of helpfulness. Discussions of responses follow.

Ellen is a 30-year-old woman who is referred to you by her therapist because "she has a serious depression and needs medication before she can benefit from therapy." Ellen recounts that she has struggled with depression since "forever." Her father was strict but could be warm and encouraging at times. He kept a tight fist on the family money and activities. Her mother was chronically depressed and angry and was mostly uninvolved with Ellen and her siblings. Ellen's grandfather was alcoholic and physically abused Ellen's mother.

As a child, Ellen was very anxious and struggled with making friends. As an adolescent, she continued to be very anxious about school and friends, but this was more often expressed with anger. Home became a battleground on a daily basis, with Ellen angrily (to the point of yelling, screaming, and slamming doors) refusing her parents' demands before shutting down for days, refusing to go to school or to do anything around the house. Ellen's friend group from grade school (the "nerds") rejected her in high school because of her anger. She did make a few friends in high school, but her friends used drugs heavily, and Ellen eventually came to use marijuana daily and binge drink on the weekends, a pattern that persists to this day. She has experimented with other drugs but never used these regularly.

Ellen attempted to go to university but found herself overwhelmed by her courses and dropped out in her first semester. She moved out on her own due to ongoing conflict with her parents. She has attempted multiple jobs in the service industry ("I don't have a problem getting jobs; I just keep getting screwed over, so I quit") and is currently unemployed. Her parents are supporting her financially but threaten to pull their support if she doesn't "get her act together and get a real job."

Ellen has had several intimate relationships with men and women. She currently identifies as gay and is in a relationship with a partner whom she describes as "the best thing that ever happened to me." The relationship has been rocky because of Ellen's intense anger in response to even minor disappointments and her constant need for her partner's reassurance that she will not leave. Recently the two have been in conflict because Ellen's partner would like to have children, whereas Ellen is ambivalent about children. She thinks she would like to have them eventually, but right now "I can barely take care of myself, so I don't know how I would take care of a child."

Ellen had several admissions as a teen for suicidality and depression. One of these admissions was for 5 months, during which time she was given the diagnosis of BPD. Although she agrees that she meets most of the criteria, she does not like the diagnosis because "my mom kept shoving it down my throat—it proved to her that I was the problem."

Ellen currently meets criteria for a major depressive episode, which seems to have started around the time that her partner started talking about wanting to have a child. She continues to use marijuana, about 1 g at bedtime "to help with sleep," and tells you "it is really the only thing that helps me anyway." She binge drinks on the weekends—"I don't really mean to, but when we go out I get really anxious. I have a couple to loosen up, then I lose control." When Ellen drinks, she is likely to fight with her part-

ner, and the couple have broken up several times. Following a breakup, Ellen will usually cut and on a couple of occasions has overdosed on Tylenol.
She is usually remorseful and frightened by the overdoses and will tell her
partner about them, ultimately presenting to the emergency department
at her partner's insistence. However, on a couple of occasions, when her
partner did not return home after a fight and Ellen was convinced her partner no longer cared about her, she did not go to the emergency department
and slept off the overdose, "not really caring whether I live or die."

At her partner's insistence, Ellen agreed to "get help" and started working with her current psychologist about 5 months ago. She likes the psychologist and looks forward to and attends her appointments regularly.
However, Ellen has not improved. She has little motivation or energy and
spends most of her days holed up in the apartment that she shares with
her partner. She recognizes that she is irritable with her partner and that
her repeated angry attacks when her partner asks her to help out are not
good for the relationship. At the same time, she reports that "I can't help
myself" and that her only reprieve in the day is when she smokes marijuana at night and tries to sleep.

Ellen has seen several psychiatrists over the years and has tried many
antidepressants. She has never found antidepressants to be much help,
and some resulted in more irritability, so she stopped them. For a while
she took prescribed benzodiazepines and really felt they helped but overdosed on them in combination with alcohol, leading her family physician
to refuse to prescribe these again. During the assessment, Ellen reports being anxious for "help right now" but appears to be somewhat ambivalent
about medications.

Your assessment is that Ellen meets criteria for a current major depressive episode in the context of lifelong dysthymia. She also has marijuana
and alcohol use disorder and likely generalized anxiety disorder and social
phobia. You agree with the diagnosis of BPD.

When you start to discuss your impression with Ellen, you notice that
she seems mildly interested in the depression and anxiety diagnoses, is
uncomfortable with the BPD diagnosis, and shuts down when you indicate you are concerned about her marijuana and alcohol use. [**Decision
Point 1**] Ellen reminds you that her mom previously "latched onto" the
BPD diagnosis and blamed "all my problems" on BPD. In response to your
asking how it made her feel when her mom latched onto the BPD diagnosis, Ellen responds, "It really pissed me off—there were lots of problems,
and they weren't all because of me." You validate that it makes sense that
she would be angry about this, and she seems to settle. When you ask if
she ever looked at the BPD criteria to see what she thought about this, she
responds, "Yeah, it fits. Not all of them, but most of them do." [**Decision
Point 2**]

Ellen is in agreement with leaving the "BPD and alcohol and pot stuff
alone since I don't think it is the major problem" but might be willing to
try an antidepressant. You review the list of what has been tried previously.
Ellen is not sure that anything helped but was using alcohol and marijuana more heavily when she was taking antidepressants and did not take

the medication regularly. You suggest a trial of escitalopram, and she agrees somewhat reluctantly. You comment on the reluctance and she responds, "I don't really think this is going to work. I don't like pills. I don't really believe in them."

You tell Ellen that you also do not want her to be taking something that is not helping her and are pleased that she is a bit skeptical about medications because it makes it less likely that she will take something that is not helping. At the same time, you remind her that despite 5 months of therapy with a therapist she likes, she has not seen the improvement she was hoping for. You indicate that you cannot give guarantees about medication. However, given that she appears to have a depression that is moderate in intensity, she might see some benefit from the antidepressant, which, in turn, could help her start experiencing benefit from her therapy. She agrees to give it a try. [**Decision Point 3**]

Ellen says that she would like to have more energy, not feel like sleeping all the time, and have more motivation to get out of the house. She is journaling for her therapist and is willing to rate these symptoms daily from 0 (no motivation, no energy) to 5 (normal motivation, normal energy). Over the next couple of months, you see Ellen three times. On her own, she is able to cut down her marijuana use (a couple of puffs at night) and has had only one episode of binge drinking to intoxication; she states, "My partner doesn't like me doing it anyway." She thinks the antidepressant has had some effect: "Maybe I am not so hopeless anymore. Maybe I have a bit more energy." She had stopped the antidepressant for a couple of weeks, and both you and she noticed that her depression seemed to get worse during that time, so she started taking it again. During this time, Ellen spoke to her partner with the help of her therapist about her ambivalence surrounding the issue of having children. Her partner was willing to put this discussion on hold for now. Ellen's anger remains about the same, but she is not interested in looking at the anger right now. The suicidal thinking has "moved to the back of my mind." Ellen decides to keep taking the antidepressant, and you refer her back to her family physician for medication renewals.

Two years later, Ellen is referred back to you. She has continued to struggle, but despite this, she started a small business cleaning houses. Her relationship has been rocky, with several short breakups. The issue of having children is still on the "back burner." Ellen is aware that her partner is not happy about the "children problem" and worries constantly that she will end the relationship. Ellen's difficulties with interpersonal hypersensitivity continue, and any suggestion that her partner is unhappy with her or is not taking her feelings into account (e.g., chewing loudly when Ellen has told her time and time again that this makes her "crazy") results in Ellen quickly becoming overwhelmed with anger and attacking her partner or storming out of the apartment. On a couple of occasions, she has broken objects by throwing them. Ellen and her therapist have addressed this in therapy, and Ellen is comfortable with the idea that she responds more intensely to these situations than others would. At the same time, it just makes her angrier when her partner tells her she is "overreacting" and "needs to settle down," making her feel that the problems that got her irritated in the first place get minimized and ignored and "it becomes all about my anger." She worries that her group of friends is secretly thinking that her partner would be better off without her, although no one has said this out loud.

Ellen has continued to take the antidepressant. She thinks it helps "a bit—maybe for my anxiety and my mood." When she has stopped taking it, she has seemed to get more depressed. She does not think it helps with her anger or with how sensitive she is with her partner. The marijuana use is occasional ("can't do it if I am working"), and she rarely drinks. She continues to have suicidal thinking—usually in response to problems with her partner—but has not acted on these thoughts since you last saw her. You check with Ellen to see what she would like help with now, and she identifies her anger as her main concern. [**Decision Point 4**]

Ellen agrees to speak with her psychologist about focusing on anger in therapy. She is also interested in a trial of omega-3 fatty acid. Monitoring shows moderate improvement in anger. Ellen's relationship troubles continue, but she feels a little better because she is noticing she has more control of her anger: "I still lose my cool, but it's not happening as much, and I am better able to use the techniques that I worked on with my therapist."

Six months later you get an urgent request from Ellen's therapist. For the past 2 weeks, Ellen has "not been doing well at all." Ellen had been suspicious because her partner was spending a lot of time away from the apartment. She read her partner's phone texts and discovered that her partner was seeing someone else and was planning on having a child. She confronted her partner about this, and the partner admitted to the affair. She said she had not told Ellen because she still loved her and was afraid the news would devastate her. In her appointments, Ellen was shut down emotionally and struggled with describing what she was feeling, something that she had been able to do easily for a while. She kept stating that she "couldn't be helped." She was drinking and smoking marijuana daily and had cut herself a few times. She reported intense suicidal ideation and was unclear about a plan. At the last appointment, the therapist insisted that Ellen be seen in the emergency department and advocated for admission. However, Ellen denied suicidal ideation and was released. The emergency record indicated that Ellen was at "chronic suicide risk." The therapist is worried about Ellen because she has not been following her crisis plan (calling the therapist before she cuts), and the therapist cannot get Ellen to talk about finding new housing.

When you see Ellen, she presents as her therapist described. She is unkempt, and her answers are vague. She had stopped her medications after her visit to the hospital because "they weren't working." She endorses all of the symptoms of a major depressive episode and is not eating or sleeping. She has cut several times and continues to endorse suicidal ideation. Although she does not have a clear plan, she does have a "stash" of several weeks of medication. She has not been to work in the past 2 weeks. Her housing is stable—her partner has not moved out yet because she is concerned about Ellen. [**Decision Point 5**]

Ellen returns to see you after a 2-week admission to hospital. She is well groomed and dressed. She is able to make some eye contact. She says that she is "coping," is able to sleep a bit better, and has an appetite, but she is not happy because she has already gained 5 pounds on quetiapine ER 150 mg/day at bedtime. You ask about work and relationships. She has not returned to work, and her finances are poor. She is planning to live with her parents again "until I get back on my feet, if that ever happens!" She is very critical of her ex ("She screwed me over and found someone else") and admits to being "pretty irritable with everyone and everything." You ask Ellen what she would like addressed now, and she responds, "My sleep and my anger, I guess."

You ask Ellen whether she feels the quetiapine ER is helping with her sleep and anger. She thinks it may be helping, but she is not willing to continue taking it because of the weight gain. [**Decision Point 6**]

Given her uncertainty about its helpfulness and concerns regarding its side-effect profile, you and Ellen agree to taper her use of quetiapine while she continues to take the antidepressant. She again becomes adherent to her medication regimen and believes that the medications "do help" with her depressed mood. In the months following Ellen's hospitalization, her partner moves out, and Ellen's mood again worsens. In your sessions, you discuss the possibility of increasing her antidepressant but also discuss the factors contributing to her mood, particularly this most recent significant interpersonal stressor, and what other things she can do to manage her mood. Although Ellen recognizes her mood is likely impacted by the breakup, she has difficulty suggesting any solutions other than changing her medications saying, "That's the only thing that's helped me besides pot, and you say I shouldn't have that." You remind her of the change she noticed in her mood and energy level when she was working consistently. You suggest this may be the most important change she could make for herself.

In the subsequent years you work with Ellen, your encouragement of her employment is a constant theme and becomes something you can joke about together.

Decision Points: Alternative Responses

Rate each response in terms of its level of helpfulness with a rating of 1 (will be helpful), 2 (possibly helpful, continuing reservations), or 3 (not helpful—or even harmful).

1. On the basis of Ellen's reactions to your diagnostic impressions, what is the best way to proceed?

    A. Decide to focus solely on the potential benefits of antidepressants for Ellen's mood and anxiety symptoms because she seems uninterested in talking about the BPD or her substance use.

B. Highlight that in the face of ongoing substance use, the benefits of antidepressants are likely to be limited.

C. Reflect on what you have observed when giving Ellen feedback: "You seem uncomfortable when I mentioned borderline personality disorder. Can you tell me a bit more about that?"

2. In light of Ellen's experiences with the BPD diagnosis, which is the best way to proceed?

A. Suggest that you leave the BPD and marijuana use for now and attempt a trial of antidepressants for the anxiety and depression. If she does not respond, you can try talking about the BPD and marijuana use again.

B. Indicate that you recognize that she is uncomfortable with this diagnosis and that understanding BPD and its treatment might help you collaborate on coming up with a treatment plan together.

C. Ask Ellen what she knows about BPD.

3. In response to Ellen's willingness to try antidepressant medication, you

A. Prescribe the medication, mentioning potential side effects but indicating that it is generally well tolerated, hoping to minimize Ellen's focus on the negative aspects of the medication.

B. Indicate to Ellen that it is important for her to be clear about her expectations of the antidepressant and that she monitor her target symptoms on a daily basis. You also suggest that she read up on the medication and call you if she has any questions about it.

C. Review side effects and indicate to Ellen that if this medication does not work, there are many other helpful medications that can be tried.

4. To attempt to address Ellen's anger, you

A. Suggest raising the dose of escitalopram, considering that Ellen has had some benefit and her dose has been low (10 mg/day).

B. Indicate that the preferred and likely most effective way to address anger is with psychotherapy. In addition, it might be helpful to consider a trial of omega-3 fatty acids, as research has shown some benefit for anger, irritability and suicidality.

C. Suggest a trial of an atypical antipsychotic such as quetiapine ER up to 150 mg/day or olanzapine 5–10 mg/day, emphasizing that these medications have only been investigated for short-term use (8–12 weeks) and that they have significant side effects, including weight gain and possibly an increase in suicidality.

5. In response to Ellen's most recent presentation, you

A. Diagnose a major depressive episode of severe intensity and advocate for hospital admission and possibly electroconvulsive therapy.
B. Recognize that Ellen is at high risk of suicide—she is not taking her medications and is experiencing a major depressive episode; she has relapsed to alcohol and marijuana use; and she has experienced a major relationship loss. She is not engaged in problem solving and is not using her crisis plan. You advocate for a short admission to provide her with support. You recommend that she restart her antidepressant and suggest a brief (3- to 4-week) trial of an atypical antipsychotic. Because she is not sleeping or eating, you suggest a trial of quetiapine ER, starting at 50 mg/day at bedtime and gradually increased as clinically indicated up to 150 mg/day.
C. Recognize that, given Ellen's chronic suicidality, hospitalization is unlikely to be of benefit. You suggest she restart her antidepressant and recommend a trial of atypical antipsychotic. Given that Ellen will need to take an antipsychotic for a prolonged period of time, you recommend aripiprazole because it has less propensity for weight gain.

6. Given Ellen's comments about quetiapine, you

A. Reduce and stop quetiapine ER, and ask Ellen to monitor her symptom targets: sleep and anger.
B. Advocate that Ellen continue taking quetiapine because it is helping.
C. Talk to Ellen about the importance of getting her life back on track and advocate that she return to work part-time. Explain that most of Ellen's improvement so far can be credited to her efforts at dealing with the separation from her partner and rebuilding her life. Indicate that medications may be playing a role, but it will be important to continue monitoring the target

symptoms to be certain. Suggest that the quetiapine be tapered, and ask Ellen to monitor her symptom targets: sleep and anger.

Decision Points: Discussion

Numbers within brackets indicate level of helpfulness ratings.

1. On the basis of Ellen's reactions to your diagnostic impressions, what is the best way to proceed?

    A. Decide to focus solely on the potential benefits of antidepressants for Ellen's mood and anxiety symptoms because she seems uninterested in talking about the BPD or her substance use. [3] (While antidepressants may be helpful, focusing solely on the potential benefits of medications will likely result in unrealistic expectations of medication and will send the message that you are not concerned about her BPD and substance use.)

    B. Highlight that in the face of ongoing substance use, the benefits of antidepressants are likely to be limited. [2] (Although this is true, it may come across as a lecture, and given Ellen's interpersonal hypersensitivity, she may feel you are disapproving of her and may become defensive and angry.)

    C. Reflect on what you have observed when giving Ellen feedback: "You seem uncomfortable when I mentioned borderline personality disorder. Can you tell me a bit more about that?" [1] (Being curious about Ellen's thoughts regarding the BPD diagnosis will enable a discussion of her feelings about the diagnosis [respond to negative attitudes with curiosity and reassurance] and will likely improve your alliance with Ellen, paving the way for acceptance of the diagnosis.)

2. In light of Ellen's experiences with the BPD diagnosis, which is the best way to proceed?

    A. Suggest that you leave the BPD and marijuana use for now and attempt a trial of antidepressants for the anxiety and depression. If she does not respond, you can try talking about the BPD and marijuana use again. [1] (This is a good example of avoiding a dichotomous stance. You have balanced your concern about Ellen's depression and the possibility that antidepressants may be helpful while at the same time leaving the door open for further discussion about BPD and marijuana use.)

B. Indicate that you recognize that she is uncomfortable with this diagnosis and that understanding BPD and its treatment might help you collaborate on coming up with a treatment plan together. [2] (Providing psychoeducation on BPD might help Ellen to be more willing to accept the diagnosis, but Ellen is still leery of the diagnosis, and psychoeducation may be received reluctantly if at all. In addition, you would like Ellen to consider an antidepressant, and psychoeducation on BPD with a reluctant patient will not achieve this goal.)

C. Ask Ellen what she knows about BPD. [2] (This response will engage Ellen more than option B; however, similar to option B, it will not help you meet your goal of encouraging Ellen to consider a trial of antidepressants.)

3. In response to Ellen's willingness to try antidepressant medication, you

A. Prescribe the medication, mentioning potential side effects but indicating that it is generally well tolerated, hoping to minimize Ellen's focus on the negative aspects of the medication. [2] (This response may be true but is not balanced and does not encourage Ellen to become an active participant in the decision about medications.)

B. Indicate to Ellen that it is important for her to be clear about her expectations of the antidepressant and that she monitor her target symptoms on a daily basis. You also suggest that she read up on the medication and call you if she has any questions about it. [1] (This response encourages Ellen to become an active participant in deciding whether or not to start this medication and to actively monitor the effects of the medication.)

C. Review side effects and indicate to Ellen that if this medication does not work, there are many other helpful medications that can be tried. [3] (It is helpful to review side effects, but expectations for antidepressants in the treatment of depression in BPD need to be tempered by research that suggests modest benefits at most. In addition, suggesting that there are many other medications that can be tried may shift Ellen's focus to finding the "right" medication and away from the hard work of psychotherapy.)

4. To attempt to address Ellen's anger, you

   A. Suggest raising the dose of escitalopram, considering that Ellen has had some benefit and her dose has been low (10 mg/day). [3] (The research on effectiveness of SSRIs on anger suggests a small benefit. Ellen is unlikely to see much improvement in the anger with a higher dose of an SSRI.)

   B. Indicate that the preferred and likely most effective way to address anger is with psychotherapy. In addition, it might be helpful to consider a trial of omega-3 fatty acids, as research has shown some benefit for anger, irritability and suicidality. [1] (This would be the best choice as it directs Ellen to psychotherapy, which has been shown to reduce anger in BPD and omega-3 fatty acids are safe in the long term.)

   C. Suggest a trial of an atypical antipsychotic such as quetiapine ER up to 150 mg/day or olanzapine 5–10 mg/day, emphasizing that these medications have only been investigated for short-term use (8–12 weeks) and that they have significant side effects, including weight gain and possibly an increase in suicidality. [2] (While there is evidence to support this option, the evidence is only for short-term use. Ellen's difficulty with anger has been present for years. If it is effective, Ellen may opt to stay with this medication, tolerating the side effects and risks; however, a better way to proceed would be option B as it has better evidence for effectiveness and safety in the long term.)

5. In response to Ellen's most recent presentation, you

   A. Diagnose a major depressive episode of severe intensity and advocate for hospital admission and possibly electroconvulsive therapy. [3] (It is reasonable to consider hospital admission, but an insistence on electroconvulsive therapy is misplaced because the main beneficial impact of hospitalization is likely to be increased support, teaching self-soothing skills, and helping Ellen come to terms with the loss of her relationship.)

   B. Recognize that Ellen is at high risk of suicide—she is not taking her medications and is experiencing a major depressive episode; she has relapsed to alcohol and marijuana use; and she has experienced a major relationship loss. She is not engaged in problem solving and is not using her crisis plan. You advocate for a short admission to provide her with support. You recommend that she restart her antidepressant and suggest a brief (3- to 4-week) trial of an atypical antipsychotic. Because she is not sleeping or eating, you suggest a trial of quetiapine ER, starting at 50 mg/day at bedtime and gradually increased as clinically indicated up to 150 mg/day. [1] (Although hospitalization can be used inappropriately for asylum or as a way to avoid distress, it is important to be thoughtful about hospitalization. Short-term hospitalization can be helpful when risk is acutely elevated in the face of significant interpersonal loss, current substance use, and untreated depression. Short-term use of antipsychotics may help with borderline symptoms, in particular anger, impulsive aggression, and cognitive perceptual features.)

C. Recognize that, given Ellen's chronic suicidality, hospitalization is unlikely to be of benefit. You suggest she restart her antidepressant and recommend a trial of atypical antipsychotic. Given that Ellen will need to take an antipsychotic for a prolonged period of time, you recommend aripiprazole because it has less propensity for weight gain. [3] (This approach to hospitalization is not consistent with GPM, which advocates for a thoughtful, balanced approach that includes weighing risks and benefits of hospitalization.)

6. Given Ellen's comments about quetiapine, you

A. Reduce and stop quetiapine ER, and ask Ellen to monitor her symptom targets: sleep and anger. [2] (This response is reasonable and will prevent polypharmacy, but it is unlikely that all of Ellen's improvement is due to the quetiapine, and symptoms such as anger and poor sleep likely will improve more with returning to work and building friendships.)

B. Advocate that Ellen continue taking quetiapine because it is helping. [3] (Although the quetiapine seems to have had an effect on Ellen's symptoms, the risks associated with this medication, particularly weight gain, are real. Ellen is unlikely to take the quetiapine regularly but may acquiesce to your providing the prescription in order to please you.)

C. Talk to Ellen about the importance of getting her life back on track and advocate that she return to work part-time. Explain that most of Ellen's improvement so far can be credited to her efforts at dealing with the separation from her partner and rebuilding her life. Indicate that medications may be playing a role, but it will be important to continue monitoring the target symptoms to be certain. Suggest that the quetiapine be tapered, and ask Ellen to monitor her symptom targets: sleep and anger. [1] (This response keeps at the forefront of treatment the interventions that have been and will be most helpful in remitting her BPD symptoms, while allowing for thoughtful prescribing of medications.)

Conclusion

Patients with BPD in acute distress pose a significant challenge to psychopharmacologists, who are forced to reconcile urges or demands to prescribe with limited evidence for pharmacotherapy of BPD and lack of FDA-approved options. A GPM-based approach rooted in a strong therapeutic alliance, reasonable expectations of medication effectiveness, and assessment of relevant case factors and comorbidity can help curb the risks of reactive prescribing and psychiatric polypharmacy and provide a much-needed road map for psychopharmacologists who are faced with patients with BPD in their practice.

References

Amad A, Thomas P, Perez-Rodriguez MM: Borderline personality disorder and oxytocin: review of clinical trials and future directions. Curr Pharm Des 21(23):3311–3316, 2015 26088114

American Psychiatric Association: Diagnostic and Statistical Manual of Mental Disorders, 4th Edition, Text Revision. Washington, DC, American Psychiatric Association, 2000

American Psychiatric Association: Practice guideline for the treatment of patients with borderline personality disorder. Am J Psychiatry 158(10 suppl):1–52, 2001 11665545

Arbabi M, Hafizi S, Ansari S, et al: High frequency TMS for the management of borderline personality disorder: a case report. Asian J Psychiatr 6(6):614–617, 2013 24309885

Bellino S, Paradiso E, Bozzatello P, et al: Efficacy and tolerability of duloxetine in the treatment of patients with borderline personality disorder: a pilot study. J Psychopharmacol 24(3):333–339, 2010 18719047

Binks CA, Fenton M, McCarthy L, et al: Pharmacological interventions for people with borderline personality disorder. Cochrane Database Syst Rev 25(1):CD005653, 2006 16437535

Black DW, Zanarini MC, Romine A, et al: Comparison of low and moderate dosages of extended-release quetiapine in borderline personality disorder: a randomized, double-blind, placebo-controlled trial. Am J Psychiatry 171(11):1174–1182, 2014 24968985

Cailhol L, Roussignol B, Klein R, et al: Borderline personality disorder and rTMS: a pilot trial. Psychiatry Res 216(1):155–157, 2014 24503285

Crawford MJ, Sanatinia R, Barrett B, et al: Lamotrigine for people with borderline personality disorder: a RCT. Health Technol Assess 22(17):1–68, 2018 29651981

Cristea IA, Gentili C, Cotet CD, et al: Efficacy of psychotherapies for borderline personality disorder: a systematic review and meta-analysis. JAMA Psychiatry 74(4):319–238, 2017 28249086

Deckman T, DeWall CN, Way B, et al: Can marijuana reduce social pain? Soc Psychol Personal Sci 5(2):131–139, 2014

Dewall CN, Macdonald G, Webster GD, et al: Acetaminophen reduces social pain: behavioral and neural evidence. Psychol Sci 21(7):931–937, 2010 20548058

Duggan C, Huband N, Smailagic N, et al: The use of pharmacological treatments for people with personality disorder: a systematic review of randomized controlled trials. Personality and Mental Health 2(3):119–170, 2008

Feffer K, Peters SK, Bhui K, et al: Successful dorsomedial prefrontal rTMS for major depression in borderline personality disorder: three cases. Brain Stimulat 10(3):716–717, 2017 28196679

Golubchik P, Sever J, Zalsman G, et al: Methylphenidate in the treatment of female adolescents with cooccurrence of attention deficit/hyperactivity disorder and borderline personality disorder: a preliminary open-label trial. Int Clin Psychopharmacol 23(4):228–231, 2008 18446088

Gunderson, JG, Choi-Kain LW: Medication management for patients with borderline personality disorder. Am J Psychiatry 175(8):709–711, 2018 30064243

Hallahan B, Hibbeln JR, Davis JM, et al: Omega-3 fatty acid supplementation in patients with recurrent self-harm: single-centre double-blind randomised controlled trial. Br J Psychiatry 190:118–122, 2007 17267927

Hancock-Johnson E, Griffiths C, Picchioni M: A focused systematic review of pharmacological treatment for borderline personality disorder. CNS Drugs 31(5):345–356, 2017 28353141

Herpertz SC, Zanarini M, Schulz CS, et al: World Federation of Societies of Biological Psychiatry (WFSBP) guidelines for biological treatment of personality disorders. World J Biol Psychiatry 8(4):212–244, 2007 17963189

Hörz S, Zanarini MC, Frankenburg FR, et al: Ten-year use of mental health services by patients with borderline personality disorder and with other Axis II disorders. Psychiatr Serv 61(6):612–616, 2010 20513685

Ingenhoven T, Lafay P, Rinne T, et al: Effectiveness of pharmacotherapy for severe personality disorders: meta-analyses of randomized controlled trials. J Clin Psychiatry 71(1):14–25, 2010 19778496

Keuroghlian AS, Gunderson JG, Pagano ME, et al: Interactions of borderline personality disorder and anxiety disorders over 10 years. J Clin Psychiatry 76(11):1529–1534, 2015 26114336

Lieb K, Völlm B, Rücker G, et al: Pharmacotherapy for borderline personality disorder: Cochrane Systematic Review of Randomised Trials. Br J Psychiatry 196(1):4–12, 2010 20044651

McMain SF, Links PS, Gnam WH, et al: A randomized trial of dialectical behavior therapy versus general psychiatric management for borderline personality disorder. Am J Psychiatry 166(12):1365–1374, 2009 19755574

Mercer D, Douglass AB, Links PS: Meta-analyses of mood stabilizers, antidepressants and antipsychotics in the treatment of borderline personality disorder: effectiveness for depression and anger symptoms. J Pers Disord 23(2):156–174, 2009 19379093

National Health and Medical Research Council: Clinical Practice Guideline for the Management of Borderline Personality Disorder. Melbourne. National Health and Medical Research Council, 2012

National Institute for Health and Care Excellence. Borderline Personality Disorder: Recognition and Management (6-Year Review). London, National Institute for Health and Care Excellence, 2015

National Institute for Health and Clinical Excellence: Borderline Personality Disorder: Treatment and Management. Report No CG78. London, National Institute for Health and Clinical Excellence, 2009

Nosè M, Cipriani A, Biancosino B, et al: Efficacy of pharmacotherapy against core traits of borderline personality disorder: meta-analysis of randomized controlled trials. Int Clin Psychopharmacol 21(6):345–353, 2006 17012981

Prada P, Nicastro R, Zimmermann J, et al: Addition of methylphenidate to intensive dialectical behaviour therapy for patients suffering from comorbid borderline personality disorder and ADHD: a naturalistic study. Atten Defic Hyperact Disord 7(3):199–209, 2015 25634471

Reich DB, Zanarini MC, Bieri KA: A preliminary study of lamotrigine in the treatment of affective instability in borderline personality disorder. Int Clin Psychopharmacol 24(5):270–275, 2009 19636254

Shamay-Tsoory SG, Fischer M, Dvash J, et al: Intranasal administration of oxytocin increases envy and schadenfreude (gloating). Biol Psychiatry 66(9):864–870, 2009 19640508

Silk KR: The process of managing medications in patients with borderline personality disorder. J Psychiatr Pract 17(5):311–319, 2011 21926526

Stoffers J, Lieb K: Pharmacotherapy for borderline personality disorder—current evidence and recent trends. Curr Psychiatry Rep 17(1):534, 2015 25413640

Stoffers J, Völlm BA, Rücker G, et al: Pharmacological interventions for borderline personality disorder. Cochrane Database Syst Rev 6(6):CD005653, 2010 20556762

Tritt K, Nickel C, Lahmann C, et al: Lamotrigine treatment of aggression in female borderline-patients: a randomized, double-blind, placebo-controlled study. J Psychopharmacol 19(3):287–291, 2005 15888514

Vita A, De Peri L, Sacchetti E: Antipsychotics, antidepressants, anticonvulsants, and placebo on the symptom dimensions of borderline personality disorder: a meta-analysis of randomized controlled and open-label trials. J Clin Psychopharmacol 31(5):613–624, 2011 21869691

Yovell Y, Bar G, Mashiah M, et al: Ultra-low-dose buprenorphine as a time-limited treatment for severe suicidal ideation: a randomized controlled trial. Am J Psychiatry 173(5):491–498, 2016 26684923

Zanarini MC, Frankenburg FR: Omega-3 fatty acid treatment of women with borderline personality disorder: a double-blind, placebo-controlled pilot study. Am J Psychiatry 160(1):167–169, 2003 12505817

Zanarini MC, Schulz SC, Detke HC, et al: A dose comparison of olanzapine for the treatment of borderline personality disorder: a 12-week randomized, double-blind, placebo-controlled study. J Clin Psychiatry 72(10):1353–1362, 2011 21535995

Zanarini MC, Schulz SC, Detke H, et al: Open-label treatment with olanzapine for patients with borderline personality disorder. J Clin Psychopharmacol 32(3):398–402, 2012 22544004

Chapter 10

Psychotherapy Supervisors

Claire Brickell, M.D.
John G. Gunderson, M.D.

Good psychiatric management (GPM) is designed to be a commonsense, pared-down approach to the complex problems and comorbidities of borderline personality disorder (BPD). It distills a considerable body of knowledge regarding BPD. The clinical expertise of its developers is digested into a pragmatic treatment that early career clinicians can use to scaffold their approach to these challenging patients in the absence of extended experience. Still, GPM therapy does need to be taught and learned. Supervision is perhaps the most important source of such learning, especially for those early in their careers or inexperienced in treating patients with BPD.

A major advantage for training GPM to residents is that this model adopts basic standards of modern psychiatry: the disorder is seen as a biomedical condition; medications should be prescribed; and clinicians are invited to use their judgment about adding family and group modalities. Supervisors are in a position to have an enduring influence over supervisees and the way they deliver care. In this chapter, we describe how the traditional supervision for psychodynamic psychotherapy should be modified to help trainees learn the GPM model.

GPM is itself a principle-driven approach: it does not prescribe what to say or when to say it, but rather describes a stance to take with the patient that promotes an understanding of the diagnosis, accountability for change, and achievement of better functioning in the real world. Supervision in GPM requires that the supervising clinician be familiar and comfortable with this model's distinguishing features:

1. *Case management:* The focus is on the patient's life outside of therapy, not primarily on the patient's psychology. This means that GPM supervisors should encourage supervisees to *focus on the patient's presenting situational problems,* as opposed to working to better understand the patient's development or the "meaning" of a particular symptom or behavior. Also, supervisors should encourage supervisees to use practical, real-world interventions that could help their patients' social adaptation (e.g., assistance with housing).

2. *Psychoeducation:* Patients and families are informed about BPD and what to expect from its treatment. Encourage supervisees to start from a foundation of good psychoeducation and to *create a shared understanding of the BPD diagnosis.* Often, this is a useful form of treatment in and of itself, and trainees frequently overlook it. Good supervision begins by exploring whether the supervisee has adequate knowledge about the disorder's diagnosis, its course of gradual improvement, its heritability, and the modest role of medications in its treatment. Once such knowledge is attained, then supervisors help students learn ways to convey this knowledge to their patients.

3. *Interpersonal hypersensitivity:* Supervisors need to help trainees make explicit and consistent efforts to connect the symptomatic emotions and behaviors of the patient with BPD to interpersonal stressors. Supervisees are encouraged to forego open-ended explanation for stressors and, instead, to actively ferret out interpersonal stressors. They should learn to teach their patients about the *link between interpersonal stress and behaviors.*

4. *Goals:* In GPM, the primary goals are successes in work and partnerships. Unlike in the practice of psychopharmacology, symptom reduction is a secondary goal. Also, in contrast to psychodynamic therapies, improving empathy and integrating aggression are secondary goals. Supervisors need to keep these distinctions in mind when teaching supervisees how to talk to their patients about goals, expectations, and progress. In GPM, patients are encouraged to assume responsibility for and gain control over the course of their lives—that is, GPM emphasizes agency and accountability.

5. *Duration and intensity:* In GPM, duration and intensity depend on whether the patient is improving. From a GPM perspective, a patient who is doing poorly should not be seen more often—an increase of an unhelpful intervention is likely to be even more ineffective. The patient's failure to improve should prompt an exploration of the reasons and possibly even a consultation by the supervisor.

   Supervisors of GPM tell trainees to enlist their patients with BPD to collaborate in considering whether their therapy—or its components, such as medications—are effective. Supervisors teach supervisees to monitor whether or not the therapy is useful. The value of actively monitoring improvements was recently demonstrated in a medication trial (Gunderson and Choi-Kain, 2018). There is a well-established reason to think that the satisfaction of patients with BPD with their treatments is an unreliable indication of its value (Cowdry and Gardner 1988).

6. *Multimodality:* Medication management is an integrated albeit *adjunctive* modality. Similarly, the addition of group therapies and family coaching are integrated into treatment when these are judged to be helpful. Referring the patient to an additional treater may be useful, but this often proves unnecessary and impractical. It is not uncommon that supervisees need to be taught to consider other treatment modalities; many residents have little training or familiarity with the value of other modalities. Again, this becomes a task for the GPM supervisor.

Keeping these principles in mind helps GPM supervisors guide supervisees through the initial stages of both caring for a patient with BPD and learning the GPM approach to treatment.

Case Vignette

The following case description includes decision points, each of which has several alternative responses listed at the end of the case. The reader will rate each alternative response in terms of its level of helpfulness. Discussions of responses follow.

> Supervision with Dr. Julie Collins begins at the beginning of her fourth year of residency. She is a polite, deferential young woman who is pleasant and reserved. She has recently been assigned a patient with BPD—a 25-year-old woman named Betsy—and would like you to supervise her work. Dr. Collins tells you that the prospect of working with a patient with BPD makes her nervous, because she has heard such patients can be volatile and difficult to manage. She confesses that she has actually tried to avoid them but that now she is planning to return after graduation to her hometown, where she will need to be able to treat them. She will begin work in a community health clinic where, as one of few psychiatrists in a small town, she is likely to see many patients with BPD. She hopes that her work with Betsy will help her feel more competent and comfortable managing the disorder. You tell her that you share this hope.
>
> Dr. Collins begins by summarizing what she has learned during her intake interview. Betsy has never attempted suicide but did cut herself regularly when she was a teenager. She has struggled with binge eating and purging and at present frequently overspends when buying clothes online. Betsy had matriculated at a reputable out-of-state university, but after a falling out with the other students on her dormitory hallway, she started drinking more and stopped going to class. This led her to transfer to another school closer to home, where she also struggled to make friends. She was placed on medical leave after revealing to her dormitory counselor that she was having thoughts of suicide. Her parents withdrew her from school, helped her find an apartment, and supported her while she completed an associate's degree in veterinary technology. Betsy was diagnosed with BPD by a therapist she saw immediately after leaving college. Since that time, Betsy has seen two different therapists, but Dr. Collins has not learned much about their treatments.
>
> Betsy is currently living in an apartment and working as a technician in a local veterinary practice. She complains that her job barely pays enough to cover her living expenses. She dreams of getting married and eventually having children. When Dr. Collins explores the topic, Betsy reveals that she has recently had a string of short-lived romantic relationships. She says that she appreciates her parents' continued financial support but resents how "judgmental" and critical her father is about her disappointing level of achievements. She tells Dr. Collins that she feels sad and insecure much of the time and that she would like to develop more self-confidence.
>
> You think that Dr. Collins, as a future community mental health provider, would be well suited to learn a nonintensive, practical approach—GPM. You explain that the GPM treatment model offers a way to structure the treatment that you expect will help her feel more competent and comfortable. You give Dr. Collins the GPM handbook (Gunderson and Links 2014) to read before your next supervisory session. [**Decision Point 1**]

You tell Dr. Collins that she should orient Betsy to the implications of the BPD diagnosis and provide Betsy with some foundational psychoeducation about the disorder's etiology, course, and treatment. You also encourage her to inform Betsy about her interpersonal sensitivity and the fact that this makes any perceived rejection or even innocent separation feel like abandonment, an interpretation that undermines her ability to sustain relationships. You remind Dr. Collins to be active in asking questions, pointing out Betsy's avoidance when it occurs, and to keep Betsy focused on reaching her legitimate long-term goals of marriage and children. You also stress the importance of Dr. Collins developing a formulation of the case, meaning developing hypotheses about how Betsy developed her BPD and what is perpetuating her symptoms.

Over the next several weeks, Dr. Collins obtains some additional information about Betsy's important relationships. Her father is a lawyer who was mostly absent during her childhood while working long hours building a successful practice. Her two older sisters have followed in his footsteps by working hard and achieving vocational success. Betsy believes that they look down on her for not finishing college. She occasionally spends time with her oldest sister, who is married and living in a nearby suburb, but Betsy says that she always comes away feeling bad about herself and jealous of her sister for "having it all." Betsy is closest to her mother, who shares her interest in horseback riding and love of animals. She and her mother speak multiple times per day. Betsy tells Dr. Collins that she finds it comforting "just to hear Mom's voice" but also admits that they argue frequently. Betsy finds it particularly irritating when her mother either gives her advice or seems to dismiss her concerns by telling her to "just look on the bright side."

Betsy remains in sporadic contact with two friends from high school but otherwise has few female friends. She is most excited and invested in a recent relationship with Dan, one of the veterinarians at work, who is 10 years her senior and recently divorced. They have recently begun an active sexual relationship, but they purposefully try to keep their romantic relationship secret from other staff.

As you get to know Dr. Collins better, you are impressed by her warmth and the genuine interest that she is taking in Betsy. She took your advice seriously about learning to provide psychoeducation about BPD and has quickly gained a comfortable grasp of the diagnosis of BPD and conveyed this well to Betsy, who was appreciative. Together, you and Dr. Collins develop the working formulation that Betsy is angry about being inadequately cared for (by her father, who was absent, and by her mother, who does not understand her misery) and is afraid that she cannot live up to the standards of her family. Therefore, she is fearful of becoming independent and has sabotaged her own progress (e.g., not going to class and leaving school). Rather than working to improve her own self-reliance, she is hoping to find a husband whom she hopes will help her feel worthwhile. This is a major reason why she is attracted to the veterinarian who is older and financially well established.

In the resident clinic, supervisors are asked to periodically review videotapes of their supervisees' therapy sessions. In the first one you see from Dr. Collins, Betsy is insistent in wanting reassurance from Dr. Collins about her boyfriend, Dan. Betsy wonders whether or not he really loves her and worries that he might be seeing someone else. She wants to keep him happy and makes herself constantly available to him, even if it means staying up very late at night or interrupting her workday. She recently spent a large amount of money buying "cuter" clothes that she thinks might appeal to him. Dan, however, seems to be increasingly short with her. She is afraid he is getting bored. As Betsy is talking, Dr. Collins initially listens intently and asks clarifying questions. Yet when she tries to gently raise questions about whether Dan is a good choice, Betsy responds irritably, saying that Dr. Collins "just doesn't understand" how important Dan is to her. As Dr. Collins's supervisor, you think that Betsy is probably speaking to Dr. Collins in a similar way to how she speaks with her mother.

You give Dr. Collins feedback that she seems to be reluctant to challenge Betsy's excessive investment in getting Dan to like her. Dr. Collins considers this and admits that she does feel tentative around Betsy. She is both afraid of making Betsy angry and unsure of how much she should impose her negative opinion about the relationship with Dan on her patient. [**Decision Point 2**]

You counter that Dr. Collins should recognize that she may have a responsibility to point out when the choices that Betsy is making (e.g., Dan) are unhealthy—much like an internist would recommend that a diabetic patient stay away from sugar. You propose that Dr. Collins would feel more confident telling Betsy her opinion about her workplace romance if Dr. Collins would explain why she disapproves. You ask her to outline her thoughts on this subject before you and Dr. Collins meet again. Dr. Collins returns having outlined several reasons why she does not think this romance is a good idea: it violates important workplace boundaries, it preoccupies Betsy to the point that she is falling behind on her work, it is a way to avoid becoming independent that will fuel her self-hate, and it is encouraging her habit of overspending. Plus, her boyfriend does not seem to be treating her that well. [**Decision Point 3**]

You suggest that Dr. Collins help Betsy keep a focus on making progress toward her own stated goals. Betsy sought therapy hoping to feel less insecure yet is embroiled in a relationship that diminishes her self-esteem and fuels her fears of rejection. Betsy wants to get married and have a family, but by virtue of sacrificing her self-care, she makes herself unappealing as a long-term partner.

After discussing in supervision the discrepancy between Betsy's goals and her behavior, Dr. Collins feels emboldened to raise some of her own concerns. She points out to Betsy that she is overaccommodating to Dan and therefore damaging her own self-respect. She also encourages Betsy to develop female friendships. Together they come up with a plan for Betsy to join a book club. When you next review a videotaped therapy session, you notice that Dr. Collins is more active in steering the content of the session. Notably, although Betsy persists in wanting to talk about Dan,

Dr. Collins interrupts this to point out that her preoccupation with him is at the expense of her own growth. She inquires about the book club and then notes how Betsy's failure to follow through on this departs from their plan. Betsy seems irritated but also shamed.

Over the next several months, Dr. Collins tells you that she feels increasingly connected to and affectionate toward Betsy. Her appreciation for Betsy's sense of humor has grown, as has her understanding of just how toxic Betsy feels. She updates the case formulation to include the fact that Betsy is repulsed by how angry and jealous she can become, especially with her family. She is afraid to assert herself with other people (e.g., Dan) for fear that what she perceives to be her ugly, angry self will show through and she will then be abandoned.

Dr. Collins formulates the interpretation that Betsy's sense of being "bad" is fueling her reluctance to assert herself more with her boyfriend, and she tells Betsy that give-and-take, including disagreements and criticisms, is part of healthy relationships. Over the next several months, she works with Betsy to call her mother less, socialize more, and set better boundaries with her boyfriend. She also helps Betsy curb her spending and sell some of her extra clothing online.

As her supervisor, you tell Dr. Collins she is doing a good job. Dr. Collins tells Betsy that she is proud of the progress she is making. When Betsy learns that her older sister is pregnant, Dr. Collins voices her fear that this will trigger jealousy and could lead to excess spending or maybe even self-harm. Betsy is not interested in talking much about this and professes to be happy for her sister. Dr. Collins does not press the point any further.

Shortly afterward, Dr. Collins asks for your help in filling out forms to help Betsy reenroll in her health insurance. When you inquire further, Dr. Collins tells you that Betsy has been increasingly contacting her between sessions for help interfacing with agencies such as her credit card company, her cell phone carrier, and now the insurance company. Dr. Collins tells you that she would ordinarily not get involved in a patient's life in this way but says that she has done this with Betsy because she thinks such case management activities are a valued aspect of what she has learned about the GPM approach. You ask Dr. Collins how she feels about Betsy's requests for assistance. She admits that they have becoming trying and time-consuming. When Dr. Collins has tried to discuss these requests in session, Betsy gets angry with Dr. Collins's questioning her need for assistance. Betsy tells Dr. Collins, "I already feel bad enough about not being able to complete these tasks. I just wish you would help me without rubbing my nose in it." Dr. Collins sheepishly tells you that she at first felt guilty, but now she is starting to feel "a little bit resentful." She is also confused because Betsy had seemed so organized and on top of activities like this earlier in their treatment. Betsy recently asked if they could meet twice weekly, and Dr. Collins wonders if it would be a good idea to do this so that they can work on these logistical tasks within sessions. [**Decision Point 4**]

You immediately validate Dr. Collins's feelings of resentment, pointing out that the requests Betsy is making are particularly irritating because Dr.

Collins believes the patient can do them herself. She tells you that your validation is a relief and describes how uncomfortable it feels to be angry with a person who is a patient that she generally really likes and feels protective of. You also tell Dr. Collins that her instinctive conscientiousness has not served her well—she has failed to ask Betsy why these requests are coming up now and what they mean in interpersonal terms. As a GPM therapist, she should endeavor to be helpful, not to offer help without considering the implications. You ask Dr. Collins to consider the case further and develop an interpersonal formulation of what is going on for Betsy.

At your next session, Dr. Collins appears uncharacteristically uncomfortable, shifting frequently in her seat as the two of you talk. When you ask whether something is bothering her, she confesses that she is confused by your instructions. She says that you told her to actually get involved with helping Betsy lead a better life outside of treatment, but after doing this she now feels like she is being chastised for not holding firmer boundaries. [**Decision Point 5**]

You tell Dr. Collins that you are glad she expressed her confusion and that you can see the role you played in it. You clarify that working with Betsy to secure health insurance coverage or manage her credit card bills might in fact under some circumstances be essential case management work. The problem here is that Dr. Collins is doing work she has good reason to believe Betsy has been and could be doing herself. Moreover, she has not explored what it means and has not used supervision to discuss this important activity. You remind Dr. Collins that, according to the construct of interpersonal hypersensitivity, patients with BPD cannot tolerate a perceived withdrawal of support. They panic and attempt to replace that support, often resorting to self-defeating or self-destructive methods. Thus, Betsy must be asking for help because she feels under threat of abandonment. Is Betsy seeking additional caretaking because she feels somehow displaced by her sister's pregnancy? Does she feel uncertain of her relationship with Dr. Collins and in need of a way to judge whether her doctor really cares? Is she seeking additional attention from Dr. Collins to help her tolerate less frequent contact with Dan and her mother?

Dr. Collins admits that Betsy's casual reaction to her sister's pregnancy may have been too good to be true. After discussing the situation with you, Dr. Collins worries that she may have been too quick to praise Betsy's "progress" in expressing support for her sister. You agree that this may have increased Betsy's reluctance to directly express anger or jealousy and caused her to fear rejection from Dr. Collins if her shameful reaction were found out. You regret that, as her supervisor, you did not pick up on the unlikelihood of Betsy's stated acceptance of her sister's pregnancy and did not encourage Dr. Collins to question this at the time. You tell Dr. Collins that, rather than adding a second weekly session, she should first talk to Betsy about what prompts her intersession requests for help.

Over the next several weeks, Dr. Collins brings up the issue of intersession contact repeatedly with Betsy. At first, Betsy just expresses shame at her behavior and promises to stop it immediately. Keeping in mind her recent supervisory session, Dr. Collins tells Betsy that she is sure there are good reasons why she needs more support and offers the suggestion that Betsy might be more jealous of her sister than she is able to admit. Gradually, Betsy becomes more willing to engage in the conversation. She tells Dr. Collins that not only is she jealous of her sister, but because her mother is preoccupied by the forthcoming grandchild, Betsy is worried about losing her place as the baby of the family. Her mother is so excited that Betsy fears she will be forgotten. Betsy says she feared Dr. Collins would be disappointed with her for reverting to old behavior and "not acting like an adult."

Dr. Collins tells you that although she was uncertain about helping Betsy, her inherent reluctance to anger her patients made it hard for her to question Betsy's requests. It was also hard for her to persist in her questioning when Betsy expressed shame—she had to wrestle with feeling that she was being cruel or rubbing Betsy's face in something embarrassing. She eventually found it very rewarding when Betsy opened up more about her jealousy and her fears.

As your supervision progresses, Dr. Collins becomes more comfortable predicting what will help Betsy feel better and what will stress her out. She needs less prompting to confront Betsy about her avoidance or her dependent behavior. She is able to make real progress with helping Betsy rely less on her mother and her boyfriend by enriching her social circle more. Similarly, as her supervisor, you learn to anticipate when Dr. Collins's instinctive reserve is an asset or when you should recommend she be more challenging. She has gotten more comfortable expressing confusion or requesting clarification immediately if something you say is unclear. Six months into supervision, you and Dr. Collins both feel more confident in her ability to be a useful therapist to Betsy and to subsequent patients with BPD.

Decision Points: Alternative Responses

Rate each response in terms of its level of helpfulness with a rating of 1 (will be helpful), 2 (possibly helpful, continuing reservations), or 3 (not helpful—or even harmful).

1. To help Dr. Collins establish a GPM framework for her therapy with Betsy, you should

   A. Instruct her to review the diagnostic criteria for BPD and the construct of interpersonal hypersensitivity with Betsy.
   B. Direct Dr. Collins to obtain additional developmental history before proceeding with treatment.
   C. Instruct Dr. Collins to negotiate a treatment contract, including an agreement not to self-injure or binge and purge.
   D. Encourage Dr. Collins to actively focus on Betsy's situational stressors.
   E. Recommend that Dr. Collins urge Betsy to enter group therapy.

2. In response to Dr. Collins's reservations about voicing her disapproval of Betsy's romance with Dan, you should

   A. Respect Dr. Collins's wish not to give direct advice but encourage her to ask more challenging questions that will bring the relationship's limitations to light.
   B. Explain to Dr. Collins that her choice to avoid a conflict with Betsy is problematic.
   C. Tell Dr. Collins that you are disappointed that she is not willing to be more directive with Betsy.

3. In response to Dr. Collins's rationale for stating her negative opinion on Betsy's romance, you

   A. Share your opinion that Betsy's boyfriend is exploiting her need for acceptance.
   B. Advise Dr. Collins to question Betsy about whether Dan offers a reasonable pathway to attain a stable marriage and have children.

4. At this point, you can most effectively support Dr. Collins by

   A. Reminding her that therapy is difficult and taxing work that requires support when one gets angry with a patient.
   B. Helping Dr. Collins fill out the paperwork that Betsy sent.
   C. Asking Dr. Collins to take a step back to try to understand why Betsy has an increased need for intersession assistance.
   D. Inviting Dr. Collins to clarify the pros and cons of adding a second weekly session.

5. In response to Dr. Collins's confusion, you should

   A. Remind Dr. Collins that maintaining appropriate boundaries is an essential part of treating BPD and helping Betsy.
   B. Apologize and tell her you can understand why your messages seem contradictory.

Decision Points: Discussion

Numbers within brackets indicate level of helpfulness ratings.

1. To help Dr. Collins establish a GPM framework for her therapy with Betsy, you should

A. Instruct her to review the diagnostic criteria for BPD and the construct of interpersonal hypersensitivity with Betsy. [1] (GPM therapy builds from a shared understanding of the diagnosis of BPD and the ways in which interpersonal hypersensitivity predicts and explains behavior.)

B. Direct Dr. Collins to obtain additional developmental history before proceeding with treatment. [2] (Do not encourage history taking at the expense of addressing Betsy's current life stressors, especially her important relationships. The fact that she is seeking help probably means she has a current interpersonal stressor.)

C. Instruct Dr. Collins to negotiate a treatment contract, including an agreement not to self-injure or binge and purge. [3] (GPM argues for taking up the issue of self-destructive behavior as part of the treatment, rather than prenegotiating a treatment contract about this or other issues.)

D. Encourage Dr. Collins to actively focus on Betsy's situational stressors. [1] (Fourth-year residents who typically have been trained in psychodynamic psychotherapy will not have been encouraged to be as active, directive, and case-management focused as in GPM.)

E. Recommend that Dr. Collins urge Betsy to enter group therapy. [3] (Groups are certainly a desirable part of many GPM treatments, but you and Dr. Collins do not yet have enough information about Betsy and her social handicaps to make such a recommendation at this time. It would be particularly useful for her to be aware of how and why she has struggled to have friends.)

2. In response to Dr. Collins's reservations about voicing her disapproval of Betsy's romance with Dan, you should

A. Respect Dr. Collins's wish not to give direct advice but encourage her to ask more challenging questions that will bring the relationship's limitations to light. [2] (Asking questions that will help Betsy see the problems in the relationship with Dan is a good strategy. However, in contrast to more traditional psychodynamic therapies, GPM encourages therapists to use their experience and wisdom to give advice. This is much like doctors would in other specialties. If Betsy gets angry, as she did, then that becomes a potentially valuable issue that needs to be addressed. In that case it might lead to productive insights about her hostile and dependent relationship with her mother.)

   B. Explain to Dr. Collins that her choice to avoid a conflict with Betsy is problematic. [1] (Dr. Collins may lose credibility if she does not voice disapproval of this relationship and the relationship subsequently goes poorly [which is likely]. Betsy's wish to please Dan exemplifies how Betsy seeks care from other people at the expense of her self-reliance and self-respect. Dr. Collins's relationship with Betsy will become healthier if she can express disagreement and then show Betsy how she can manage anger.)

   C. Tell Dr. Collins that you are disappointed that she is not willing to be more directive with Betsy. [3] (This statement is too shaming to be helpful. It is understandable for someone at Dr. Collins's stage in training to be reluctant to make judgments about the viability of a patient's relationship. She may have been taught that it would be incorrect to share her opinion on the matter. You want to help Dr. Collins feel more confident in giving her patient advice.)

3. In response to Dr. Collins's rationale for stating her negative opinion about Betsy's romance, you

   A. Share your opinion that Betsy's boyfriend is exploiting her need for acceptance. [2] (This interpretation may be true and useful for Betsy to understand, but it runs the risk of being harmful. For Betsy to blame Dan or to feel victimized would be less helpful than taking responsibility for abdicating her self-respect in order for her to attain a potential caretaker.)

   B. Advise Dr. Collins to question Betsy about whether Dan offers a reasonable pathway to attain a stable marriage and have children. [1] (This approach reminds Betsy of her goals but then invites Betsy to look into the many risky and potentially self-damaging aspects—which Dr. Collins is clearly very aware of—in regard to Betsy's relationship with Dan.)

4. At this point, you can most effectively support Dr. Collins by

   A. Reminding her that therapy is difficult and taxing work that requires support when one gets angry with a patient. [3] (You should validate Dr. Collins's resentment toward Betsy, but Dr. Collins needs help in managing Betsy's requests better. Most critically, Dr. Collins has not explored the stressors [probably interpersonal] that prompt Betsy's problematic behavior. You need to help her address this.)

B. Helping Dr. Collins fill out the paperwork that Betsy sent. [3] Doing so would miss an important opportunity to address how Dr. Collins's request for help overlooks her feelings of frustration—just as Betsy's requests for added help probably do. Moreover, helping Dr. Collins reinforces her sense of inadequacy just as Dr. Collins's helping Betsy would reinforce the patient's inadequacy.)

C. Asking Dr. Collins to take a step back to try to understand why Betsy has an increased need for intersession assistance. [1] (GPM suggests that the onset of a symptom is usually prompted by interpersonal adversities, such as Betsy's problems with anger [e.g., her jealousy of her sister] and her loss of interpersonal supports. This is important; trainees often react to the particular problem at hand without remembering to use their case formulation.)

D. Inviting Dr. Collins to clarify the pros and cons of adding a second weekly session. [2] (Making a list of pros and cons is a useful way to approach a difficult decision, but, as noted, you and Dr. Collins first need to figure out what is driving Betsy's request. As a general rule, GPM would not advocate a second weekly session unless a patient is using therapy uncommonly well.)

5. In response to Dr. Collins's confusion, you should

A. Remind Dr. Collins that maintaining appropriate boundaries is an essential part of treating BPD and helping Betsy. [3] (This is true but will only aggravate Dr. Collins's feelings of not being understood. It is more important to address the confusion of Dr. Collins and the inconsistency of your message.)

B. Apologize and tell her you can understand why your messages seem contradictory. [1] (This response recognizes your contribution to Dr. Collins's confusion and validates her complaint. It also models the way a GPM therapist should "lean in" to a patient's disapproval and readily acknowledge one's own contribution.)

Conclusion

In this chapter, we identify the distinctive features of GPM that require psychodynamic supervisors to make adaptations in order to train their students. A GPM supervisor, in particular, should endeavor to increase a sense of optimism and comfort in treating BPD. He or she should not only teach the principles of GPM but also exemplify the GPM approach by being active, thoughtful, flexible, pragmatic, and ready to acknowledge mistakes. Being a GPM supervisor, just like being a "good enough" GPM therapist, relies heavily on common sense and a strong knowledge base about BPD. The case vignette illustrates how supervisors need to make sure supervisees know about the role of genetics in BPD and its expected course of improvement and then communicate this to their patients with BPD. Supervisees are directed to recognize that when symptoms recur, they are triggered by adverse interpersonal events, and they are expected to actively search for interpersonal stressors. The vignette also illustrates the use of giving supervisees homework, just as GPM therapists are encouraged to give homework to patients.

It is important for modern psychotherapy supervisors to learn how to teach GPM. It is simply not feasible without standard training programs to teach the specialist modules such as dialectical behavior therapy, mentalization-based treatment, or transference-focused psychotherapy (Bernanke and McCommon 2018; Choi-Kain et al. 2016). They require too much time. In contrast, training supervisees in GPM is feasible, but to do so requires adjustments in standard psychotherapy supervision (Bernanke and McCommon 2018). These adjustments are significant but are quite consistent with the good psychiatric management that needs to be taught in emergency departments, hospitals, diagnostic evaluations, and consultation services.

For psychiatry residents, GPM comfortably incorporates medication management. This is important given that most psychiatrists are primarily involved in medication management (Mojtabai and Olfson 2010). With adjustments similar to those outlined for psychiatry supervisors, supervisors in medication clinics can also teach GPM.

In a recent article, Bernanke and McCommon (2018) pointed out that teaching GPM fulfills the requirements of the Accreditation Council for Graduate Medical Education. Specifically, GPM fulfills the requirement for training in supportive psychotherapy while building on the learning otherwise received in psychodynamic therapy and, we would add, in case management.

As noted in the introduction, clinicians who see the value of teaching GPM but feel inadequately trained to do so with confidence need to become familiar with and knowledgeable about GPM. We have two suggestions. First, clinicians who have already had extensive experience managing patients with BPD will likely find by reading the GPM handbook (Gunderson and Links 2014) that they are already, albeit unwittingly, competent to teach other clinicians their version of GPM. GPM is above all a distillation of clinical experience, and experienced clinicians usually feel their practices are validated (Keuroghlian et al. 2016). Even these clinicians will probably have refinements to their practices after becoming familiar with GPM. Second, for supervisors who have been immersed in psychodynamic therapy or who do not have much case management experience with patients with BPD, attending a GPM workshop will quickly help shift their attitudes (e.g., if a patient isn't getting better, this needs to be marked and explained) and their supervisory techniques (e.g., tell their trainees to convey their knowledge base to share their practical advice). GPM workshops are about to become available online without charge (see Appendix A, "Additional Resources"; http://hms.harvard.edu/BPD). Supervisors who want to teach GPM or students who want to learn GPM are encouraged to make use of this resource.

References

Bernanke J, McCommon B: Training in good psychiatric management for borderline personality disorder in residency: an aide to learning supportive psychotherapy for challenging-to-treat patients. Psychodyn Psychiatry 46(2):181–200, 2018 29809114

Choi-Kain LW, Albert EB, Gunderson JG: Evidence-based treatments for borderline personality disorder: implementation, integration, and stepped care. Harv Rev Psychiatry 24(5):342–356, 2016 27603742

Cowdry RW, Gardner DL: Pharmacotherapy of borderline personality disorder. Alprazolam, carbamazepine, trifluoperazine, and tranylcypromine. Arch Gen Psychiatry 45(2):111–119, 1988 3276280

Gunderson JG, Choi-Kain LW: Medication management for patients with borderline personality disorder. Am J Psychiatry 175(8):709–711, 2018 30064243

Gunderson JG, Links PS: Handbook of Good Psychiatric Management for Borderline Personality Disorder. Washington, DC, American Psychiatric Publishing, 2014

Keuroghlian AS, Palmer BA, Choi-Kain LW, et al: The effect of attending good psychiatric management (GPM) workshops on attitudes toward patients with borderline personality disorder. J Pers Disord 30(4):567–576, 2016 26111249

Mojtabai R, Olfson M: National trends in psychotropic medication polypharmacy in office-based psychiatry. Arch Gen Psychiatry 67(1):26–36, 2010 20048220

PART III

Implementation and Integration

Chapter 11

Implementation of Good Psychiatric Management in 10 Sessions

Patrick Charbon, M.D.

Ueli Kramer, Ph.D.

Jessica Droz, M.D.

Stéphane Kolly, M.D.

For many years, borderline personality disorder (BPD) has been considered a long-term debilitating disorder with little improvement expected from treatment. In the 1990s, however, dialectical behavior therapy

(DBT) showed evidence of therapeutic effects after a 1-year period (Linehan et al. 1993). Other therapeutic modalities (transference-focused and mentalization-based treatments) have since shown evidence of efficacy as well (e.g., Bateman and Fonagy 2001; Clarkin et al. 2001). Most of these studies have demonstrated effects using multiple intensive sessions per week over the course of 1 or more years, so they are quite rigorous and demanding on both the clinician and the patient. The time frame of 1 year is more pragmatic because of research funding and feasibility. In fact, it is probable that certain types of progress should be expected within this relatively brief time frame, whereas other types of progress may necessitate a lengthier treatment (Choi-Kain et al. 2010; Tracie Shea et al. 2009; Zanarini et al. 2010). For example, impulsivity symptoms remit in a shorter time frame than affective temperamental symptoms (Zanarini et al. 2016).

A limitation of these evidence-based treatments is that they require highly skilled and trained therapists, as well as highly motivated patients and therapists, making the treatments difficult to implement and accessible only to select patients and therapists. Accessibility and generalizability are priorities of treatments using good psychiatric management (GPM) principles (Gunderson 2016).

Short-term treatments for BPD have been used across different contexts using several therapeutic models. A particularly well-studied population for brief treatments is adolescents (Chanen and McCutcheon 2013; Chanen et al. 2007b, 2008). This population is at higher risk of poor psychosocial functioning than patients with Axis I pathology (Chanen et al. 2007a). Furthermore, for many patients with BPD, heavy use of psychiatric resources (two or more sessions per week) and medications may have already started by the time they reach their 20s (Zanarini et al. 2001). Early and time-limited interventions for subsyndromal or full-blown BPD have demonstrated a reduction in psychopathology, including parasuicide, and improvement at 24-month follow-up (Chanen and McCutcheon 2013).

Brief treatments lasting between 1 and 3 months for adult BPD show a partial regression of symptoms across different domains (i.e., mood, emotion dysregulation, subjective stress, parasuicidality, maladaptive behavior), but functional impairment and a low quality of life persist (Gratz et al. 2006). A brief version of the DBT skills group component over 20 weeks demonstrated sustained (i.e., >32 weeks) reductions in anger and distress tolerance and improvement in emotion regulation (McMain et al. 2017). A 3-week intensive suicidality-focused DBT treatment for suicidal patients had a significant effect on the reduction of hopelessness (McQuillan et al. 2005). These studies' findings indicate that short time-focused interventions may be helpful in reducing impulsivity-related symptoms as well as in improving some aspects of patients' relationships. This is not surprising, because impulsivity and relational difficulties can be diminished with detailed diagnostic disclosure and psychoeducation (Zanarini and Frankenburg 2008).

A 10-Session Brief GPM Intervention: From Diagnosis to Psychotherapy

This chapter describes our experience with GPM brief interventions for BPD in a psychiatric outpatient university clinic in Lausanne, Switzerland. Switzerland has a strong tradition of integrating psychiatry with psychotherapy. Since the 1950s, the title of a psychiatrist is both "psychiatrist and psychotherapist" and requires double training. This integrative tradition also applies to integration of different theories and approaches. Most institutional consultation centers offer a great variety of psychotherapeutic approaches: psychodynamic, cognitive, behavioral, family systemic, and humanistic. Our team is interdisciplinary and composed of nurses, social workers, medical residents, and psychologists. Psychologists and medical doctors learn psychotherapy and psychiatry in our department. As a public outpatient clinic, it serves the general population. Our short-term GPM-based service is integrated in a non-BPD-specialized general setting, and our work has to be intelligible for other specialized partners in the institution.

GPM fits perfectly within this context because it is transmittable and accessible to residents, nurses, and social workers and is thus a useful tool to provide coherence to a multidisciplinary team (Kramer et al. 2017a). In Switzerland, it corresponds to the concept of integrated psychotherapeutic psychiatric treatment (IPPT), which is commonly used and accepted by insurance companies and medical administrations. IPPT includes pragmatic interventions that draw inspiration from psychotherapy theories and psychiatric guidelines. As such, it clearly differentiates itself from formal psychotherapy. IPPT represents the frame, whereas GPM can be a specialized clinical content. Because GPM is diagnostically oriented, it is easily accepted in a general psychiatric context, where it becomes a useful tool to foster both a psychosocial and a relational understanding.

A large number of psychotherapists do private practice in Lausanne, and patients are referred because they require a specialized treatment or an interdisciplinary or crisis intervention. Given this context, the consulting patients tend to have a mix of psychiatric problems and social impairments. Most of them are referred to the outpatient clinic by a first-line service (e.g., emergency service, psychiatric first-line facilities, hospital, other specialized services). We treat patients ages 18–65 years. Some patients with BPD who come to our clinic have been previously informed about a personality disorder diagnosis (or a suspicion thereof), usually without much explanation about the diagnosis or its impact on their life.

Over the past years, by trying to respond to an increasing demand in the community for appropriate treatment, we have started offering a brief intervention for all outpatients as part of a stepped care approach. Generally speaking, brief interventions may represent a useful public health intervention by giving access to more available time-limited treatments. They give the opportunity for more patients to be treated in a "good enough" initial treatment. This seems to have specific advantages for patients with BPD.

More specifically, for patients with BPD, a time-limited therapeutic proposition has the advantages of focusing on treatment goals and avoiding treatments that go on and on without a clear time frame. This prevents the scattering of therapeutic efforts and unrealistic expectations, such as the constant availability of the therapist, which can perpetuate a lack of change. Instead, time-limited interventions imply an anticipated separation and thus activate abandonment anxiety and rejection sensitivity that will be manifest during the 10 sessions and that can then be addressed and discussed within the framework of interpersonal hypersensitivity (Gunderson and Lyons-Ruth 2008).

Our structured 10-session intervention helps patients with BPD to move from a state of chaotic painful feelings, often caused by perceived rejection from caretakers, to a state where they can have a better understanding of their problems. Patients with BPD can then formulate a more coherent therapeutic plan, which is generally associated with a greater motivation to change. Our 10-session intervention also helps to establish a BPD diagnosis in situations in which many clinicians avoid it because they believe it is premature to disclose a BPD diagnosis during a relational crisis or in which they mistakenly think another diagnosis (DSM-5; American Psychiatric Association 2013) is the main diagnosis (including in patients whose other pathology is seen as resistant to treatment; Zimmerman and Mattia 1999). Failure to give the diagnosis of BPD is often the result of insufficient information or fear of stigma (Sisti et al. 2016).

What Is the 10-Session Intervention?

The 10-session intervention is a GPM-inspired, time-limited, personality disorder–oriented intervention that can be used as either a specialized assessment or a brief therapy. The goals of the intervention are to actively involve the patient in understanding the diagnostic process, to introduce psychoeducation progressively, and to promote mentalization. Therefore, across the intervention, the diagnostic process shifts from the imposition of a medical "expert" point of view to the proposal of an active collaboration and thinking about each patient's actual problems and needs.

Structured tools (e.g., Structured Clinical Interview for DSM-5 Personality Disorders [SCID-5-PD; First et al. 2016]) are used to foster the patient's awareness and active collaboration. Comorbidities are discussed, first as they may require specific treatment, and second as they may represent a future threat to the treatment. Psychoeducation and the patient's integration of the links between symptoms and his or her life problems help to motivate and structure the request for a future treatment. Developing an interpersonal alliance, containing abandonment anxiety, exploring problems, and psychoeducation can be done without being excessively supportive. On the contrary, the patient's recognition of problems may foster the process of collaboration and the crucial therapeutic alliance.

In regard to interpersonal hypersensitivity (Gunderson and Lyons-Ruth 2008), one can predict that a brief intervention, because it is explicitly time limited, will evoke in the patient feelings of abandonment and/or rejection and may eventually activate pathological attachment processes, manifested as excessive calls, suicidal threats, and the like. As these behaviors emerge and become activated, we believe that they become accessible to early change if the therapist constructively addresses them. This intervention is intended to be a short-term specialized treatment and should be developed in that direction.

As we have a broad spectrum of patients with BPD, we have tried to fine-tune our 10-session interventions depending on the needs of the patient. The choice between one intervention and another is made during the first session (Table 11–1).

We differentiate between two different types of 10-session interventions with distinct clinical consequences: the 10-session assessment and the 10-session therapy (Table 11–1). Both involve once-weekly sessions. The 10-session assessment is helpful in establishing a well-informed treatment plan, whereas the 10-session therapy is used as a brief structured intervention for acute symptom management and solution-oriented treatment.

The 10-Session Assessment

The 10-session assessment is a time-limited global evaluation for patients with BPD who have impeded social functioning or longer-evolving symptoms. This intervention aims to establish a well-informed treatment plan, by integrating diagnostics in a therapeutically oriented hierarchy and establishing a therapeutic frame that takes into account comorbid diagno-

TABLE 11–1. **Two versions of 10-session good psychiatric management: assessment and therapy**

	10-Session assessment	10-Session therapy
Indications	Patients with acute or long-term symptoms, comorbidities, and maladaptive behaviors leading to social functioning impairment	Patients with acute symptoms or crisis symptoms who have enough psychological motivation and do not want to engage in a long psychiatric treatment
Goals	Propose an adequate treatment as needed	Avoid becoming a chronic psychiatric patient
Abandonment fears and rejection sensitivity	Mostly documented while exploring the patient's history and actual real-life relations	Mostly manifested toward the therapy frame and primary clinician
Work on interpersonal relationships	Exploring relationships in the assessment may be helpful to prevent dropout	Exploring relationships in the therapy may be helpful to prevent dropout
	Exploring real life, work, relations, previous treatments provides examples for psychoeducation about interpersonal hypersensitivity	Exploring relationships in therapy provides examples for psychoeducation about interpersonal hypersensitivity
Use of psychoeducation	Fosters engagement in future treatment and alliance	Provides a canvas for future self-help or to improve use of care

ses, relational contexts, and existing therapeutic networks (Table 11–2). It fosters a better comprehension of the role of BPD pathology in resistance to well-administered treatments of comorbid pathology and more generally to factors adverse to therapeutic progress.

This assessment is indicated for patients with severe or complex BPD pathology with comorbidities, which may be frequently misdiagnosed. Such misdiagnosis would likely prevent amelioration of comorbid pathology and positive treatment outcomes. The aim of the 10-session assessment

TABLE 11–2. Goals of 10-session assessment

1.	Diagnostic	Identify personality disorders (including in patients receiving only Axis I treatment without sufficient amelioration) and comorbid pathology, with use of reality-focused multimodal assessment.
2.	Psychopathological working hypothesis	Produce an articulated framework for future treatment, integrating and hierarchizing primary, secondary, and comorbid problems (e.g., depression, posttraumatic stress disorder).
3.	Personalized treatment indication (stepped care)	Offer a coherent treatment, integrating diagnosis, motivation, and potential obstacles to treatment.
4.	Therapeutic alliance	Promote the patient's motivation for change and valuation of treatment.

is prevention of inadequate or excessive use of highly specialized treatments and promotion of selective use of long-term resources. It is useful for diagnosing comorbidity, which is crucial to successful psychotherapeutic treatment. It is also aimed at giving a precise indication of treatment needs and goals.

The 10-session assessment facilitates orientation to an adapted treatment, such as the stepped care model (see Appendix B; Choi-Kain et al. 2016). This practice favors adequate use of limited therapeutic resources. This 10-session assessment is easy to implement in a medically oriented psychiatric institution and can be understood as a pretreatment that can prepare the patient for longer-term treatment when indicated.

Case Vignette 1: The 10-Session Assessment

Colleen is a 30-year-old patient who was discharged from her first inpatient treatment a week prior to her consultation with an outpatient therapist. She had never been diagnosed with a psychiatric disorder, but she reported that she had been using marijuana for several years. She had split up with her boyfriend 6 months before the consultation and said that she had just gone through a "rough" year. She was admitted to the hospital because of suicidal threats in the context of intense arguments with her ex-boyfriend. She reported to the therapist that when she smoked marijuana, she experienced increased well-being and release of internal tensions; reduction of sleep and increased mental and physical activity; and increased impulsivity and irritability in interpersonal contexts (mostly with her boyfriend). On the basis of this clinical presentation, the therapist diagnosed Colleen with bipolar affective disorder, which the patient initially rejected but then accepted in a quite convinced, almost rigid, manner.

Colleen came to the first interview with the outpatient therapist and declared that she had "bipolar disorder" and had been told she needed to see a psychiatrist for the monitoring of her lamotrigine treatment. She declared that she was not interested in "spending too much time talking about her life." The therapist expressed some astonishment and invited Colleen to elaborate a bit on her life, at which point Colleen started to cry. She mentioned being at the end of her rope and now being psychiatrically ill on top of that. Everything seemed lost. She had lost her job and her boyfriend through an interpersonal crisis that had led her to the inpatient treatment. She said, "I am 30 and I feel like I have no future. Who will ever want to be in a relationship with me when I am bipolar and will have to take meds for the rest of my life? All my friends have stable relationships.... Why won't it work out for me? Honestly, I still think about killing myself."

A 10-session assessment was offered to Colleen at the end of the initial session. The therapist made the following suggestion:

> I can see that your suffering is immense. There are still areas we have not completely understood. How is it that you were able to function fairly well over the years in a quite stable relationship and then after this relationship ended, you stumbled and got diagnosed with "bipolar disorder"? I want both of us to keep searching for the best explanation for your psychological difficulties, and I am not sure for now what the best diagnosis is. We will use these 10 sessions to clarify this. Is that okay for you?

The process of assessment was informed by GPM principles and involved a specific focus on the differential diagnosis between bipolar disorder and BPD. Two sessions (out of 10) were dedicated to clarifying the symptoms and case history to find out that the so-called manic symptoms were being induced by heavy marijuana consumption, which had increased as a consequence of Colleen's feeling rejected by her ex-boyfriend. In subsequent sessions, it emerged that Colleen in reality presented with the clinical features of BPD, with intense fear of abandonment, identity problems, marked impulsivity patterns, suicidal threats, and several affective symptoms. At the final session of the brief intervention, therapist and patient discussed this diagnosis while acknowledging that the inpatient team seemed to have misdiagnosed the patient's condition. Explaining the misdiagnosis represented a particularly challenging clinical dilemma.

> Clinician: You know, a diagnosis helps us to bring together and understand all the problems you describe. On the basis of your descriptions, we can say that the acceleration of your thoughts and behaviors was induced by your marijuana

consumption. You smoked much more during these past months because you had an internal feeling of not existing anymore, of having no future, and of being left alone by your boyfriend and by everybody else, including your parents and your friends. Is this correct?

Colleen: Yes, absolutely.

Clinician: So, it is unclear whether the diagnosis of bipolar disorder that you were given is accurate.

Colleen: Are you saying that I am not bipolar? I can't believe it. Everybody tells me I'm bipolar and that I need to take that medication all my life now.

Clinician: Yes, I understand that my colleagues at the hospital made the hypothesis that you may suffer from bipolar disorder. But remember, we took several sessions here to really find out what the core problems are, and they turned out to be inconsistent with bipolar disorder.

Colleen: I am so lost.... [cries] This is so confusing.

Clinician: Yes, this does seem a bit confusing, and I understand that you want to know what you suffer from. [The therapist reviews all of Colleen's borderline symptoms again in detail.] So, based on all of this, a diagnosis of borderline personality disorder (BPD) would actually better summarize these problems. Have you already heard of this diagnosis?"

Colleen: No, I am not sure.

Clinician: Well, it is a condition that may explain the problems you are experiencing—in particular why you are so sensitive to interpersonal rejection. It may also explain why it is so important for you to know what diagnosis you have, so you feel more confident about who you really are.

Colleen: Yes.

Clinician: And this condition *is* treatable. I want us now to think about what this may mean for your treatment from today on. The central treatment for overcoming problems related to BPD is psychotherapy, not medication. I will refer you to a colleague who offers specialized treatments for BPD and he, with you, will decide what themes you have to work on to get better and whether or not lamotrigine is still the appropriate medication. For now, I'd suggest you continue lamotrigine until you talk about it with him.

Colleen: You know what? I have talked to all these psychiatrists and nurses at the hospital, and everybody was trying to convince me that I am bipolar, but deep inside, I knew that label did not describe me. Then I came to see you, and you really understood me and gave me hope. I know that I can trust you now and that I can always come back to you if I have questions. Thank you so much.

Clinician: You are very welcome.

Colleen left the session relieved and started a structured psychotherapy 2 months later. Based on reports from her new therapist, we know that Colleen worked very hard in her psychotherapy, was committed to change, and per medical decision, stopped taking lamotrigine no more than 3 weeks later. She found a new job, worked through her abandonment issues, and was able to reclaim her life. No further inpatient treatment was necessary.

The 10-Session Therapy

The 10-session therapy is a time-limited intervention for patients with moderate, mild, or subsyndromal BPD symptoms and relatively good social functioning. It can be used as a brief structured intervention during a crisis when short-term intervention could be expected to prevent a symptomatic exacerbation.

There is an explicit agreement between patient and therapist that the therapy will stop after 10 sessions. The goal of a 10-session therapy should be to help patients better manage interpersonal relations by helping them avoid social isolation and its consequences and by promoting a better relational life with the help of psychoeducation focused on interpersonal hypersensitivity (Table 11–3). Adequate early short-term therapy may help reduce further relationship-induced problems and avoid use of harmful interventions (e.g., unnecessary medications). It is important to notice that symptoms most susceptible to being responsive to a short-term treatment are those frequently associated with the "bad reputation" of patients with BPD, such as self-harm and suicidality.

In the 10-session therapy setting, the predictable and imposed end-of-treatment separation is, according to interpersonal hypersensitivity theory, likely to induce feelings of abandonment and rejection in the patient, revealing emptiness and aloneness experiences. Maladaptive behaviors aimed at restoring attachment are likely to be manifest. This situation will require constant evaluation to determine whether the behaviors should be directly addressed to maintain the therapeutic movement because they could cause a premature end of therapeutic work and thus represent an actual threat to the treatment. Working through these potential relational crises can help patients with BPD link their symptoms to interpersonal stressors and thereby confirm what they have learned through psychoeducation based on interpersonal hypersensitivity. This therapeutic experience can help foster better affective and cognitive integration.

Comorbidities will be explored in a way to help the patient have a healthier life and seek specialized help if needed. Psychoeducation will be given in a way that can be integrated by the patient and used later. Explo-

TABLE 11–3.   Goals of 10-session therapy

1.	Clarification of medical diagnosis	Comprehend symptoms in medical terms, as well as links between BPD and real-life problems; explain false beliefs about BPD.
2.	Meaningful psychiatric diagnosis	Recognize links between borderline personality disorder diagnosis as a medical construct and the patient's real-life problems.
3.	Cognitive and affective integration of the diagnosis	Recognize importance of affective and cognitive integration of interpersonal hypersensitivity in patient's interpersonal life, outside and inside the therapy.
4.	Emphasize importance of adequate goals outside of therapy (e.g., work and love)	Comprehend and integrate good psychiatric management principles in real life.

Note.   BPD=borderline personality disorder.

ration and psychoeducation about comorbidities are supportive aspects of the 10-session GPM therapy.

Case Vignette 2:   10-Session Therapy

Paul is a 22-year-old engineering student. He moved from his parents' home 2 years ago to attend college. His studies are going well, and his goal for after graduation is to work with his father in his engineering consulting company. He was in a romantic relationship for a year with a young student he met at a party, but when he had a discussion with her about sharing an apartment, he had the feeling she started to progressively distance herself from him. He then expressed suicidal ideas and was so angry with her that he insulted her in front of her friends. He apologized 2 days later, but she said she never wanted to see him again.

After that, Paul drank heavily for a few days and realized one morning that he had driven home drunk after a party. Before that, Paul had consumed alcohol and cannabis only occasionally. He took some ecstasy one evening but did not want to take any after that. Afraid of his behavior, he made an appointment for psychiatric consultation at a student health clinic.

Paul explained that his girlfriend did not show any signs of joy when he suggested that they could share an apartment. He felt rejected when she answered her phone in his presence while he was expecting her to show feeling toward him. He immediately felt angry toward the friend who was calling her on the phone, feeling that she was more important to his girlfriend than he was.

Paul felt depressed but did not want any medication. He stayed with his parents for a week in a nearby city and rapidly got better. When he came back, he decided to stop meeting the psychologist, arguing that it would divert his attention and energy from his studies and that he wished to prepare for his exams. Later, he passed his exams and had another romantic relationship, although he felt that he did not invest as much in this relationship as in the previous one.

He went to a concert with a friend and saw his ex-girlfriend kissing another student. The next night, he texted her hateful and impolite messages and wrote a letter in which he accused her of being an evil person. He came back to consultation 10 months later and was admitted to our specialized unit. Paul said that he needed help but was afraid of being put on medication and did not want to become a psychiatric patient. Nevertheless, he wished he could speak to someone, because when he tries to talk about his problems to friends, and particularly about sad feelings and occasional suicidal thoughts, he feels like they distance themselves from him.

Paul: It's scary to think that I might have BPD.... I've heard that it's a chronic disease, and besides, it's always the bad guys in the movies who have it.

Clinician: It might be useful for you to have some information about the way BPD is understood today. First, BPD is a disorder that is likely to remit within 10 years. People with BPD usually get better when they understand the interpersonal sources of their symptoms. Some people with BPD then organize their lives so that they have fewer relational interactions and avoid interpersonal stress, which does not produce the best outcome.

Paul: You know, when I go out with friends, I very often come home earlier because I know that if I stay longer with them, I may become sad, angry...all sorts of things that I don't want to show my friends and that may provoke some interpersonal crisis. I want to become more comfortable and better able to enjoy spending time with my friends.

Clinician: You said before that you did not want to become a psychiatric patient, and I think this is very legitimate. On the other hand, having a little help can make your life easier. Getting help with your problems does not necessarily require long-term treatment.

The clinician then proposed a 10-session therapy. At the second session, the therapist took a brief personal history.

Clinician: We have quickly gone through your personal history, but I realize I do not know much about your emotional side.

Paul: I am not comfortable talking about my emotions and love life.... But in general, I'd say I am not too happy about either. When I have feelings for a girl, they are so strong that I cannot talk to my friends about them, so I usually end up keeping them to myself. Every time I want to confess my feelings to a girl, the same thing happens. As soon as she hears I have a crush on her, she pushes me away and avoids seeing me.

These sorts of situations make me think that I'm uninteresting and that no girl will ever like me.

Clinician: I would like to understand better how it feels to be in this situation when you try to share your strong feelings and feel rejected. [Paul becomes tense, sweats, and seems uncomfortable.]

Paul: In fact, I feel very angry when that happens to me. [Pause] You are going to think that I'm crazy, or that I'm a bad person. Probably you think, "Oh that guy is a nasty person with girls...." What are you thinking of me?

Clinician: I think I may understand what you are talking about—that you can have very strong feelings, sometimes so strong that you don't really know what to do with them, and that when you share these feelings you feel rejected, so much so that you become furious with the person whom you feel rejected by. And I am wondering if what you are speaking about is not happening right now between you and me: you feel rejected by me because you think I could have bad ideas about you.

Paul: This is what is happening now. I think you see me as a bad person.

Clinician: That very much reminds me of something we understand about painful relations that people with BPD can experience. It is called *interpersonal hypersensitivity*, and I think learning about it could help you understand how these feelings happen in your life, as has happened right now between you and me.

Suggested Interventions Within the 10-Session Model of GPM

We offer some specific interventions in this section. Clinicians should not expect to comply precisely with these formulations, but our information may be helpful as guidelines for some therapists.

Presenting the 10-Session Intervention to Other Professionals

The 10-session intervention is a specialized assessment or therapy that is aimed at documenting and informing the patient about his or her personality disorder and its consequences, as well as assessing potential comorbidities. It is also aimed at helping the patient have enough time during the intervention to understand and link the diagnosis of personality disorder with its life consequences. A 10-session intervention is time limited. It can be the only intervention or can lead to specialized treatment in our unit or in private practice.

Presenting the 10-Session Intervention to Patients

The 10-session intervention is not a usual medical process in which patients are passive and receive the diagnosis as a result of the doctor's work. In this intervention, you, the patient, will be the investigator, and the clinician will help you with that work through some structured and some less structured procedures. The aim of the 10-session intervention is to explore your personality functioning and the influence it may have on your life, the way you think, your behavior, and your relationships.

Content of the 10-Session Intervention: By Session

The 10-session intervention is a once-a-week multimodal approach with a primary clinician (medical doctor or psychologist). It is composed of some structured content (e.g., use of Mini-International Neuropsychiatric Interview [MINI; Lecrubier et al. 1997], SCID-5-PD [First et al. 2016]), some partly structured content (psychoeducation), and some less structured content (first session, exploration of relational conflicts).

First Session.   The aim of the first session is to meet the patient and explore his or her difficulties. The session is constructed around supportive and open-ended questions. The clinician actively investigates problems, with a focus on patterns of relational problems (private life, work, previous treatments). Repetitive alliance ruptures between the clinician and patient in this first session may indicate a major threat to continuing with further sessions and thus should be addressed. At the end of this session, a first rendition of the clinician's formulation of the patient's problems is offered, and the frame of the 10-session intervention and its content are set. If the proposition is a 10-session therapy, the clinician will announce that the remaining number of sessions will be exactly 9.

Further Sessions.   Further sessions follow GPM guidelines, and they are mostly centered on real life, relational crises, treatment breakdowns, and major changes in interests and goals. We use interpersonal hypersensitivity as a frame for investigation and, later on, for recovery and psychoeducation. Comorbidities and medical problems are rigorously investigated; a structured psychiatric interview (e.g., MINI, SCID-5-PD) may be used. It is particularly important to investigate topics some patients try to put aside, such as addictions, interpersonal issues, or economic problems, and important not to share the patient's denial of theses aspects. When useful, other professionals can participate in the investigation. We make extensive use of specialized resources (e.g., social workers, psychiatric nurses), including resources outside the unit (e.g., addressing addiction, attention-deficit/

hyperactivity disorder, trauma, migration). Families and relatives are frequently invited to be part of the process. Diagnostic disclosure and discussion are mandatory, integrated with discussion about the relationship between the patient's personality disorder and comorbidities and their effects on the patient's life. We discuss the diagnosis with the patient and sometimes the relatives (e.g., when a young patient is living with or dependent on parents). The goal is not only to deliver a medical diagnosis but also to build an individualized working hypothesis that integrates in a meaningful way the BPD diagnosis, comorbidities, and problems in real life. This formulation most of all must make sense for the patient.

Focus on Real Life. We are interested in the patient's daily life outside of treatment because it will provide a lot of information on social functioning (work, disability, schema use, autonomy) and interpersonal issues (conflicts, relational stressors, resources). A review of the patient's financial difficulties with a social worker helps us understand real-life problems and eventually provide specialized support.

Psychoeducation. Psychoeducation is used as a productive way to help the patient understand and reduce symptoms. It can be used in a supportive way, as something the patient can learn in a short time and find useful in real life. Psychoeducation enables the patient to make sense of clinical manifestations by throwing light on interpersonal and attachment conflicts. It helps establish hope that recovery is possible, even likely (Table 11–4).

Psychoeducation may also include explorations that show the importance of negative affects on real life, the ways in which "symptoms" can be used to justify a passive life, or the fact that externalizing problems or responsibilities on others is self-defeating. Psychoeducation helps prevent excessive hope regarding "passive" pharmacological treatment and helps to actively engage the patient in treatment.

Expectation of Change. Some improvement is expected quite early during intervention. We observe whether or not the patient uses early psychoeducation to promote some change, which reveals either motivation or resistance that should then be addressed. It is difficult to evaluate motivation for change in a few sessions, and a 10-session intervention may be long enough to evaluate whether a patient makes use of psychoeducation and what his or her potential is for active engagement in a future treatment.

Our clinical observations, supported by research reported in the section "Empirical Evidence," indicate that the most predictable changes in a 10-session GPM intervention are amelioration of self-harm behaviors, better recognition of the influence of interpersonal factors in symptoms,

---

TABLE 11–4.   Psychoeducation: content

---

1. Nature and natural course of borderline personality disorder
2. Interpersonal hypersensitivity and its consequences in real life
3. Importance of change in real life
4. Build a life, prioritizing work before romantic relationships
5. What helps and what does not (e.g., information on treatments, nonprofessional help, useful behaviors to prevent crisis)
6. Expectations about therapy and about medication

---

amelioration of subjective distress, and improved attitude toward treatment interventions.

Formulation of an Integrated Diagnostic and Working Hypothesis.
In the 10-session assessment, the goal of the formulation of a hypothesis is to inform the patient's decision either to engage in further treatment or to end treatment. We observe that some patients decide to go on with a treatment, inside or outside our institution, whereas others do not pursue more.

In the 10-session intervention, the goal is to give patients a meaningful understanding of their problems, especially of relational problems, in a way they can identify with and use later on with the goal of having a better life. More useful than the diagnosis itself is a working hypothesis, which combines BPD-specific contents (e.g., elements of interpersonal hypersensitivity), the relationship of BPD to comorbidities and to current problems, and the recognition of relational triggers in current crises and conflicts. This understanding is both cognitive (through psychoeducation) and emotional (through active exploration of relational problems in personal history or during the intervention).

Last Session.   The last session with the patient, sometimes accompanied by relatives, consists of a review of the assessment as made by the clinician and of what the patient has gained in knowledge about himself or herself. Clinician and patient make a joint decision to continue or end the intervention. At that point, goals and tools of additional treatment are discussed in detail.

Empirical Evidence

A series of studies empirically investigated whether a brief version of GPM relieves initial BPD symptoms. It was observed that the rate of change was greatest during the first 4 months of treatment (e.g., McMain et al. 2009).

In terms of pre/post changes on self-reported general symptoms (i.e., distress, interpersonal, social role domains), BPD symptoms, and interpersonal problems, we observed a medium pre/post effect for brief 10-session GPM in two distinct samples (total N=99; Kramer et al. 2011, 2014). In a randomized controlled trial, we studied whether the add-on component of an individualized case formulation consistent with the plan analysis method produced additional pre/post symptom decrease. The main analysis showed that this was the case only for general symptoms, not for the specific BPD symptoms (and only marginally for interpersonal problems). This result indicated that brief GPM is "good enough" for reducing initial BPD symptoms but may be improved on the more general levels of change in patients' distress. Interestingly, these differences did not hold up to the analysis at 6 months' follow-up, where the general symptom level improved on average to a similar extent in both conditions (Kramer et al. 2017c). Thus, the pattern of change found in another study (i.e., Mc-Main et al. 2009) was shown here: strong initial symptom decrease followed by a plateaued evolution over time. It is noteworthy that we found a marginal prediction between the treatment frequency and symptom decrease after 6 months of follow-up: the fewer sessions per week, the better the outcome. This surprising result may speak to a flexible approach in handling missing sessions in the very beginning of treatment for patients with BPD. Our in-depth process analyses yielded pre/post process ameliorations in the levels of emotional processing (Berthoud et al. 2017), coping effectiveness (Kramer et al. 2017b), and biased thinking (Keller et al. 2018), with some specific advantages in the prediction of outcome for the enhanced intervention component. Finally, we analyzed the therapist adherence to GPM principles, using the GPM Adherence Scale, and demonstrated high adherence; the level of adherence was linked with the symptom change at the end of brief GPM (Kolly et al. 2016), suggesting that the overall use of GPM stance may be a potential candidate for an effective intervention ingredient.

Conclusion

The 10-session GPM-based intervention can be conveniently integrated into a psychiatric outpatient organization. It is helpful to introduce psychotherapy along with psychiatric procedures and to organize care by providing coordination between different professions of different theoretical backgrounds. Short interventions aim to be cost-effective by offering a good enough treatment for most patients and avoiding excessive use of highly specialized treatments (and thus augmenting accessibility to patients who need them). A 10-session GPM-based intervention has a strong educational value and helps highly specialized clinicians to work with and transmit their experience to patients and trainees in a limited time.

References

American Psychiatric Association: Diagnostic and Statistical Manual of Mental Disorders, 4th Edition, Text Revision. Washington, DC, American Psychiatric Association, 2000

American Psychiatric Association: Diagnostic and Statistical Manual of Mental Disorders, 5th Edition. Arlington, VA, American Psychiatric Association, 2013

Bateman A, Fonagy P: Treatment of borderline personality disorder with psycho-analytically oriented partial hospitalization: an 18-month follow-up. Am J Psychiatry 158(1):36–42, 2001 11136631

Berthoud L, Pascual-Leone A, Caspar F, et al: Leaving distress behind: a randomized controlled study on change in emotional processing in borderline personality disorder. Psychiatry 80(2):139–154, 2017 28767333

Chanen AM, McCutcheon L: Prevention and early intervention for borderline personality disorder: current status and recent evidence. Br J Psychiatry Suppl 54:s24–s29, 2013 23288497

Chanen AM, Jovev M, Jackson HJ: Adaptive functioning and psychiatric symptoms in adolescents with borderline personality disorder. J Clin Psychiatry 68(2):297–306, 2007a 17335330

Chanen AM, McCutcheon LK, Jovev M, et al: Prevention and early intervention for borderline personality disorder. Med J Aust 187(7 suppl):S18–S21, 2007b 17908019

Chanen AM, Jackson HJ, McCutcheon LK, et al: Early intervention for adolescents with borderline personality disorder using cognitive analytic therapy: randomised controlled trial. Br J Psychiatry 193(6):477–484, 2008 19043151

Choi-Kain LW, Zanarini MC, Frankenburg FR, et al: A longitudinal study of the 10-year course of interpersonal features in borderline personality disorder. J Pers Disord 24(3):365–376, 2010 20545500

Choi-Kain LW, Albert EB, Gunderson JG: Evidence-based treatments for borderline personality disorder: implementation, integration, and stepped care. Harv Rev Psychiatry 24(5):342–356, 2016 27603742

Clarkin JF, Foelsch PA, Levy KN, et al: The development of a psychodynamic treatment for patients with borderline personality disorder: a preliminary study of behavioral change. J Pers Disord 15(6):487–495, 2001 11778390

First MB, Williams JWB, Benjamin LS, Spitzer RL, et al: Structured Clinical Interview for DSM-5 Personality Disorders (SCID-5-PD). Arlington, VA, American Psychiatric Press, 2016

Gratz KL, Lacroce DM, Gunderson JG: Measuring changes in symptoms relevant to borderline personality disorder following short-term treatment across partial hospital and intensive outpatient levels of care. J Psychiatr Pract 12(3):153–159, 2006 16732134

Gunderson JG: The emergence of a generalist model to meet public health needs for patients with borderline personality disorder. Am J Psychiatry 173(5):452–458, 2016 27133405

Gunderson JG, Lyons-Ruth K: BPD's interpersonal hypersensitivity phenotype: a gene-environment-developmental model. J Pers Disord 22(1):22–41, 2008 18312121

Keller S, Stelmaszczyk K, Kolly S, et al: Change in biased thinking in a treatment based on the motive-oriented therapeutic relationship for borderline personality disorder. J Pers Disord 32(suppl):75–92, 2018 29388899

Kolly S, Despland JN, de Roten Y, et al: Therapist adherence to good psychiatric practice in a short-term treatment for borderline personality disorder. J Nerv Ment Dis 204(7):489–493, 2016 27187770

Kramer U, Berger T, Kolly S, et al: Effects of motive-oriented therapeutic relationship in early-phase treatment of borderline personality disorder: a pilot study of a randomized trial. J Nerv Ment Dis 199(4):244–250, 2011 21451348

Kramer U, Kolly S, Berthoud L, et al: Effects of motive-oriented therapeutic relationship in a ten-session general psychiatric treatment of borderline personality disorder: a randomized controlled trial. Psychother Psychosom 83(3):176–186, 2014 24752034

Kramer U, Charbon P, Despland JN, et al: "Good enough" training in clinical practice for BPD? Swiss Archives of Neurology, Psychiatry and Psychotherapy 168(8):241, 2017a

Kramer U, Keller S, Caspar F, et al: Early change in coping strategies in responsive treatments for borderline personality disorder: a mediation analysis. J Consult Clin Psychol 85(5):530–535, 2017b 28425747

Kramer U, Stulz N, Berthoud L, et al: The shorter the better? A follow-up analysis of 10-session psychiatric treatment including the motive-oriented therapeutic relationship for borderline personality disorder. Psychother Res 27(3):362–370, 2017c 26684670

Lecrubier Y, Sheehan DV, Weiller E, et al: The Mini International Neuropsychiatric Interview (MINI). A short diagnostic structured interview: reliability and validity according to the CIDI. Eur Psychiatry 12(5):224–231, 1997

Linehan MM, Heard HL, Armstrong HE: Naturalistic follow-up of a behavioral treatment for chronically parasuicidal borderline patients. Arch Gen Psychiatry 50(12):971–974, 1993 8250683

McMain SF, Links PS, Gnam WH, et al: A randomized trial of dialectical behavior therapy versus general psychiatric management for borderline personality disorder. Am J Psychiatry 166(12):1365–1374, 2009 19755574

McMain SF, Guimond T, Barnhart R, et al: A randomized trial of brief dialectical behaviour therapy skills training in suicidal patients suffering from borderline disorder. Acta Psychiatr Scand 135(2):138–148, 2017 27858962

McQuillan A, Nicastro R, Guenot F, et al: Intensive dialectical behavior therapy for outpatients with borderline personality disorder who are in crisis. Psychiatr Serv 56(2):193–197, 2005 15703347

Sisti D, Segal AG, Siegel AM, et al: Diagnosing, disclosing, and documenting borderline personality disorder: a survey of psychiatrists' practices. J Pers Disord 30(6):848–856, 2016 26623537

Tracie Shea M, Edelen MO, Pinto A, et al: Improvement in borderline personality disorder in relationship to age. Acta Psychiatr Scand 119(2):143–148, 2009 18851719

Zanarini MC, Frankenburg FR: A preliminary, randomized trial of psychoeducation for women with borderline personality disorder. J Pers Disord 22(3):284–290, 2008 18540800

Zanarini MC, Frankenburg FR, Khera GS, et al: Treatment histories of borderline inpatients. Compr Psychiatry 42(2):144–150, 2001 11244151

Zanarini MC, Frankenburg FR, Reich DB, et al: The 10-year course of psychosocial functioning among patients with borderline personality disorder and Axis II comparison subjects. Acta Psychiatr Scand 122(2):103–109, 2010 20199493

Zanarini MC, Frankenburg FR, Reich DB, et al: Fluidity of the subsyndromal phenomenology of borderline personality disorder over 16 years of prospective follow-up. Am J Psychiatry 173(7):688–694, 2016 26869248

Zimmerman M, Mattia JI: Differences between clinical and research practices in diagnosing borderline personality disorder. Am J Psychiatry 156(10):1570–1574, 1999 10518168

Chapter 12

Implementation of Good Psychiatric Management for Narcissistic Personality Disorder

GOOD ENOUGH OR NOT GOOD ENOUGH?

Igor Weinberg, Ph.D.
Ellen F. Finch, B.A.
Lois W. Choi-Kain, M.D., M.Ed.

Personality disorders are prevalent and complicate the course of many major psychiatric illnesses (Tyrer et al. 2016). In the general population, about 10% of individuals meet criteria for at least one personality disorder, and in psychiatric settings, the proportion of the clinical population with at least one personality disorder is as high as 50% (Torgersen 2012; Zimmerman et al. 2008). Personality disorders are associated with significant morbidity (e.g., Zanarini et al. 2004), mortality (e.g., Oldham 2006), dysfunction (Gunderson et al. 2011; Zanarini et al. 2010), and costs to the individuals, their families, and society (Bateman and Fonagy 2003; van Asselt et al. 2007). Personality disorders contribute to persistence of depression (Newton-Howes et al. 2006), anxiety disorder (Skodol et al. 2014), and substance use disorders (Skodol et al. 1999).

Despite the prevalence and clinical significance of personality disorders, treatments for personality disorders other than borderline remain largely undefined and unavailable. Earlier conceptualizations of personality disorders in terms of pathological defenses, primitive object relations, or unconsolidated fragile sense of self dictated long-term treatments. Those were expensive, lasted many years, and required a highly trained professional—usually a psychoanalytically trained therapist—to deliver them. The extensive nature of the training required for the professionals before they reach competence in treating patients with personality disorders is at odds with the clinical reality in which patients with personality disorders are rarely seeking these specialized treatments but predominantly come to the attention of medical, psychiatric, or legal systems because of comorbid conditions (DSM-5; American Psychiatric Association 2013) or psychosocial consequences of personality disorders. They are more likely to seek help from general practitioners, social workers, or therapists available in the community. If they are lucky, they will get a referral to a specialist who is trained in modalities designed for personality disorders. More commonly, though, they drop out of treatment; are misdiagnosed and receive ineffective or, at times, harmful treatments; or are labeled as "untreatable" patients. Consequently, they become even less likely to seek professional help in the future.

The development of a significant research literature and varied evidence-based treatments (EBTs) for borderline personality disorder (BPD) has catalyzed a sea change in enhanced recognition and treatment for patients who were previously (more heavily) stigmatized and deemed beyond help. Dialectical behavior therapy (DBT; Linehan 1993) was the first EBT for BPD. Although subsequent EBTs for BPD became shorter and less costly, they still required extensive training of the professionals, thus limiting availability of these treatments. Good psychiatric management (GPM; Gunderson and Links 2014), developed originally as "general" psychiatric management by Gunderson and Links (2008), provides a hopeful alternative as an empirically validated treatment (McMain et al. 2009,

2012) that requires relatively minimal training and therefore is more feasible outside of specialized treatment settings. Consequently, GPM is a likely candidate for an intervention that can be delivered in settings where patients with any personality disorder naturally seek help.

To what degree EBTs for BPD apply to the treatment of other personality disorders is still largely unknown. DBT is the most widely known and available treatment for BPD, but its utility in treating other personality disorders has not been studied in a methodologically rigorous way. Personality disorders share common factors (Sharp et al. 2015), which suggests that unified treatment protocols for different personality disorders may be possible. Mentalization-based treatment (MBT; Bateman and Fonagy 1999), schema-focused therapy (SFT; Giesen-Bloo et al. 2006), and transference-focused psychotherapy (TFP; Clarkin et al. 2007) are more broadly designed to address personality disorders generally, with a focus on dysfunctional interpersonal patterns and poor self-management capacities. However, the evidentiary base that validates these approaches for personality disorders other than BPD is still just developing. A multicenter trial of SFT for Cluster C (avoidant, dependent, obsessive-compulsive), paranoid, histrionic, and narcissistic personality disorders showed general improvement in personality disorder symptoms, social adjustment, and quality of life (Bamelis et al. 2014; Bateman et al. 2016). SFT training is not widely available in the United States, which limits its utility to the generalist clinician.

GPM's framework relies on basic interventions that can be adjusted to the differing findings regarding and features of separate personality disorders. GPM's fundamental features include making a diagnosis using DSM-5 symptoms (American Psychiatric Association 2013); psychoeducation about heritability, course, and model of core vulnerabilities; goal setting; accountability for change (with "getting a life" as an overarching goal); informed management of comorbidities; and conservative use of hospitalization and medications. These fundamentals constitute good treatment for many diagnostic entities as an entry-level approach to good psychiatric care.

Although a large trial to test GPM for personality disorders other than BPD is needed, we begin by outlining how we can extend principles of GPM to treat narcissistic personality disorder (NPD) in this chapter. NPD is another prevalent, sometimes fatal, and complicating co-occurring diagnosis that renders the treatment of other psychiatric and medical conditions more complex. Our goals are twofold: Our first aim is to illustrate the way in which GPM provides a map for plain old "good" psychiatric management. It is a recipe for good medical care broadly and psychiatric care specifically. The second is to provide a feasible basic approach for clinical professionals who are bound to have patients with NPD in their practice settings. We hope this feeds into a movement to "make NPD the new BPD" (L. W. Choi-Kain, "Introduction to TFP for NPD" 3-day training, Borderline Personality Disorder Training Institute, April 2017) and destigmatize NPD in both clinical and research domains.

GPM for Narcissistic Personality Disorder: Good Enough or Not Good Enough?

NPD is characterized by persistent patterns of grandiose self-perception, fantasies of unlimited success, sense of specialness, and exploitative, non-empathic relations with others (American Psychiatric Association 2013). Compared with BPD, NPD has been the focus of a much more limited body of empirical research, although attention to this condition has been increasing in the past decade. Simple PubMed searches for the terms *borderline personality* and *narcissistic personality* result in more than a 20-fold increase in the number of papers for BPD versus NPD. Estimation of prevalence is obfuscated by fluidity and variability in clinical manifestations of NPD across patients and within the same patient. The prevalence of NPD in the general population is as high as 6% (Stinson et al. 2008) when the NPD assessment relies only on evaluation of symptomatic criteria. When readjusted to account for subjective distress and functional impairment, this figure deflates to 1% (Trull et al. 2013). These findings parallel the distinction of the broad concept of *pathological narcissism*, defined as maladaptive patterns of regulation of self-esteem (Reich 1960), versus the narrower concept of NPD as defined in DSM-5, which depicts a specific syndrome of personality characteristics. Patients with NPD typically present with numerous comorbid conditions, most typically with mood disorders, anxiety disorders, or substance use disorders (Stinson et al. 2008). Not only do these conditions complicate the clinical presentation and course of NPD, but also NPD confers a lower risk of recovery from any comorbid conditions (Jansson et al. 2008). NPD is typically associated with an increased risk of suicide, marital dysfunction, and vocational difficulties (for a review, see Ronningstam and Weinberg 2015). These challenges call for an effective intervention for patients with NPD. A number of such specialized treatments have been reported in the literature (Diamond and Meehan 2013; Young et al. 1993), although none were subjected to empirical testing and training; a long process is required to adherently deliver these treatments.

In this chapter, we present our adaptation of GPM to the treatment of the patient with NPD. Given a wide range of presentations of pathological narcissism, we focus more specifically on NPD as depicted in the DSM-5 main criteria (not the alternative model proposed in Section III of DSM-5). The DSM variant is the most paradigmatic recognizable manifestation of pathological narcissism that is also associated with subjective distress and functional impairment. We believe that GPM can be used to help patients with NPD modify some of the maladaptive behaviors and develop more effective ways of maintaining self-esteem, relating to others, and improving their functioning. Similarly, we believe that most clinicians can readily identify these patients and use a GPM framework to stabilize treatment through a predictable and relatable structure. GPM provides a basic protocol of good clinical management for any psychiatric disorder, starting with diagnosis, psychoeducation, and case management. It is pragmatic, goal oriented, easy to learn, and adaptable for most clinical settings, including acute settings such as inpatient hospitals. GPM's nonintensive, flexible format allows for greater implementation as a gateway treatment. More specialized treatment, when desired and available, can be pursued. At the same time, this approach of applied GPM for NPD provides good enough definitive treatment, which otherwise does not exist in a simple, coherent way. GPM holds the patient accountable for reaching goals, with an imperative to change, while also fostering an alliance around a shared sense of why problems occur for the patient in his or her life as well as in the treatment relationship.

Diagnosis and Psychoeducation

Avoidance of diagnostic disclosure of personality disorders, through a practice of "Axis II deferred," has been harmful to patients with BPD, who for many years receive treatments for other co-occurring or misdiagnosed problems that do not respond to treatment, and thus recovery from NPD is delayed. Although there is still not adequate clarity and scope of empirical evidence surrounding the phenomenology, biology, course, and treatment of NPD, there is a DSM-based diagnosis, and growing research suggests that it is a reliable diagnosis and that the disorder sometimes improves and can respond to treatment. It is not yet known how well treatment can ameliorate this disorder because it is not often diagnosed and is only rarely the focus of manualized psychotherapeutic treatments.

The GPM approach to diagnosis involves simply reviewing NPD criteria in DSM. When reviewing the diagnostic criteria for NPD with a patient, the GPM-informed clinician frames symptoms as related to a central difficulty with regulating self-esteem. When symptoms are posed in that context, more sympathy and collaboration in identifying the way criteria apply to the patient is possible; the goal is posed as improvement of the patient's capacity to manage his or her difficulties. The medicalizing attitude frames the problem more objectively as the main motive for clinician and patient interaction, with the goal of managing a set of vulnerabilities that are the genesis of the symptoms of the disease. For the patient with NPD, looking at personal or character flaws may feel too subjective and critical. GPM diffuses that treatment obstacle with its psychoeducational case management focus. A central resource for clinicians, patients, and families is a pamphlet called "Narcissistic Personality Disorder Basics" (Ronningstam 2016). Clinicians can give this pamphlet, written in a patient-centered, clear, and optimistic way, to patients and collaboratively review it in session.

Intrapsychic Coherence Model

Whereas patients with BPD are vulnerable to the availability of others (Gunderson 1984), we believe that the Achilles' heel of patients with NPD is availability of support for their unstable self-esteem. Figure 12–1 and Table 12–1 illustrate this vulnerability in more detail.

The top circle in Figure 12–1 corresponds to *compensated* narcissism. In such a state, the patient is typically holding a belief of self-sufficiency (Modell 1975). He or she is asymptomatic and yet presents with a sense of disconnection from self and others. While not in distress at this stage, the narcissistic patient describes diffuse existential distress. The patient wants to be envied and presents as such, but also envies others. Owing to an underdeveloped connection to oneself and related problems of empathy, the patient with NPD has limited and unstable means of relating to others. However, if the patient encounters significant threat to the self-esteem, the fragile compensation collapses and the patient regresses to the next level— *threatened* self-esteem (Baumeister et al. 1993). In such a state, the patient is frantically trying to return to the compensated state through ineffective strategies such as self-aggrandizing, devaluation of others, and aggressive and even sadistic behaviors. This is a typical presentation for "grandiose narcissism" (Kernberg 1984). Other patients adopt a self-loathing stance designed to invite others to reassure them against these self-devaluing statements. Such a patient with NPD demands that he or she as well as other people "live up" to his or her standards. Simultaneously, the self-shaming creates an illusion of control over the threat to self-esteem by anticipating the worst-case scenarios. This at least may allow the patient with NPD to claim a "most aggrieved" position. This is a more typical presenta-

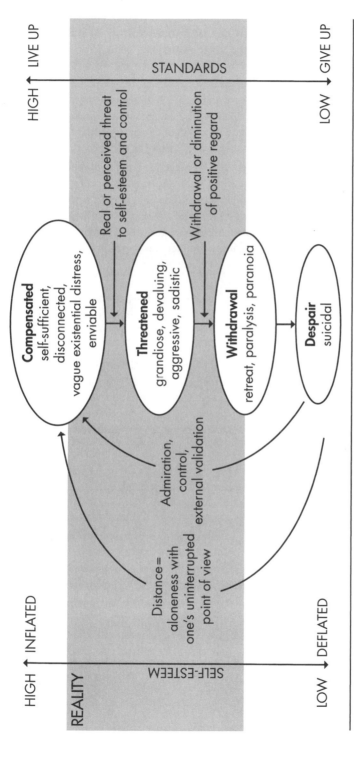

FIGURE 12–1. Good psychiatric management's intrapsychic coherence model of narcissistic personality disorder.

Source. Developed by L.W. Choi-Kain, I. Weinberg, E. F. Finch, B. McCommon, and R.H. Hersh. Presented at the Narcissistic Personality Disorder Conference at McLean's Borderline Personality Disorders Training Institute, March 2018.

TABLE 12–1.   **Oscillations in the phenomenology of narcissistic personality disorder (NPD)**

State	Description
Compensated	Without threats or injuries to self-esteem, the patient with NPD is self-sufficient and compensated. However, the patient remains disconnected from the self and others and likely experiences vague existential distress.
Threatened	When faced with real or perceived threats to self-esteem or control, a threatened state emerges. The prototypical grandiosity of NPD involves self-aggrandizement, devaluation of others, and aggressive or sadistic behaviors in an attempt to preserve superiority. Demanding and entitled behaviors are enacted to promote "living up" to standards either by self or others.
Withdrawal	If the tendencies of the threatened state promote withdrawal of positive regard from others, the patient responds by socially retreating into a state of paralysis or paranoia. The patient isolates himself or herself from relationships and real-life pursuits.
Despair	When the patient falls further into decompensation and loses hope of returning to self-sufficiency and meeting his or her high self-expectations, the patient becomes suicidal. This regression can be rapid and associated with "giving up" on standards when "living up" to standards feels impossible.

Compensatory phenomenon	Description
Admiration and external validation	Receiving admiration and external validation from others is congruent with the patient's narcissistic view of self and promotes the reinstatement of inflated self-esteem, even if it is about the extent of his or her despair and desperation. This admiration or validation may be provoked by serious suicidality, when others are shocked or amazed by the extent of the patient's suffering or seriousness of despair.
Distance	When withdrawn, the patient is alone with his or her own narcissistic point of view. Failures and opinions of others no longer influence the patient's sense of self, and the patient's uninterrupted narcissism can reinstate self-esteem.

tion for "closet narcissists" (Masterson 1993). In the short term, these frantic strategies for restitution of the self-sufficient state create an illusion of self-esteem and of self-sufficiency. These two upper states (see Figure 12–1) are associated with *inflated* self-esteem, which remains fragile and easily shattered by reality. In the long term, the patient with NPD pushes significant others away and withdraws from the desperately needed regard from others because the patient's behavior sours the realistic responses of those interacting with the patient. This leads to further regression, and the patient with NPD presents with even further *depleted and decompensated* narcissism (Svrakić 1987). This is where the patient experiences a deflation of self-esteem and starts to give up on the high standards for self and others, thus further regressing to the next state of *withdrawal*. In that state (i.e. withdrawal), the patient presents with paranoia and paralysis and retreats from relationships or real-life pursuits (Steiner 1993). In that state, the patient is retreating into a state of total aloneness with his or her interrupted and unchallenged point of view, also described as intolerance of the alternative perspectives (Britton 2004). When these attempts fail still further and the patient loses hope to ever return to the *compensated*, self-sufficient state, the patient regresses to the state of *despair* (Figure 12–1), and the danger of suicide becomes imminent (Maltsberger 2004). Such regressions can be quite rapid and unfold following relatively circumscribed life events, making assessment of the patient difficult, unless the subjective experiences of the patient can be accessed and taken into account. Such mercurial shifts between compensated and decompensated states explain "surprise suicides" that are typical of patients with NPD.

Recompensation in patients with NPD can be achieved by two pathways. The first one is related to receiving *admiration and external validation* from others or gaining a sense of control over previously stressful events that led to the decompensation. In such cases, a clinician can help a fragile patient with NPD "return" from the deeply decompensated states through empathic validation in therapy, experience of success or admiration, or development of an action plan that increases a sense of control. Environmental interventions that remove sources of stress can be helpful as well. A second pathway involves a retreat into an uninterrupted sense of self or *one's uninterrupted point of view*, where like the Greek mythological figure Narcissus, the patient can be alone in his or her own world, unfettered by the intrusions of reality or other people. At once, he or she is the projectionist and sole audience in his or her own theater (Akhtar and Thomson 1982; Johnson 1977). In these cases, the clinician can provide the patient *space* while also remaining available.

TABLE 12–2.   Narcissistic personality disorder features that call for modification of good psychiatric management

Self-regulation by avoidance of others, not by seeking contact (Diamond and Meehan 2013)

Need for autonomy and control that interferes with dependency (Ronningstam 2017)

Primary vulnerability—success/failure and power/powerlessness (Twenge and Campbell 2010)

Lack of internal motivation for treatment (Kernberg 2007)

Propensity to leave treatment prematurely (Ellison et al. 2013)

Application of GPM Principles to Treatment of Patients With Narcissistic Personality Disorder

Overall, in our experience, GPM offers a useful framework for treatment of NPD. However, a number of NPD features call for modification of the standard GPM treatment to make it "good enough" for treatment of patients with NPD. Table 12–2 summarizes these features, and Table 12–3 presents GPM elements in the treatment of patients with NPD.

Diagnostic Disclosure

Diagnostic disclosure is one of the cornerstones of GPM. In work with patients with BPD, it involves ascertaining the diagnosis, usually by a collaborative review of the diagnostic criteria, provision of the explanation regarding the diagnostic criteria, explanation of the interpersonal coherence model (see Appendix C), and validation of the patient's difficulties through the lenses of the developmental narrative. For patients with NPD, this model applies with two major modifications. First, the clinician is using the *intrapsychic* coherence model (see Figure 12–1 and Table 12–1) and not the *interpersonal* coherence model, as in work with patients with BPD. Second, the clinician is advised to "take an inside view" of the patient's difficulties instead of focusing exclusively on the external manifestations of the disorder. As mentioned previously, Ronningstam's (2016) "Narcissistic Personality Disorder Basics" is a comprehensive, reader-friendly resource that can be the basis of GPM's collaborative approach to making a diagnosis.

TABLE 12–3. Elements of good psychiatric management for narcissistic personality disorder

---

1. Diagnostic disclosure—essential first step
2. Psychoeducation—genetics, course, vulnerability
3. Case management—focus on life outside of treatment
4. Progress—determines duration and intensity of treatment
5. Treatment—psychodynamic (motives, feelings) and behavioral (contingency, accountability)
6. Multimodality—"it takes a village"
7. Managing safety (suicidality)—collaborative but patients are in charge of their own safety

---

Psychoeducation

The importance of psychoeducation is hard to overestimate given its immediate contribution to the treatment alliance and reduction of shame (Rubovszcky et al. 2006; Zanarini and Frankenburg 2008). Compared with studies of BPD, fewer studies of NPD are available to address these areas of psychoeducation, making overall conclusions regarding NPD more tentative. Studies report that heritability of NPD is 71% (Torgersen et al. 2012)—a high figure suggesting a substantial contribution of genetic (as opposed to environmental) factors. The prevalence of NPD is estimated at 1% (Trull et al. 2013), which is similar to that of BPD. Sensitivity to success and failure was examined in empirical studies (Baumeister et al. 1993), and findings suggested that helping the patient develop strategies to manage such vulnerability is likely to be helpful. Preliminary imaging studies confirmed that patients with NPD display physiological abnormalities, such as abnormalities in the right hemisphere (Schulze et al. 2013), and such abnormalities can be meaningfully connected to the phenomenological characteristics of patients with NPD (Schore 1999; Weinberg 2000). Prospectively, improvements in patients with NPD were documented (Ronningstam et al. 1995), indicating that despite high heritability, NPD is amenable to change. Unlike for BPD, there are no empirically validated treatments for NPD, although most specialized treatments for NPD reported clinical success in ameliorating NPD symptoms (for a review, see Ronningstam and Weinberg 2015). These are hopeful messages that are likely to help destigmatize the disorder in the eyes of the patient, reduce shame, and help build the alliance. An important addition to GPM for NPD is psychoeducation regarding risks of dropping out from treatment and the importance of staying in treatment despite the urges to quit.

Psychoeducation can extend from where diagnostic disclosure leaves off. An in-depth discussion of the intrapsychic coherence model (see Figure 12–1 and Table 12–1) allows the clinician and patient to review how the different states and interactive triggers apply to what the patient experiences. Clinicians can use the model to also predict where they can "lean in," as they do in cases of BPD when a patie'nt is most available for the advisement of others (Figure 12–2). Clinicians can instruct the patient to expect that they can work together in the fluctuations between states of compensation, threats to the patient's feelings of control and competence, and last in transitions to withdrawal. Emphasizing mastery and control, elements the patient will more likely to be willing to invest in, can help. Also, focusing on *stabilizing* self-esteem as a goal can appeal to the patient with NPD who might not easily align with attending to his or her "flaws" or "vulnerabilities."

Another powerful process that helps some patients with NPD recompensate involves confrontation with reality that challenges the unrealistic and dysfunctional nature of the grandiose beliefs. Such confrontation helps many patients with NPD, especially when they are accompanied by support from others, to modify and adjust their grandiose beliefs (Ronningstam et al. 1995).

As part of psychoeducation, clinicians can deliver important therapeutic messages to the patient. Table 12–4 lists areas of psychoeducation in GPM for BPD, with messages adapted to the concerns of patients with NPD.

Case Management

Case management is another cornerstone of standard GPM. It helps the patient identify and maintain focus on life-related goals. Treatment emphasizes goals of improvement in the vocational sphere and deemphasizes the importance of romantic relationships. It emphasizes accountability, thus aiming at increasing the patient's self-reliance. In working with patients with BPD, the therapist is advised to take a skeptical stance regarding overreliance and the need for dependence on others. In keeping with the pragmatic style of the treatment, the therapist anticipates challenges, such as the patient's propensity to develop crises in response to the therapist's decreased availability.

For patients with NPD, the same GPM principles of case management are helpful, with the following modifications: First, the therapist has to help the patient identify goals that are realistic and not based on grandi-

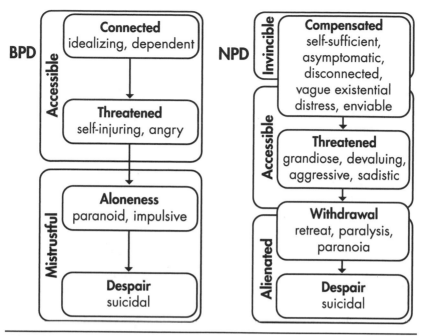

FIGURE 12–2. Accessibility to interventions in the symptomatic oscillations of borderline personality disorder (BPD) versus narcissistic personality disorder (NPD).

Source.   Presented by L. W. Choi-Kain and E. F. Finch at the Narcissistic Personality Disorder Conference at McLean's Borderline Personality Disorders Training Institute, March 2018.

TABLE 12–4.   Psychoeducation used in good psychiatric management and therapeutic messages adapted for narcissistic personality disorder

Area of psychoeducation	Message
Heritability	"It is not your fault."
Prevalence	"You are not alone."
Vulnerability	"Be proactive; anticipate difficulties."
Physiological basis	"The difficulties are real, not made up."
Naturalistic course	"Improvements happen over time."
Available treatments	"Treatments can help."

ose self. Second, in addition to focusing on vocational rehabilitation, in work with patients with NPD, the therapist is likely to target interpersonal dysfunctional style, such as isolation, devaluation, or inattention to others. Third, the therapist of the patient with NPD is advised to be skeptical regarding *overreliance on self.* Fourth, the therapist is advised to stay attuned to possible unworkable arrangements in therapy that the patient with NPD might suggest or adopt, such as nonpayment for therapy or expectation to conduct therapy through electronic media at any time of day and night. Finally, the therapist of patients with NPD should anticipate typical challenges, such as the patient's dropping out of therapy when the initial crisis is over or when vulnerabilities surface in treatment.

Progress Is Expected: Treatment Continues If There Is Progress

An essential component of GPM is that its very continuation is contingent on the patient's progress and fair investment in the therapy; the therapy stops if such progress does not take place. Therefore, both expectation and facilitation of changes are built into the GPM framework.

This principle is especially relevant in work with patients with NPD, to safeguard against the risk of "nontreatment treatment"—a patient's retreat into pseudo self-understanding that is not accompanied by change (Steiner 1993). Real progress is possible in NPD, but it can be anticipated to be slower than with BPD patients. In work with patients with NPD, it is helpful to identify how avoidance interferes with pursuit of the treatment goals.

Treatment—Psychodynamic and Behavioral

GPM flexibly integrates both psychodynamic understanding of the patient's motives and feelings and the importance of behavioral interventions, including contingency management. A number of modifications are relevant in work with patients with NPD. First, therapists should avoid excessive empathy that leads to avoidance of action. Second, therapists are advised to promote curiosity and to question pathological certainty (Britton and Steiner 1994). Third, use of contingencies and emphasis on real-life consequences of behaviors help the patient to develop a realistic sense of agency and self-esteem—an adaptive alternative to the sense of grandiosity that is based on fantasies of absolute control and invincibility. Finally, when patients with NPD present with significant antisocial elements, use of external contingencies becomes a sine qua non of effective treatment (Salekin 2002).

TABLE 12–5. Unique characteristics of suicidality in patients with narcissistic personality disorder

Absence of major psychopathology

Low impulsivity

Lack of communication

Lack of overt distress due to dissociation

Sense of meaninglessness

Some suicidal thinking that is paradoxically self-protective

Grandiose fantasies that fuel suicidal action

Multimodality

GPM can be flexibly implemented along with other treatments. For patients with NPD, such treatments may include group therapy (Alonso 1992), couples therapy (Links and Stockwell 2001), family therapy (Harman and Waldo 2004), and behavior therapy (Turkat 1990). Pharmacotherapy can be integrated as well, usually to address comorbid disorders, although specialized pharmacological treatments for NPD have not been tested.

Managing Suicidality

Completed suicide is one of the most tragic outcomes for some unfortunate patients with NPD. Although the exact prevalence rate of suicide in NPD has not been tested, studies confirm that NPD increases risk of both attempted and completed suicides (for a review, see Ronningstam and Weinberg 2015). Some of the characteristics of suicide in patients with NPD overlap with those in patients with BPD (e.g., suicide in response to unbearable emotional pain). Other features make suicide in patients with NPD unique. To borrow a phrase coined by Alan Apter (Apter et al. 1993), we think that many suicides in patients with NPD can be called "death without warning"—they catch the therapist by surprise and shock. Table 12–5 summarizes unique features of suicidality in patients with NPD (for a review, see Ronningstam and Weinberg 2015).

Usually suicidal risk in patients with NPD can be understood in terms of the balance between risk factors (i.e., substance use, mood disorder, dissociation, shame, humiliation, rage, failures, job loss, legal or medical problems, aging) and protective factors (i.e., successes, promotions, signs of recognition, good crisis management skills, low-dose neuroleptics, brief hospitalizations) (for a review, see Ronningstam and Weinberg 2015). Table 12–6 summarizes GPM principles of managing safety in patients with NPD.

The following case vignette illustrates the application of these GPM principles to the treatment of NPD.

Case Vignette

The following case description includes decision points, each of which has several alternative responses listed at the end of the case. The reader will rate each alternative response in terms of its level of helpfulness. Discussions of responses follow.

> Justin is a 24-year-old single white man who came to treatment with you after taking numerous medical leaves from college. He felt trapped in a pernicious circle of returning to college, procrastinating, not going to classes, ruminating about failing, smoking marijuana, and consequently failing classes. He would then go home for treatment, develop further "insight" regarding this cycle, and return to school only to face his Sisyphean plight all over again. He described feelings of depression and self-doubt, although he presented with a flair for grandiosity and contempt while talking about his dreams of becoming a world-renowned architect in the future. He reported that previous treatments with a prominent psychopharmacologist and a famous analyst "accomplished nothing" besides adding a phrase "treatment resistant" to his diagnosis of depression. [**Decision Points 1 and 2**]
>
> Early in treatment Justin developed a pattern of avoiding asking for help; instead, he would describe in painstaking detail how he had come up with solutions to existing problems. [**Decision Points 3 and 4**] Justin came to a therapy session and described difficulties following through with meeting the deadline to submit a paper at the class he took at the local community college. [**Decision Point 5**]
>
> As Justin was progressing in treatment, he started sharing that at times he was thinking that he could always kill himself if he could not succeed in life. He mentioned that these thoughts usually made him more hopeful and made him feel more in control. However, he never acted on these thoughts, and he denied suicidal plans. [**Decision Point 6**]
>
> Justin continues in treatment. With your help, he is able to start focusing on the other ways that he can manage realistic control in his life. For example, he becomes more consistent with taking tests and turning in school assignments. In your sessions, he reckons with the less satisfying grades he receives and practices simply following through on tasks, intermittently able to acknowledge his fear of failure. Justin stops taking medical leave from college, and although he remains somewhat socially isolated, he regularly attends a local chess league.

TABLE 12–6. **Good psychiatric management principles of managing safety in patients with narcissistic personality disorder**

---

1. Express concern—do not ignore or derogate.
2. Assess risk—differentiate self-sustaining from imminent suicidal preoccupation.
3. Ask what the patient thinks could help.
4. Hospitalize reluctantly.
5. Clarify precipitants—assume role of self-esteem–relevant life events or failures.
6. Be clear about your limits—do not be omniscient or tolerate pathological uncertainty (e.g., say to patient, "If you cannot call me when you are suicidal, I have no way to tell what radio silence means").
7. Explore the meaning of suicidal behavior vis-à-vis treatment goals. Consider whether patient is using therapy enough to move toward accomplishing the goals.
8. Develop safety plan (Stanley et al. 2018).
9. Seek consultation.

Decision Points: Alternative Responses

Rate each response in terms of its level of helpfulness with a rating of 1 (will be helpful), 2 (possibly helpful, continuing reservations), or 3 (not helpful—or even harmful).

1. You should intervene as follows regarding Justin's diagnosis:

   A. Avoid diagnosing further disorders until his depression and substance use remit because these disorders obfuscate diagnostic clarifications.
   B. Assess NPD but avoid discussing this new diagnosis with Justin in order to protect his already fragile self-esteem that has suffered so many blows.
   C. Assess NPD and tell Justin that he meets the criteria for NPD; then simply refer Justin to the Internet if he has further questions.
   D. Assess NPD collaboratively with Justin and then spend time providing information about it; advise Justin to avoid using the Internet because of the unreliable nature of such information.

2. While you are providing psychoeducation to Justin, it will be helpful to say,

   A. "There is a lot of research on NPD, and today we have very clear practices for how to treat this disorder."
   B. "We know that NPD can improve over time and that treatment is likely to help. However, it will take a lot of hard work and staying in therapy despite the difficulties."
   C. "With the right treatment, your NPD can be fully resolved."
   D. "There is so little research on NPD that we should stick to what we know about treatment of your depression before we target NPD."

3. You can effectively use case management principles by intervening as follows:

   A. Express praise for and admiration of Justin's efforts, thereby hoping to build his fragile self-esteem.
   B. Offer an interpretation that Justin is treating you as irrelevant or useless.
   C. Note to Justin that although he is adequately solving these problems, you are skeptical of whether he will ask for help with problems for which he has no solutions.
   D. Dismiss this behavior of Justin's as an expression of self-aggrandizement and change the subject.

4. The following recommendation regarding session frequency is likely to help Justin in treatment:

   A. Schedule sessions as frequently as possible to help Justin process his failures.
   B. If Justin stops making progress, increase session frequency to resolve negative feelings that are likely reasons for that stalemate.
   C. If Justin stops making progress, interpret that as Justin's attempts to defeat your efforts.
   D. Increase treatment frequency once Justin demonstrates progress in completing assignments in a class at the local community college.

5. Within a dynamic-behavioral framework of GPM, you could intervene by saying the following:

    A. "You could schedule time every day to work on this paper."

    B. "I think you are so afraid of failure that you are afraid to work on the paper."

    C. "Let's not meet until you finish the paper."

    D. "I can understand that it is difficult for you to start your paper because you are afraid of failure. By scheduling times to work on the paper and then actually writing the paper during these times, you can develop confidence in your ability to work despite your fear of failure—the reason for your difficulties in college."

6. You could do the following:

    A. Help Justin to identify the function of these thoughts (e.g., maintaining sense of control) and to identify when these thoughts help him stay in control and when they propel him to plan suicide.

    B. Tell Justin that his treatment cannot continue until he makes a full commitment to staying alive.

    C. Ask Justin to monitor these thoughts daily.

    D. Hospitalize Justin until he has no thoughts of suicide.

Decision Points: Discussion

Numbers within brackets indicate level of helpfulness ratings.

1. You should intervene as follows regarding Justin's diagnosis:

    A. Avoid diagnosing further disorders until his depression and substance use remit because these disorders obfuscate diagnostic clarifications. [3] (This response is overly conservative and invites inattention to NPD, which is one of the reasons for the persistence of other comorbid disorders despite treatment. This has been a likely reason for Justin's lack of improvement in prior treatments.)

    B. Assess NPD but avoid discussing this new diagnosis with Justin in order to protect his already fragile self-esteem that has suffered so many blows. [2] (This response does not help Justin develop understanding of his difficulties, including previous treatment failures, and does not allow him to formulate treatment goals around these issues.)

    C. Assess NPD and tell Justin that he meets the criteria for NPD; then simply refer Justin to the Internet if he has further questions. [2] (This response exposes Justin to the danger of reading overly negative and uninformed accounts of NPD. Providing psychoeducation formally is a part of treatment and is associated with improvements in symptoms, in contrast to research the patient does on his own.)

  D. Assess NPD collaboratively with Justin and then spend time providing information about it; advise Justin to avoid using the Internet because of the unreliable nature of such information. [1] (This response is consistent with GPM and provides Justin with important psychoeducation. This collaborative process allows clinician and patient to develop a shared understanding of the patient's difficulties and frames the goals and expectations of treatment.)

2. While you are providing psychoeducation to Justin, it will be helpful to say,

  A. "There is a lot of research on NPD, and today we have very clear practices for how to treat this disorder." [2] (Although some significant research on NPD exists, clear practices have not been formed. This response represents unrealistic optimism and misinforms Justin regarding the strength of the scientific basis for treatment or the actual prognosis. Although this type of optimism is justified for BPD, it is not yet applicable to NPD.)

  B. "We know that NPD can improve over time and that treatment is likely to help. However, it will take a lot of hard work and staying in therapy despite the difficulties." [1] (This response is consistent with the GPM approach of realistic and pragmatic reassurance. It is balanced, and it invites Justin to take a proactive role.)

  C. "With the right treatment, your NPD can be fully resolved." [2] (Similar to response A, this response is overly optimistic and misinforms Justin regarding his prognosis.)

  D. "There is so little research on NPD that we should stick to what we know about treatment of your depression before we target NPD." [3] (This response is plagued by an overly pessimistic stance that, in reality, withholds from Justin effective interventions that target NPD.)

3. You can effectively use case management principles by intervening as follows:

A. Express praise for and admiration of Justin's efforts, thereby hoping to build his fragile self-esteem. [2] (This approach incorporates a misguided use of empathy that aims to build Justin's self-esteem, even though it is not based on the reality of his progress because it neglects his awareness of difficulties.)
B. Offer an interpretation that Justin is treating you as irrelevant or useless. [3] (This response is too confrontational, and although it could be accurate intellectually, it centers the therapy on the therapist-patient relationship rather than the pursuit of the goals of treatment.)
C. Note that Justin is solving these problems but remain skeptical whether he is asking for help for problems that he has no solutions for. [1] (This response is more in line with GPM in its simple description of the situation. It provides frank feedback in a supportive manner and invites Justin to look at his difficulty and limitations.)
D. Dismiss this behavior of Justin's as an expression of self-aggrandizement and change the subject. [3] (This reaction represents a typical countertransference enactment that clinicians often struggle with vis-à-vis the patient with NPD—dismissal of Justin's experiences altogether because they stem from narcissistic dynamics.)

4. The following recommendation regarding session frequency is likely to help Justin in treatment:

A. Schedule sessions as frequently as possible to help Justin process his failures. [3] (A common tendency among therapists is to increase session frequency in response to poor progress. This tactic is contraindicated in GPM because it inadvertently reinforces the impasse.)
B. If Justin stops making progress, increase session frequency to resolve negative feelings that are likely reasons for that stalemate. [3] (This response is contraindicated in GPM for a similar reason as given in response A.)
C. If Justin stops making progress, interpret that as Justin's attempts to defeat your efforts. [3] (This response uses deep interpretations of the transference [therapist-patient relationship], with the hope of shifting Justin into a more productive state. This is likely a high-risk, high-gain intervention [Gabbard et al. 1994] with some patients; however, it focuses the treatment around the therapy relationship instead of the pursuit of treat-

ment goals. Although this intervention may be effective in other modalities, it is not encouraged in GPM.)

D. Increase treatment frequency once Justin demonstrates progress in completing assignments in a class at the local community college. [1] (This response is GPM adherent in that it emphasizes that treatment is increased if the patient is making gains. The better the treatment is working, the more it can be made available in the service of the patient building his life outside of treatment.)

5. Within a dynamic-behavioral framework of GPM, you could intervene by saying the following:

A. "You could schedule time every day to work on this paper." [2] (This response is a behavioral intervention that should be implemented only after the clinician and patient sort out what the difficulties are and what they have to do with the symptoms of NPD on which they are working.)

B. "I think you are so afraid of failure that you are afraid to work on the paper." [3] (Therapist and patient have not collaboratively looked at what the underlying problem or obstacle is, and interpreting this authoritatively without collaboration is too omnipotent a stance for a GPM clinician.)

C. "Let's not meet until you finish the paper." [2] (This response uses contingencies, but it actually may be too punitive and fails to meet Justin where he is at and help him address the issues at hand. Given his NPD diagnosis, this may threaten him and destabilize him further.)

D. "I can understand that it is difficult for you to start your paper because you are afraid of failure. By scheduling times to work on the paper and then actually writing the paper during these times, you can develop confidence in your ability to work despite your fear of failure—the reason for your difficulties in college." [1] (This message expresses empathic understanding, suggests a behavioral intervention, and, importantly, links the intervention to the core issues of self-esteem and development of self-confidence—the ultimate treatment goals.)

6. You could do the following:

A. Help Justin to identify the function of these thoughts (e.g., maintaining sense of control) and to identify when these thoughts help him stay in control and when they propel him to plan suicide. [1] (The examination of what happens intrapsychically to drive suicidal thinking is fully consistent with GPM and the clinical presentation of Justin.)

B. Tell Justin that his treatment cannot continue until he makes a full commitment to staying alive. [3] (Safety contracting is not an effective intervention and cannot replace safety assessment. The clinician should evaluate whether these suicidal thoughts indicate actual suicidal preoccupation or a desire to end one's life. In this case, however, Justin seems to use thoughts of suicide for self-sustaining purposes, to self-validate the severity of his adversity.)

C. Ask Justin to monitor these thoughts daily. [2] (Having Justin be responsible for tracking and assessing his level of suicidality is advocated only after the clinician and patient go through a chain analysis to understand why Justin is feeling suicidal.)

D. Hospitalize Justin until he has no thoughts of suicide. [3] (This response is inconsistent with the level of risk, because Justin lacks the intent or plan to kill himself.)

Conclusion

In this chapter, we applied the principles, structure, and tasks framed within GPM for BPD to NPD, a prevalent, sometimes fatal, and complex personality disorder. NPD has yet to be adequately studied and characterized in terms of longitudinal course, genetics, neurobiology, and treatment to reach the same status of BPD. Whether or not that will occur remains to be seen. However, we hope that with our research and clinical colleagues, we can "make NPD the new BPD"—that is, destigmatize NPD by understanding it more objectively and clearly. GPM provides an entry-level, basic framework for organizing what we do know to date about NPD as it is framed in DSM. Perhaps the tremendous sea change in attitudes toward NPD can be catalyzed as it was for BPD and thereby help patients, clinicians, and families do better in their efforts toward symptom management and recovery.

References

Akhtar S, Thomson JA Jr: Overview: narcissistic personality disorder. Am J Psychiatry 139(1):12–20, 1982 7034551

Alonso A: The shattered mirror: treatment of a group of narcissistic patients. Group 16(4):210–219, 1992

American Psychiatric Association: Diagnostic and Statistical Manual of Mental Disorders, 5th Edition. Arlington, VA, American Psychiatric Association, 2013

Apter A, Bleich A, King RA, et al: Death without warning? A clinical postmortem study of suicide in 43 Israeli adolescent males. Arch Gen Psychiatry 50(2):138–142, 1993 8427554

Bamelis LL, Evers SM, Spinhoven P, et al: Results of a multicenter randomized controlled trial of the clinical effectiveness of schema therapy for personality disorders. Am J Psychiatry 171(3):305–322, 2014 24322378

Bateman A, Fonagy P: Effectiveness of partial hospitalization in the treatment of borderline personality disorder: a randomized controlled trial. Am J Psychiatry 156(10):1563–1569, 1999 10518167

Bateman A, Fonagy P: Health service utilization costs for borderline personality disorder patients treated with psychoanalytically oriented partial hospitalization versus general psychiatric care. Am J Psychiatry 160(1):169–171, 2003 12505818

Bateman A, O'Connell J, Lorenzini N, et al: A randomised controlled trial of mentalization-based treatment versus structured clinical management for patients with comorbid borderline personality disorder and antisocial personality disorder. BMC Psychiatry 16:304, 2016 27577562

Baumeister RF, Heatherton TF, Tice DM: When ego threats lead to self-regulation failure: negative consequences of high self-esteem. J Pers Soc Psychol 64(1):141–156, 1993 8421250

Britton R: Subjectivity, objectivity, and triangular space. Psychoanal Q 73(1):47–61, 2004 14750465

Britton R, Steiner J: Interpretation: selected fact or overvalued idea? Int J Psychoanal 75 (Pt 5–6):1069–1078, 1994 7713646

Clarkin JF, Levy KN, Lenzenweger MF, et al: Evaluating three treatments for borderline personality disorder: a multiwave study. Am J Psychiatry 164(6):922–928, 2007 17541052

Diamond D, Meehan KB: Attachment and object relations in patients with narcissistic personality disorder: implications for therapeutic process and outcome. J Clin Psychol 69(11):1148–1159, 2013 23996275

Ellison WD, Levy KN, Cain NM, et al: The impact of pathological narcissism on psychotherapy utilization, initial symptom severity, and early treatment symptom change: a naturalistic investigation. J Pers Assess 95(3):291–300, 2013 23186259

Gabbard GO, Horwitz L, Allen JG, et al: Transference interpretation in the psychotherapy of borderline patients: a high-risk, high-gain phenomenon. Harv Rev Psychiatry 2(2):59–69, 1994 9384884

Giesen-Bloo J, van Dyck R, Spinhoven P, et al: Outpatient psychotherapy for borderline personality disorder: randomized trial of schema-focused therapy vs transference-focused psychotherapy. Arch Gen Psychiatry 63(6):649–658, 2006 16754838

Gunderson JG: Borderline Personality Disorder. Washington, DC, American Psychiatric Press, 1984

Gunderson JG, Links PS: Borderline Personality Disorder: A Clinical Guide, 2nd Edition. Washington, DC, American Psychiatric Publishing, 2008

Gunderson JG, Links PS: Handbook of Good Psychiatric Management for Borderline Personality Disorder. Washington, DC, American Psychiatric Publishing, 2014

Gunderson JG, Stout RL, McGlashan TH, et al: Ten-year course of borderline personality disorder: psychopathology and function from the Collaborative Longitudinal Personality Disorders Study. Arch Gen Psychiatry 68(8):827–837, 2011 21464343

Harman MJ, Waldo M: Relationship enhancement family therapy with NPD, in Family Treatment of Personality Disorders. Edited by MacFarlane MM. New York, Haworth, 2004, pp 335–360

Jansson I, Hesse M, Fridell M: Personality disorder features as predictors of symptoms five years post-treatment. Am J Addict 17(3):172–175, 2008 18463992

Johnson FA: Psychotherapy of the alienated individuals, in The Narcissistic Condition. Edited by Nelson MC. New York, Human Sciences, 1977

Kernberg OF: Severe Personality Disorders. New Haven, CT, Yale University, 1984

Kernberg OF: The almost untreatable narcissistic patient. J Am Psychoanal Assoc 55(2):503–539, 2007 17601104

Linehan M: Cognitive-Behavioral Treatment of Borderline Personality Disorder. New York, Guilford, 1993

Links PS, Stockwell M: Is couple therapy indicated for borderline personality disorder? Am J Psychother 55(4):491–506, 2001 11824216

Maltsberger JT: The descent into suicide. Int J Psychoanal 85(Pt 3):653–667, 2004 15228702

Masterson J: The Emerging Self. New York, Brunner/Mazel, 1993

McMain SF, Links PS, Gnam WH, et al: A randomized trial of dialectical behavior therapy versus general psychiatric management for borderline personality disorder. Am J Psychiatry 166(12):1365–1374, 2009 19755574

McMain SF, Guimond T, Streiner DL, et al: Dialectical behavior therapy compared with general psychiatric management for borderline personality disorder: clinical outcomes and functioning over a 2-year follow-up. Am J Psychiatry 169(6):650–661, 2012 22581157

Modell AH: A narcissistic defence against affects and the illusion of self-sufficiency. Int J Psychoanal 56(3):275–282, 1975 1236838

Newton-Howes G, Tyrer P, Johnson T: Personality disorder and the outcome of depression: meta-analysis of published studies. Br J Psychiatry 188:13–20, 2006 16388064

Oldham JM: Borderline personality disorder and suicidality. Am J Psychiatry 163(1):20–26, 2006 16390884

Reich A: Pathologic forms of self-esteem regulation. Psychoanal Study Child 15:215–232, 1960 13740410

Ronningstam E: Narcissistic Personality Disorder Basics. New York, National Education Alliance for Borderline Personality Disorder, 2016

Ronningstam E: Intersect between self-esteem and emotion regulation in narcissistic personality disorder—implications for alliance building and treatment. Borderline Personal Disorder Emotion Dysregul 4:3, 2017 28191317

Ronningstam E, Weinberg I: Narcissism in DSM-5 Section III Model for Diagnosis of Personality Disorder. Lessons in Psychiatry, Hobart, NY, Hatherleigh Medical Education, 2015

Ronningstam E, Gunderson J, Lyons M: Changes in pathological narcissism. Am J Psychiatry 152(2):253–257, 1995 7840360

Rubovszcky GG, Gunderson JG, Weinberg I: Patients' acceptance and emotional reactions to disclosure of borderline personality disorder diagnosis. Paper presented at American Psychiatric Association Conference, Toronto, ON, Canada, 2006

Salekin RT: Psychopathy and therapeutic pessimism. Clinical lore or clinical reality? Clin Psychol Rev 22(1):79–112, 2002 11793579

Schore AN: Affect Regulation and the Origin of the Self: The Neurobiology of Emotional Development. Hillsdale, NJ, L Erlbaum, 1999

Schulze L, Dziobek I, Vater A, et al: Gray matter abnormalities in patients with narcissistic personality disorder. J Psychiatr Res 47(10):1363–1369, 2013 23777939

Sharp C, Wright AG, Fowler JC, et al: The structure of personality pathology: both general ('g') and specific ('s') factors? J Abnorm Psychol 124(2):387–398, 2015 25730515

Skodol AE, Oldham JM, Gallaher PE: Axis II comorbidity of substance use disorders among patients referred for treatment of personality disorders. Am J Psychiatry 156(5):733–738, 1999 10327906

Skodol AE, Geier T, Grant BF, et al: Personality disorders and the persistence of anxiety disorders in a nationally representative sample. Depress Anxiety 31(9):721–728, 2014 24995387

Stanley B, Brown GK, Brenner LA, et al: Comparison of the safety planning intervention with follow-up vs usual care of suicidal patients treated in the emergency department. JAMA Psychiatry 75(9):894–900, 2018 29998307

Steiner J: Psychic Retreats. London, Routledge, 1993

Stinson FS, Dawson DA, Goldstein RB, et al: Prevalence, correlates, disability, and comorbidity of DSM-IV narcissistic personality disorder: results from the Wave 2 National Epidemiologic Survey on Alcohol and Related Conditions. J Clin Psychiatry 69(7):1033–1045, 2008 18557663

Svrakić DM: Pessimistic mood in narcissistic decompensation. Am J Psychoanal 47(1):58–71, 1987 3578598

Torgersen S: Epidemiology, in The Oxford Handbook of Personality Disorders. Edited by Widiger TA. New York, Oxford University Press, 2012, pp 186–205

Torgersen S, Myers J, Reichborn-Kjennerud T, et al: The heritability of cluster B personality disorders assessed both by personal interview and questionnaire. J Pers Disord 26(6):848–866, 2012 23281671

Trull TJ, Vergés A, Wood PK, et al: The structure of DSM-IV-TR personality disorder diagnoses in NESARC: a reanalysis. J Pers Disord 27(6):727–734, 2013 23718818

Turkat LD: The Personality Disorders. New York, Pergamon Press, 1990

Twenge JM, Campbell WK: The Narcissistic Epidemic. New York, Atria Books, 2010

Tyrer P, Tyrer H, Yang M, et al: Long-term impact of temporary and persistent personality disorder on anxiety and depressive disorders. Pers Ment Health 10(2):76–83, 2016 26754031

van Asselt AD, Dirksen CD, Arntz A, et al: The cost of borderline personality disorder: societal cost of illness in BPD-patients. Eur Psychiatry 22(6):354–361, 2007 17544636

Weinberg I: The prisoners of despair: right hemisphere deficiency and suicide. Neurosci Biobehav Rev 24(8):799–815, 2000 11118607

Young JE, Klosko JS, Weishaar ME: Schema Therapy. A Practitioner's Guide. New York, Guilford, 1993

Zanarini MC, Frankenburg FR: A preliminary, randomized trial of psychoeducation for women with borderline personality disorder. J Pers Disord 22(3):284–290, 2008 18540800

Zanarini MC, Frankenburg FR, Hennen J, et al: Axis I comorbidity in patients with borderline personality disorder: 6-year follow-up and prediction of time to remission. Am J Psychiatry 161(11):2108–2114, 2004 15514413

Zanarini MC, Frankenburg FR, Reich DB, et al: Time to attainment of recovery from borderline personality disorder and stability of recovery: a 10-year prospective follow-up study. Am J Psychiatry 167(6):663–667, 2010 20395399

Zimmerman M, Chelminski I, Young D: The frequency of personality disorders in psychiatric patients. Psychiatr Clin North Am 31(3):405–420, vi, 2008 18638643

Chapter 13

Integration With Dialectical Behavior Therapy

Deanna Mercer, M.D., FRCPC

Paul S. Links, M.D., M.Sc., FRCPC

Anne K.I. Sonley, M.D., J.D.

Gabrielle Ilagan, B.A.

Lois W. Choi-Kain, M.D., M.Ed.

The good news about the current state of treatments for border-line personality disorder (BPD) is that there are numerous evidence-based manualized treatments for mental health professionals to apply in the care of their patients. Of these choices, dialectical behavior therapy (DBT; Linehan 1993) is arguably the most established and proliferated, and for good reason. It has a robust empirical basis, an efficient training system, and materials that are clinician and patient friendly. At the same time, it is an intensive treatment involving significant dedication by both clinician and patient to carry out in an *adherent* format. The system of DBT training has launched a process of certification, advocating for DBT to be practiced true to its original form. This package of intensive and comprehensive care is both ideal and difficult to implement in large systems such as the Veterans Health Administration (Landes et al. 2017), which is the largest organization through which psychology interns receive training (Association of Psychology Postdoctoral and Internship Centers 2017). However, despite its rigorous requirements, DBT has been widely implemented in eclectic forms and has become a household name associated with the diagnosis of BPD.

A relative newcomer for the treatment of BPD is general or good psychiatric management (GPM). As mentioned throughout this book, GPM integrates psychodynamic concepts and an up-to-date scientific understanding of BPD into a case management approach. GPM is suitable for a range of clinical scenarios, spanning from brief acute interactions in the emergency department to longer-term processes such as outpatient weekly therapy. Gunderson and Links (2014), the developers, specifically advocate for pragmatism and common sense over specification of the exact mode of delivery.

Both DBT and GPM are presented as options for treatments for BPD. DBT is already widespread but not entirely feasible in brief settings or when resources are constrained, and training opportunities for clinicians are limited (Choi-Kain et al. 2016). Although DBT is considered a gold standard of treatment for some patients, clinicians and patients sometimes need other treatments that blend aspects of DBT with more easily implemented and accessible options. GPM fills a niche for lower-intensity, brief approaches applicable to a wide range of health care and psychiatric settings.

These two approaches have many similarities. Like all empirically supported therapies for BPD, DBT and GPM share the following characteristics: 1) a structured manual that supports the therapist and provides recommendations for common clinical problems; 2) an attitude that encourages increased activity, proactivity, and self-agency for patients; 3) a focus on emotion processing and creating robust connections between acts and feelings; 4) a model of psychopathology that is carefully explained to the patient; and 5) an active stance by the therapist including explicit intent to validate, demonstrate empathy, and generate a strong attachment relationship (Bateman 2012). Furthermore, DBT and GPM performed equally well in a large randomized controlled trial (RCT) in terms of reducing suicidal, nonsuicidal, and self-injurious behavior; health care utilization; BPD symptoms; depression; and anger and in improving interpersonal functioning (McMain et al. 2009). Both approaches encourage similar goals, provide psychoeducation, and have specific treatment components including individual sessions, therapist supervision, and intersession contact.

Although the advent of many treatments that work for BPD is good news, for many clinicians, lack of accessibility, time, or funding limits their ability to complete the training required to provide a specialist treatment such as DBT. Therefore, this chapter aims to help the clinical professional orient to the overlaps and key differences between DBT and GPM to suggest ways to combine or sequence different components of each modality. Although these scenarios are not "empirically validated" by RCTs, they are possibly the most common applications of DBT and GPM. The case vignettes illustrate how treatment decisions are made with patients for whom standard DBT or stand-alone GPM is inaccessible or insufficient.

Points of Overlap and Departure

Formulation

Both DBT and GPM emphasize the transaction of biological and environmental factors (Gunderson and Links 2014). However, GPM places more emphasis on the contribution of medical aspects of disease such as heritability and neurobiology. According to GPM, an extremely calm and involved parent may be necessary to quell the emotional expressions, sensitivity to separation, and anger of a young person with the genetic predisposition for interpersonal hypersensitivity. GPM warns patients that perfect responsiveness by caregivers is an unrealistic expectation; therefore, patients need to learn how to manage their interpersonal hypersensitivity in a way that renders interactions more predictable. DBT focuses on the emotionally intense temperament of the individual with BPD, highlighting that the child and his or her caregivers interact in a way that reinforces the child's emotional arousal (Linehan 1993). According to DBT, persistent, invalidating responses to the emotionally sensitive individual (responses that do not acknowledge the validity within an emotionally intense response) perpetuate similar responses. As a result of this formulation, DBT focuses on teaching patients skills to manage emotion dysregulation and communicate more effectively within invalidating environments.

GPM conceptualizes the core deficit in BPD as being one of *interpersonal hypersensitivity* (see Appendix C, "Interpersonal Coherence Model"). DBT acknowledges that people with BPD seem to do well when in stable, positive relationships and poorly when in unhealthy relationships; however, DBT does not see interpersonal hypersensitivity as the primary deficit of BPD. GPM links the phenomenology of BPD to the real or perceived level of availability of significant others. According to GPM, when individuals with BPD feel "held" or attached, they may be depressed, idealizing, and rejection sensitive, but they will be able to collaborate with therapy. When faced with perceived hostility or rejection, they will feel threatened and will be at risk of reacting with anger toward themselves or the other person. At this point, a person with BPD will often seek care, and if the individual receives support, he or she will feel "held" and contained by that support. However, if the person from whom the individual with BPD is seeking support withdraws, the person with BPD will feel alone and will be at risk of dissociation, paranoid ideation, and impulsive behavior. Finally, if the containing influence of a needed other continues to be unavailable, the person with BPD will descend into despair, where he or she becomes anhedonic and suicidal.

DBT conceptualizes the core deficit of BPD as *emotion dysregulation*, which is described as the inability to regulate emotional responses to life experiences. The symptoms of BPD, such as impulsive behaviors, deficits in the development of a stable sense of self, and the inability to have stable relationships, are all thought to be consequences of emotion dysregulation. The behavioral patterns that define BPD are framed in terms of dialectical dilemmas. The core dialectic has emotional vulnerability (i.e., emotional sensitivity and intensity) at one pole and self-invalidation at the other pole. People with BPD are unable to synthesize these two extremes and as a result vacillate between one and the other, at times blaming others for failing to appreciate their vulnerability (emotional vulnerability) and at other times seeing themselves as inherently bad and the cause of all their troubles (self-invalidation). These two extreme positions reinforce each other. When the emotionally vulnerable person invalidates himself or herself in an attempt to regulate emotions, the person becomes more emotionally vulnerable, which results in further self-invalidation. The goal of the DBT therapist is to help the individual synthesize these two poles by validating the patient's emotional vulnerability and modeling validation for the patient, so that eventually the person is able to validate himself or herself. This validation and gradual attempts at change, self-management, and self-soothing are the ingredients that reduce emotional vulnerability and subsequently self-invalidation.

Goals and Mechanisms of Change

Goals are central organizing points of focus in both DBT and GPM. For both DBT and GPM clinicians, the main goal of treatment is to improve the lives of patients with BPD. Both approaches also advocate for "building a life worth living," which ultimately counteracts the wish to be dead. Both have specific techniques to address suicidal behaviors. Each promotes doing the work of therapy both in and outside of sessions, with the goal of helping patients to generalize what they have learned in therapy to the process of building meaningful work and improving relationships.

Longitudinal and treatment outcome research regarding high rates of disability and unemployment among patients with BPD informs this focus on building a life worth living within both treatments. The longest follow-up study of BPD is the McLean Study of Adult Development, which demonstrated that patients with BPD improve symptomatically, with 93% achieving *remission* (defined as no longer meeting criteria for BPD) by 10-year follow-up, but they do not improve to the same extent in terms of overall functioning, with only 50% achieving *functional recovery* (defined as having at least one supportive friendship or romantic partnership and full-time vocational engagement) at 10 years (Zanarini et al. 2010). To date, evidence-based psychotherapies for BPD have been unsuccessful in improving participation in work, school, or other productive activity. McMain et al. (2009, 2012) indicated in their RCT comparing DBT with GPM that across the entire sample, 51.8% of the participants were neither working nor attending school at the end of the follow-up period compared with 60.3% of them at the beginning of therapy. Similarly, 39.7% of participants were receiving psychiatric disability benefits before therapy and 38.8% were receiving this support at the end of follow-up.

When GPM and DBT are integrated, both therapies must maintain a focus on the patient's life outside of the therapy. In GPM, patients are directed to develop a goal for productive activity, whether volunteering or employment, as part of "getting a life." Although patients often come to therapy with the goal of improving relationships, GPM encourages first setting goals around work rather than relationships. At the start of therapy, creating a goal can be difficult for patients, and the first goal may be to learn how to set smaller, achievable goals. GPM's focus on getting a life will not be foreign to DBT therapists. In DBT, patients are encouraged to use their skills to find and maintain work; this is fostered through shaping active responses from the patient that promote thought before action, teaching the patient to manage life problems, and reinforcing the view of the patient as being capable of participating in work.

Implementation and Accessibility

In many health care settings, the implementation of DBT is limited due to the fact that the demand of patients needing services far exceeds the supply of available providers (Carmel et al. 2014; Herschell et al. 2009). As a specialized treatment, DBT requires more provider training than does GPM. Currently, GPM is taught to clinicians in 1-day workshops, and clinicians are advised to read the GPM handbook (Gunderson and Links 2014). The DBT training recommended by the Linehan Institute involves 10 days' worth of coursework, with 6–9 months of home study (Behavioral Tech 2017). Clinician consultation or supervision is also recommended. In settings where staff turnover is high and caseloads are heavy, training staff in GPM may be more practical and effective. The difference in training requirements is what essentially distinguishes DBT as a *specialist* or *expert* approach and GPM as a *basic, standard*, or *general* approach.

The number of patients that can be seen by an individual clinician also varies when comparing GPM and DBT. Depending on patient acuity, a DBT clinician generally follows between 15 and 25 patients for standard DBT treatment. At a maximum, a DBT clinician could see approximately 32 patients for standard DBT treatment at a time.[1] Given that standard DBT is generally administered for 1 year, this is 32 patients per year per clinician. To put this into perspective, the city of Ottawa, the capital of Canada, has a population of approximately 1 million people (Statistics Canada 2017). The conservative population estimate of the prevalence of BPD is 1.6% (Lenzenweger et al. 2007). That means that approximately 16,000 people in Ottawa have BPD. It would take a single clinician more than 500 years to treat that many people with standard DBT, and it would take a clinic of 12 people around 42 years.[2]

That being said, many people with BPD do not seek treatment, and symptoms can remit over time without treatment (Zanarini et al. 2010). In a study of a national household population of people in Britain with BPD, Coid et al. (2009) found that only 56% of patients with BPD access health care and only 13% have had a lifetime psychiatric admission. In a clinic with 12 clinicians providing standard DBT, it would still take 23 years

---

[1]Consultation group (2 hours)+three groups of 10–11 patients (6 hours)+32 individual sessions (32 hours)=40 hours (this is assuming an 8-hour workday and not accounting for lunch or time spent on crisis calls).

[2]16,000 people with BPD/32=500 years; 16,000 people with BPD/(12 clinicians×32 clients)=42 years.

to treat all people with BPD who access health care and 5 years to treat only the people with BPD who have had psychiatric admissions.[3]

GPM offers some flexibility to increase access for patients with BPD who do not require a specialized treatment such as DBT. GPM is easily integrated into a general outpatient program because it does not require intensive training. A generalist clinician can learn to work effectively with patients with BPD reasonably quickly while continuing to treat patients with other disorders. Also, GPM suggests seeing patients on an as-needed frequency. Newer patients might be seen weekly, whereas patients who are more stable might be seen biweekly or monthly. In addition, there is no absolute time commitment for GPM, and GPM is acceptable for intermittent treatment, further reducing the required intensity of treatment.

Although many clinicians who provide GPM will see a broad spectrum of patients, if a GPM clinician were to see only patients with BPD and saw a mix of around 50% weekly patients, 25% biweekly patients, and 25% monthly patients, the clinician would be able to treat an average of 55 patients per year.[4] Using the same figures from Ottawa as previously mentioned, in a clinic with 12 GPM clinicians, it would take around 14 years to treat the people with BPD who access health care in Ottawa and just over 3 years to treat only the people with BPD who have had a psychiatric admission.[5] This is close to double the capacity with standard DBT. Thus, having a stepped care model in which patients generally receive GPM and receive DBT only if necessary might be beneficial in public health care settings (see Appendix B, "Stepped Care Model"). Some patients may receive GPM as a foundation with components of DBT added as severity increases. Another option is to maintain a GPM psychopharmacologist when the patient begins with the full-package DBT treatment. Choosing which GPM and DBT elements to integrate will depend on the patient and the clinical scenario.

---

[3](16,000 people with BPD×0.56 of them who access health care)/(12 clinicians×32 clients)=23.3 years; (16,000 people with BPD×0.13 of them who have had psychiatric admissions)/(12 clinicians×32 clients)=5.42 years.
[4]4-hour supervision/month+27 weekly patients/month+14 biweekly patients/month+14 monthly patients/month=55 patients/month (this is assuming an 8-hour workday and not accounting for lunch or time spent on crisis calls).
[5](16,000 people with BPD×0.56 of them who access health care)/(12 clinicians×55 clients)=13.6 years; (16,000 people with BPD×0.13 of them who have had psychiatric admissions)/(12 clinicians×55 clients)=3.15 years.

Addressing Clinician Stigma

GPM addresses many commonly held myths about BPD that can fuel clinicians' negative countertransference toward patients, particularly in regard to anger and hopelessness (Table 13–1). In DBT, clinicians operate from a set of assumptions that also help to reduce stigma and frame useful ways of understanding countertransference problems (see Table 13–1).

Contracting With the Patient

Putting Self-Harm on Hold

Perhaps one of the most significant differences between DBT and GPM lies in their respective approaches to self-harm. In GPM, clinicians see self-harm as problematic, and the hope is that patients will work on finding other ways to manage triggers that lead to self-harm. However, if a patient does not agree to stop self-harming, a GPM therapist may still choose to continue to work with the patient. If self-harm does occur, the GPM clinician will explore the reasons and effects of self-harm on the person and his or her relationship with others in order to enrich the patient's understanding of the causes of self-harm (particularly interpersonal causes) and to find other ways to address the difficulties. In the case of self-harm that is dangerous or life threatening, a GPM clinician would be more insistent that the behavior be addressed. Even in this case, however, the GPM clinician has the option of continuing to work with the patient as long as the clinician 1) ensures that the patient and his or her significant others understand and accept that suicide might occur and 2) consults with another psychiatrist who confirms that there are no other viable treatment options.

In contrast, in DBT, therapy does not proceed until the patient has made a commitment to the goal of putting suicide and self-harm behaviors on hold. DBT acknowledges that patients will often be ambivalent regarding suicide and that the commitment to reducing suicide and self-harm behaviors may not be as strong as the therapist would like. In practice, a therapist will usually accept a patient's commitment to "do everything humanly possible" to put suicide on hold from week to week. DBT also requires explicit commitment by the patient to reduce behaviors that interfere with therapy—for example, not showing up for sessions. DBT therefore requires more of patients before they can start treatment. When adequate commitment to start DBT cannot be obtained from a patient, the clinician can consider a trial of GPM as an alternative.

TABLE 13–1.	Myths and Assumptions in good psychiatric management (GPM) and dialectical behavior therapy (DBT)

GPM

Myth: People with borderline personality disorder (BPD) resist treatment.
Clarification: Most seek relief from their pain, and treatment requires psychoeducation.

Myth: People with BPD angrily attack their treaters.
Clarification: Excessive anger and fearfulness of treaters are symptoms of the disorder.

Myth: People with BPD rarely get better.
Clarification: 10% remit within 6 months, 25% by a year, and 50% by 2 years. Relapses are unusual.

Myth: People with BPD get better only if given intensive treatment by experts.
Clarification: Such treatment is needed only by a subsample of patients.

Myth: Recurrent risk of suicide burdens treaters with serious liability risks.
Clarification: Excessive burden or fears of litigation are symptoms of inexperience and poorly structured treatments.

Myth: Recurrent crises require treaters to be available 24/7.
Clarification: Such a requirement is rare and may mean a different level of care is needed.

Myth: BPD traits are "character flaws" or moral deficits.
Clarification: Although individuals with BPD often see themselves as being "bad" or "evil," BPD traits are rooted in genetics and learned behaviors.

DBT

Assumptions

People with BPD are doing the best that they can.

People with BPD want to improve.

People with BPD need to do better, try harder, and be more motivated to change.

People with BPD may not have caused all of their own problems, but they have to solve them anyway.

The lives of suicidal individuals with BPD are unbearable as they are currently being lived.

People with BPD must learn new behaviors in all relevant contexts.

Patients cannot fail in therapy.

Clinicians treating patients with BPD need support.

Source. GPM myths and clarifications adapted from Gunderson and Links 2014, p. viii. DBT assumptions adapted from Linehan, MM: "Overview of Treatment: Targets, Strategies, and Assumptions in a Nutshell," in *Cognitive-Behavioral Treatment for Borderline Personality Disorder.* New York, Guilford, 1993, pp. 106–108. Republished with permission of The Guilford Press, permission conveyed through Copyright Clearance Center, Inc.

Intersession Contact

Access to the primary therapist outside regularly scheduled appointments (telephone coaching) is a requirement in standard DBT, and patients generally have access to a round-the-clock pager so that the patient's skills can be generalized to life outside of treatment encounters. Telephone coaching is available for crisis coaching, and calls can also be used for skills coaching in noncrisis situations as well as to address therapeutic ruptures. Patients are asked to call only before they self-harm and are asked not to call for 24 hours after self-harming.

In GPM, contacting the therapist outside of sessions is encouraged for crises, but it is recommended that clinicians set limits on noncrisis calls. GPM clinicians are not expected to be available at all times but are expected to address their availability with patients. GPM therefore accommodates the reality that some clinical environments do not involve availability of clinical staff after hours. When setting up treatment contracts, GPM therapists should discuss the parameters of their availability. Because crises are expected, patients must be fully informed about emergency services that are available and ways to access these services. GPM clinicians rely on patients to be responsible for their safety and make clear that dependency on the availability of others to "stay safe" is doomed to be a risky, nonoptimal solution.

Despite this discussion about availability, some patients may try to have intersession contact beyond the limits established. Difficulty with repeated calls or violations of the therapy boundaries are not the norm and typically happen only with a minority of patients. When the patient does test or break these limits, the issue must be brought up as a priority in the next session and discussed openly. Although the patient may struggle to live within these limits, the therapist must maintain them and must not take the patient's behavior personally. This struggle to make contact and test the limits is best understood as a demonstration of the underlying difficulties with interpersonal hypersensitivity and intolerance of aloneness.

Multiple Clinicians

Both DBT and GPM acknowledge that there are benefits to having more than one clinician involved in treatment and recognize that clinicians need to communicate with each other in order to provide optimal care. In standard DBT, an unimpeded flow of communication between clinicians exists only within the DBT team. The DBT "consultation to the patient" agreement means that clinicians prioritize helping the patients communicate with their outside providers themselves rather than speaking for them. If a DBT therapist wanted to discuss a patient's progress in the skills group, the conversation would likely occur with the patient present, or the patient and skills group leader might draft a progress summary together for the patient to take to the GPM therapist. The main exception to the "consultation to the patient" agreement would be if an issue arises that is important or dangerous and the therapist does not feel that the patient is able to effectively advocate for himself or herself. GPM takes a more flexible approach. Clinicians will encourage patients to assert their needs to clinicians and family members as an expected part of their treatment, and GPM clinicians will also proactively acquire permissions from patients to speak directly with other care providers.

Treatment Overview

Structure

Both GPM and DBT emphasize psychoeducation about the etiology of BPD in the early stages of treatment and require discussing the diagnosis with the patient. GPM differs from DBT somewhat in that information regarding the natural history of BPD is provided. In particular, it is highlighted that patients are expected to improve over time even *without* regular therapy.

DBT is more explicit than GPM in terms of what happens within each session and what elements are included as a part of standard treatment. Standard DBT is composed of a weekly individual therapy session, 2 hours of weekly group skills training, and therapist availability for telephone consultation (ideally 24/7). Therapists are also required to meet weekly with DBT therapists who work in the same facility for a 2-hour consultation session to review cases and receive peer consultation. GPM treatment generally occurs once per week at most, but the number of sessions is flexible. Frequency depends on whether or not treatment is effective in helping patients achieve the agreed-upon goals of treatment. In addition, GPM trainers acknowledge that GPM must be scaled to the frequency allocated by insurance companies, health care systems, and clinician caseloads. Patient attendance at any type of group is encouraged in GPM, whereas in DBT the group is limited to DBT skills training. GPM clinicians are strongly encouraged to have access to consultation either with peers or with more experienced clinicians, but weekly meetings are not mandatory.

A DBT individual therapy session opens with reviewing the patient's diary card from the previous week. The diary card is a standard way of rating daily problem behaviors or urges, intensity of emotions, lying, and use of skills. An agenda for the session is then co-created. In creating the agenda, the therapist adheres to a hierarchy of targets that need to be addressed, starting with 1) current suicidal ideation and followed by 2) suicide attempts or suicidality over the past week, 3) behaviors that interfere with the patient's ability to benefit from therapy, and 4) behaviors that interfere with the patient's quality of life. In the event of suicide or self-harm behaviors, a chain analysis is completed that involves finding out the details of what happened, including vulnerabilities and prompting events. A detailed analysis of the links between the prompting event, the problematic behavior, and the positive and negative consequences for the patient and significant others is completed. This is followed by a solution analysis in which the therapist and patient identify more skillful ways to deal with problematic events in the future. The session finishes with a summary of the session, assigning homework, and troubleshooting any anticipated obstacles to completing homework.

GPM sessions also focus on problems in coping, but the structure in each session is more flexible. GPM focuses on links to interpersonal events as the origin of emotional and behavioral difficulties. In GPM, interpersonal events, particularly rejection and fear of being alone, are presumed to have a central role in suicide and self-harm acts. A patient's statement that "nothing happened" may lead a GPM therapist to continue looking for an interpersonal event or to ponder whether loneliness was the interpersonal event. The clinician communicates to the patient that he or she will help the patient find ways to manage self-harm and suicidal behavior, but to experience significant improvement, the patient needs to work on finding better social supports in order to decrease the causes of suicide and self-harm behaviors. Also central to GPM is the process of developing a coherent narrative about one's life as a remedy to the identity diffusion inherent in BPD. The GPM clinician asks patients to write autobiographies with the purpose of helping patients to make sense of themselves and their lives (Gunderson and Links 2014).

Although DBT has a more explicit within-session structure, GPM is more explicit about expected progress with therapy over time (Table 13–2). These benchmarks of progress may be useful for DBT therapists to keep in mind as well, so as to notice when treatment is not working as expected.

Split Treatments

Because treatment of patients with BPD may call for an eclectic array of methods, there is often value in the patient's use of different providers for different aspects of care. For example, one clinician may address a partic-

TABLE 13–2. **Course of treatment with good psychiatric management**

Target area	Changes	Time	Relevant interventions
Subjective distress or dysphoria	↓ Anxiety and depression	1–3 weeks	Support, situational changes Contractual alliance Agreement on goals and roles
Behavior	↓ Self-harm, rages, and promiscuity	2–6 months	↑ Awareness of self and interpersonal triggers ↑ Problem-solving strategies Relational alliance (liking, trusting)
Interpersonal relationships	↓ Devaluation ↑ Assertiveness + Dependency[a]	6–12 months	↑ Mentalization ↑ Stability of attachment Developing stable supports outside treatment
Social function	Increased school/work/domestic responsibilities	6–18 months	↓ Decreased fear of failure and abandonment fears Coaching on social functioning
Recovery	Internalizes sense of the "good self"	24+ months	Combination of all interventions over time

Source. Adapted from Gunderson and Links 2014, p. 29.

[a]A positive and dependent relationship to the therapist has formed.

ular intervention (e.g., medication) while another may address a different intervention or need (e.g., skills training). It is simply impossible for most clinical providers to provide all the types of interventions that are helpful for a particular patient. The use of different resources to meet a patient's overall needs is of particular value with the most challenging patients with BPD. Split treatments are encouraged and may even be essential in

GPM because they mitigate idealizing tendencies that any one person can be omniscient, omnipotent, and omnipresent (Maltsberger and Buie 1974). Advantages of encouraging patients to use more than one therapist or modality include 1) patients' becoming reliant on more than one source of support, thus diluting the transference response to any one therapist; 2) lessening the risk of therapist "burnout"; and 3) enhancing the patients' connections to their communities or to the healthier aspects of themselves. Because splitting can occur between therapists, GPM requires open communication between therapists and insists that this be established as part of the original treatment contract with the patient (Links et al. 2016).

Although it is desirable to have more than one clinician involved in treatment, both GPM and DBT agree that there should be only one primary clinician. In the case of a GPM clinician providing individual therapy for a patient who is also participating in a DBT skills training group, that clinician will be expected to fulfill the role of primary therapist. It is optimal for the primary clinician to coach the patient to use DBT skills in everyday life by showing an interest in what the patient is learning in groups and encouraging him or her to apply what is learned to day-to-day life outside of therapy. In DBT as well as GPM, the primary therapist is expected to be responsible for overall treatment planning; management of crises, including suicide crisis; taking intersession calls; and making decisions about modification of treatment, including admission to higher levels of care.

Pharmacotherapy

Another structural difference between GPM and DBT is the role of the pharmacotherapist. In standard DBT, it is desired that, even when the primary therapist is a physician, the primary therapist generally does not prescribe medication. The ability to prescribe medications is considered to put the therapist in a position of power, which interferes with his or her ability to work collaboratively with the patient, particularly around the abuse of prescription medications, if this is occurring. In DBT, the patient will also be encouraged to use skills rather than medications to manage symptoms.

In contrast, medication management has a central role in GPM and is thought to be an appropriate role for a physician even if he or she is the primary therapist. A clinician following the GPM model will reinforce that medication is an adjunct to treatment that may lessen certain target symptoms and improve functioning. In addition, GPM clinicians will stress that medications are not a definitive treatment for BPD and that they have not been approved by the U.S. Food and Drug Administration for BPD symptoms.

Family Involvement

Both DBT and GPM advocate for involving family when the risk of suicide is high; however, the ways in which families are involved differ slightly. In GPM, if the patient is refusing to allow the clinician to have contact with significant others when behaviors are dangerous, it is considered a serious mistake for the clinician not to insist on contacting them. Even when dangerousness is not rated to be high, a clinician may decide that contacting the person's significant others is an important part of suicide management, such as when the patient's suicidality is occurring in relation to interactions with family members that the patient lives with and is financially dependent on. The clinician's agreeing not to involve the family can lead to the patient's idealization of the clinician or dismissal of the clinician as a weak link. In GPM, involving family members in the patient's care is also a specific goal of therapy. Although this goal is not always successful and the clinician may have to help a patient accept the reality of dysfunctional parenting, many families are relieved to be included in the care of their family member, and their involvement is often helpful.

In DBT, the involvement of the family generally occurs only with the patient's permission, and meetings with the family would generally be held jointly with the patient. DBT does not place as much emphasis as GPM on involving families or significant others in treatment; however, there are support programs that have been developed for family members, such as Family Connections through the National Education Alliance for Borderline Personality Disorder. These programs focus on providing support and psychoeducation to families who are also taught DBT skills in order to be better able to support their family member with BPD.

When to Consider Dialectical Behavior Therapy and GPM

Considering that the natural course of BPD predicts symptomatic remission for most patients without specialized care, only a minority of patients should need intensive treatments such as DBT. In the stepped care model (see Appendix B), we propose that patients who maintain moderate to severe symptoms without responsiveness to GPM should be referred to a specialized psychotherapy such as DBT (Choi-Kain et al. 2016). Within the GPM model, the patient will continue in therapy as long as change is made and the patient progresses. When a patient's suicidality is not decreasing, either because suicidal acts continue to occur more than once every 3 months or because suicidality fails to improve by 6 months, GPM therapists will openly question whether the treatment is useful. They will look for ways they may be unintentionally reinforcing suicide—for example, by giving the patient more attention during crises or stimulating suicide behaviors by being too nurturing or too distant. They will also consider asking the patient to "take suicide off the table." Following this, if there is no improvement, the therapist should insist on more-intensive multimodal treatment or refer the patient to a BPD-specific therapy.

The GPM model also outlines clear benchmarks for improvement beyond self-harm and suicidal behavior (see Table 13–2), and consideration of specialized care could also occur if these benchmarks are not being met. If benchmarks are not being met, the patient and therapist need to have a frank discussion about the lack of progress and explore the reasons why this might be occurring. If progress remains stalled, it can be useful to take one of the following steps: 1) asking for an informal peer or expert consultation (i.e., not involving the patient) with a valued colleague or mentor to try to better understand the difficulties in the therapy; 2) arranging a formal consultation (i.e., having the consultant meet with the patient) about the patient's lack of progress, particularly if there are questions about whether the therapy should continue; or 3) considering a more intensive specialized treatment such as DBT, either as a stand-alone treatment or in combination with GPM.

There are several situations in which transitioning from DBT to a GPM approach might be beneficial. For example, if it becomes clear during the assessment phase in standard DBT that stopping self-harm is not one of the patient's goals, GPM might be a better fit due to the flexibility around self-harm as a primary target. Another example is if a patient is having difficulties in a DBT skills group due to disruptive behavior, intellectual deficits, or another reason; he or she might experience a better fit with GPM, given the flexibility around participation in groups.

Although these arrangements of sequencing or integrating GPM and DBT are quite workable, this chapter has highlighted some of the challenges that might arise when the two models work in parallel. In general, the two treatments share many similarities and are quite compatible. Despite minor difference in structure and approach, there are many elements of each treatment that can enhance the other if integrated, such as GPM's focus on benchmarks of progress, "getting a life," and the role of interpersonal conflict and DBT's variety of skills and focus on the dialectic of validation and change. Possible approaches to integrating and sequencing DBT and GPM are highlighted in the following clinical vignettes.

Case Vignettes

The following descriptions of two cases include decision points, each of which has several alternative responses listed at the end of the cases. The reader will rate each alternative response in terms of its level of helpfulness. Discussions of responses follow.

Individualized Care

You are a second-year psychiatry resident on call in the emergency department on a Saturday night. At around 3:00 A.M. you are consulted regarding two cases that are being referred by the emergency physician because of suicidal ideation.

In the first chart, you find out that Marc is a 32-year-old man who is well known to the emergency department. Although he generally presents with suicidal ideation, Marc has on some occasions been brought in by police with injuries due to altercations with others. During his last visit a month ago, it was noted that he is homeless and supported by social assistance. He has been using cannabis and alcohol daily since his late 20s. The emergency physician informs you that Marc was brought to the emergency department by police after expressing, while intoxicated, that he was suicidal to bystanders in a coffee shop parking lot. The emergency physician now feels that Marc is sober and would like you to assess him.

In speaking to Marc, you find out that he has been homeless on and off since his last visit to the emergency department. Over the past 2 weeks, he had started dating a woman and was staying at her apartment. Yesterday afternoon, she broke up with him, and he began thinking about killing himself by jumping in front of the subway train. He drank a significant amount of alcohol and became argumentative and aggressive. He endorses a history, dating back to his teen years, of physical altercations with others and an inability to hold on to jobs due to outbursts of anger that he later regrets. He endorses a history of unstable interpersonal relationships, chronic feelings of emptiness, and chronic suicidal ideation, but denies any intent or plan to kill himself currently. He does not have a history of previous suicide attempts but has a history of self-harm in terms of burning himself with cigarettes as a teen. [**Decision Point 1**]

After seeing Marc, you quickly go to see the second referral, Desiree, before going to phone the attending physician to review the cases. Desiree is a 21-year-old woman who was seen early the previous day in the emergency department after overdosing on cough syrup with Tylenol. She was held in the emergency department overnight, but internal medicine does not want to admit her. She is currently cutting daily and due to her frequent overdoses involving Tylenol has developed liver damage. She has been noted to have mild intellectual delay; however, it is unclear if this is due to frequent overdoses or has been present since birth. She additionally has a history of binge drinking. She was sexually assaulted by a previous roommate a few years ago and states that since that time she has found herself in several other risky situations where she has been sexually assaulted while intoxicated. Desiree reports that she drank the cough syrup because she was worrying that she was going to lose her spot at her group home due to smoking cigarettes indoors. She states that she drank the cough syrup because she wanted a "break"; she denies any suicidal intent and states that she had only wanted to fall asleep. She would like to leave the emergency department now to go speak to the staff at the group home so she does not lose her spot. In the community, she is currently followed only by a caseworker, who is experiencing futility over the tasks of managing Desiree's care over the course of her recurrent crises. [**Decision Point 2**]

Fitting the Therapy to the Patient

You and your attending physician have not yet heard about GPM, and Marc and Desiree are both referred for specialist treatment. It takes about 6 months for them to be assessed in the BPD clinic. The clinic has created a new tiered model to reduce the wait list. All patients attend a psychoeducational group about BPD and then are assigned either to GPM or DBT, depending on what is likely to be the best fit for them. Marc will receive GPM, and Desiree will receive DBT.

Marc's Anger and Affective Lability

You are now a third-year resident, and your residency program has a newly developed requirement for residents to learn about GPM and follow at least one supervised GPM case through the BPD clinic. Marc is assigned as your patient, and you begin following him. Over the next 6 months, you develop a good therapeutic alliance. He stops using cannabis and alcohol and works with you to find stable housing by moving in with an uncle. However, his affective lability and anger increase, and he begins self-harming again by burning himself with cigarettes. He also visits the emergency department twice more with suicidal ideation after arguments with his uncle. His behaviors seem to be getting worse rather than better. In taking a careful history, his anger and affective lability do not appear to be due to an emerging bipolar disorder. [**Decision Point 3**]

Marc is very resistant to trying a medication, but he agrees that he might benefit from learning DBT strategies to help him with affect regulation and self-harm. Over the next 6 months, he attends both group DBT and weekly sessions with you. His affect regulation improves, as do his anger outbursts and self-harm. He is able to work toward getting his truck driving license, and at the end of a year you mutually agree to end therapy because he is stable and is beginning to work as a long-haul truck driver. He agrees to check in 3 months later when he returns for a maintenance visit.

Desiree's Disruptive Behavior

Another resident is doing a DBT elective in the BPD clinic and tells you that she is seeing Desiree, the patient you referred, for individual therapy. You ask how Desiree is doing, and the resident tells you that Desiree has exhibited a fair amount of commitment to stopping self-harming, and in fact, she has not self-harmed in the past month. She also appears to be using her individual sessions well. That being said, Desiree has significant difficulties in group meetings. She has significant social anxiety and has been missing groups or coming to groups noticeably intoxicated at times. She has had to be asked to leave at times because of triggering the other patients. She had refused a selective serotonin reuptake inhibitor (SSRI) to help with the social anxiety. She also does not do the homework, and there is a question as to how able she is to do it given her intellectual impairment. Despite committing several times to make changes, she continues to be quite disruptive to the group. She has now missed group three times in a row and is at risk of being dismissed from the group. [**Decision Point 4**]

Desiree misses DBT group four times in a row and is told that she can no longer continue with DBT. You are interested in taking on an additional GPM patient and agree to follow her. She has some slips initially: she comes to sessions intoxicated and she also begins overdosing again on cough syrup at times in response to what she perceives as negative interpersonal interactions in the group home. Within the first month, she stops coming to session intoxicated in response to your setting of limits and she becomes more comfortable with you. She eventually agrees to start an SSRI for social anxiety, and you work with her on making friends within her group home. She eventually makes several friends and gets a part-time job at a warehouse. Over the next 2 years, she is eventually transitioned from weekly to biweekly sessions and then to monthly, and then she is discharged.

Decision Points: Alternative Responses

Rate each response in terms of its level of helpfulness with a rating of 1 (will be helpful), 2 (possibly helpful, continuing reservations), or 3 (not helpful—or even harmful).

1. You call the attending physician to review Marc's case. What form of outpatient follow-up would you propose?

   A. Refer Marc for DBT treatment.
   B. Follow Marc yourself in the outpatient clinic using the GPM model.
   C. Discharge Marc without follow-up.
   D. Refer Marc for addictions counseling.

2. What form of outpatient follow-up would you propose for Desiree?

   A. Refer Desiree for DBT treatment.
   B. Follow Desiree yourself in the outpatient clinic using the GPM model.
   C. Discharge Desiree without follow-up.
   D. Refer Desiree for residential treatment of substance abuse.

3. Marc's self-harm and interpersonal functioning seem to be worsening rather than improving after 6 months of treatment. What will you do next?

   A. Continue with GPM.
   B. Switch Marc to the DBT program.
   C. Suggest that Marc attend a DBT group.
   D. Start a medication.

4. What do you think would be best for Desiree, given how disruptive she is in the group?

   A. Address her behavior and continue with DBT.
   B. Transition to GPM.
   C. Discharge Desiree from the DBT program.
   D. Refer Desiree for alcohol use disorder treatment.

Decision Points: Discussion

Numbers within brackets indicate level of helpfulness ratings.

1. You call the attending physician to review Marc's case. What form of outpatient follow-up would you propose?

   A. Refer Marc for DBT treatment. [2] (DBT may be helpful for Marc; however, if GPM is available, it might be the better choice from a public health perspective because specialized treatment may not be necessary for him. He has not self-harmed in several years and has never had a suicide attempt, and there are some DBT programs that might exclude him. Given that he does not have a high level of target 1, as per page 370, suicidal behavior, use of DBT as a scarce resource may not be optimal.)
   B. Follow Marc yourself in the outpatient clinic using the GPM model. [1] (This option would likely be helpful for both the res-

ident and the patient. If the resident receives training in GPM
and is supervised, this may be a good fit.)

C. Discharge Marc without follow-up. [3] (The patient is no longer
intoxicated, is not actively suicidal, and is likely appropriate for
discharge; however, he has a pattern of chronic suicidal ideation
and remains at risk. He also will likely continue to have recurrent visits to the emergency department. Outpatient treatment
for BPD may target a range of problems at once, because his
symptoms of BPD seem to get in the way of his keeping a job
and may be contributing to his substance use.)

D. Refer Marc for addictions counseling. [2] (This option might be
useful for Marc given his daily alcohol and cannabis use; however, he also appears to have many difficulties in addition to alcohol and cannabis use. DBT or GPM may be a more appropriate
option. Both DBT and GPM recommend substance use treatment if the substance use will interfere with the patient's ability
to participate in therapy. GPM recommends at least 3 months of
sobriety in the case of alcohol dependence to make BPD treatment feasible. DBT is somewhat more flexible around substance
use and has been studied to treat substance use disorders [Line-
han et al. 1999, 2002].)

2. What form of outpatient follow-up would you propose for Desiree?

A. Refer Desiree for DBT treatment. [1] (Desiree's case seems particularly severe given her liver functioning, frequent self-harm,
binge drinking, and risk of further sexual assaults. She may benefit from specialized care if it is available. Her intellectual disability is mild; however, it is important to consider given that
standard DBT requires a certain level of literacy and cognitive
functioning. However, her anxiety in social situations and her
difficulty with follow-through may make it hard for Desiree to
make the commitments required for DBT.)

B. Follow Desiree yourself in the outpatient clinic using the GPM
model. [1] (Desiree could benefit from the GPM model. Supervision by a more experienced clinician will help the resident
manage the complexity of Desiree's various problems.)

C. Discharge Desiree without follow-up. [3] (Desiree denies current active suicidal ideation; however, given her current pattern
of behavior, she remains at risk of further liver damage and possible sexual assault. Specific treatment for BPD could organize

her problems and help her cope and manage relationships in a way that diminishes the problems leading her to intermittent recurrent crises.)

D. Refer Desiree for residential treatment of substance abuse. [2] (This referral might be useful for Desiree given her binge drinking; however, she also appears to have many difficulties above and beyond drinking. DBT or GPM may be a more appropriate option. Both DBT and GPM recommend substance use treatment first if the substance use will interfere with the ability to participate in therapy; with Desiree's level of binge drinking, either GPM or DBT is likely feasible without her having substance use treatment first.)

3. Marc's self-harm and interpersonal functioning seem to be worsening rather than improving after 6 months of treatment. What will you do next?

A. Continue with GPM. [2] (This might be helpful; however, it is concerning that the treatment is at the 6-month mark and the patient's self-harm and anger are not improving. GPM would suggest having a frank discussion with Marc about the lack of progress to explore potential reasons. The therapist could ask for an informal peer or expert consultation or arrange for a formal consultation about Marc's lack of progress. Considering a more intensive specialized treatment such as DBT is another option.)

B. Switch Marc to a DBT approach. [2] (Switching to another approach might be helpful given Marc's lack of progress; however, given that the GPM therapist and the patient already have a good therapeutic alliance, this may not be the best option.)

C. Suggest that Marc attend a DBT group. [1] (If more intensive treatment is needed with more structure and accountability, then the addition of a DBT group might be a good fit. Marc could continue to see the GPM therapist while attending a DBT group.)

D. Start a medication. [2] (GPM suggests the atypical antipsychotics quetiapine extended release (ER) and olanzapine, in low doses, may be helpful in the short term for anger and impulsive aggression. As Marc's anger appears to have worsened since he stopped using alcohol and cannabis, a brief (8–12 weeks) trial of quetiapine ER or olanzapine may be an option if the patient is interested.)

4. What do you think would be best for Desiree, given how disruptive she is in the group?

A. Address her behavior and continue with DBT. [2] (It is possible that Desiree's behavior will improve; however, the behavior has already been addressed several times and she remains disruptive in the group.)

B. Transition to GPM. [1] (A transfer from DBT to GPM may be helpful both for Desiree and for maintaining the integrity of the group that has been disrupted. An individual therapist may be better able to tolerate and work with some of Desiree's disruptive behaviors, and in standard DBT, attending only individual therapy is not an option. Her intellectual disability and failure to do the homework also raise the question as to whether she may benefit from the GPM approach, which relies less on written materials and involves a certain level of paternalism.)

C. Discharge Desiree from the DBT program. [3] (Although Desiree has made some gains and has not self-harmed over the past month, she remains at high risk of these behaviors returning at this juncture if she is left without treatment.)

D. Refer Desiree for alcohol use disorder treatment. [2] (Binge drinking continues to be a problem for Desiree, and treatment for alcohol use disorder could be helpful. She continues to have a profile more complex than alcohol use disorder alone, and treatment for BPD remains important.)

Conclusion

DBT and GPM are two important evidence-based treatments for BPD. DBT is arguably a gold standard intensive outpatient treatment. DBT practitioners and patients show a degree of commitment and an exemplary knowledge of DBT skills. However, as noted, obstacles to implementing DBT in its adherent form abound (Choi-Kain et al. 2016; Landes et al. 2017). DBT skills training combined with case management has been shown to work as well as standard, full-package DBT on most outcome measures (Linehan et al. 2015; McMain et al. 2017); we feel that this is some limited evidence pointing to the utility of a stepped care model that utilizes DBT skills training as an essential basic option for patients with BPD and can be readily combined with any well-informed approach guided by basic principles of GPM. There is a likelihood that many clinicians and patients will only be able to collaborate in a pastiche of elements of different evidence-based psychotherapies for BPD. We hope this chapter provides a clearer overview of how these options can be navigated to best serve the patients and improve access to services.

References

Association of Psychology Postdoctoral and Internship Center: 2017 APPIC Match: Survey of Internship Applicants, Part 1: Summary of Survey Results. Houston, TX, Association of Psychology Postdoctoral and Internship Center, February 22, 2017. Available at: https://www.appic.org/Internships/Match/Match-Statistics/Applicant-Survey-2017-Part-1. Accessed July 23, 2018.

Bateman AW: Treating borderline personality disorder in clinical practice. Am J Psychiatry 169(6):560–563, 2012 22684591

Behavioral Tech: Level 3—Comprehensive Training in Standard DBT. Seattle, WA, Behavioral Tech: A Linehan Institute Training Program, 2017. Available at: https://behavioraltech.org/training/training-catalog/level-3. Accessed July 16, 2018.

Carmel A, Rose ML, Fruzzetti AE: Barriers and solutions to implementing dialectical behavior therapy in a public behavioral health system. Adm Policy Ment Health 41(5):608–614, 2014 23754686

Choi-Kain LW, Albert EB, Gunderson JG: Evidence-based treatments for borderline personality disorder: implementation, integration, and stepped care. Harv Rev Psychiatry 24(5):342–356, 2016 27603742

Coid J, Yang M, Bebbington P, et al: Borderline personality disorder: health service use and social functioning among a national household population. Psychol Med 39(10):1721–1731, 2009 19250579

Gunderson JG, Links PS: Handbook of Good Psychiatric Management for Borderline Personality Disorder. Washington, DC, American Psychiatric Publishing, 2014

Herschell AD, Kogan JN, Celedonia KL, et al: Understanding community mental health administrators' perspectives on dialectical behavior therapy implementation. Psychiatr Serv 60(7):989–992, 2009 19564234

Landes SJ, Rodriguez AL, Smith BN, et al: Barriers, facilitators, and benefits of implementation of dialectical behavior therapy in routine care: results from a national program evaluation survey in the Veterans Health Administration. Transl Behav Med 7(4):832–844, 2017 28168608

Lenzenweger MF, Lane MC, Loranger AW, et al: DSM-IV personality disorders in the National Comorbidity Survey Replication. Biol Psychiatry 62(6):553–564, 2007 17217923

Linehan MM: Cognitive-Behavioral Treatment of Borderline Personality Disorder. New York, Guilford, 1993

Linehan MM, Schmidt H 3rd, Dimeff LA, et al: Dialectical behavior therapy for patients with borderline personality disorder and drug-dependence. Am J Addict 8(4):279–292, 1999 10598211

Linehan MM, Dimeff LA, Reynolds SK, et al: Dialectical behavior therapy versus comprehensive validation therapy plus 12-step for the treatment of opioid dependent women meeting criteria for borderline personality disorder. Drug Alcohol Depend 67(1):13–26, 2002 12062776

Linehan MM, Korslund KE, Harned MS, et al: Dialectical behavior therapy for high suicide risk in individuals with borderline personality disorder: a randomized clinical trial and component analysis. JAMA Psychiatry 72(5):475–482, 2015 25806661

Links PS, Mercer D, Novick J: Establishing a treatment framework and therapeutic alliance, in Integrated Treatment for Personality Disorder: A Modular Approach. Edited by Livesley WJ, Dimaggio G, Clarkin JF. New York, Guilford, 2016, pp 101–122

Maltsberger JT, Buie DH: Countertransference hate in the treatment of suicidal patients. Arch Gen Psychiatry 30(5):625–633, 1974 4824197

McMain SF, Links PS, Gnam WH, et al: A randomized trial of dialectical behavior therapy versus general psychiatric management for borderline personality disorder. Am J Psychiatry 166(12):1365–1374, 2009 19755574

McMain SF, Guimond T, Streiner DL, et al: Dialectical behavior therapy compared with general psychiatric management for borderline personality disorder: clinical outcomes and functioning over a 2-year follow-up. Am J Psychiatry 169(6):650–661, 2012 22581157

McMain SF, Guimond T, Barnhart R, et al: A randomized trial of brief dialectical behaviour therapy skills training in suicidal patients suffering from borderline disorder. Acta Psychiatr Scand 135(2):138–148, 2017 27858962

Statistics Canada: Census Profile, 2016 Census. Statistics Canada Catalogue no. 98-316-X2016001. Ottawa, Ontario, Canada, Statistic Canada, November 29, 2017. Available at: https://www12.statcan.gc.ca/census-recensement/2016/dp-pd/prof/index.cfm?Lang=E. Accessed July 16, 2018.

Zanarini MC, Frankenburg FR, Reich DB, et al: Time to attainment of recovery from borderline personality disorder and stability of recovery: a 10-year prospective follow-up study. Am J Psychiatry 167(6):663–667, 2010 20395399

Chapter 14

Integration With Mentalization-Based Treatment

Brandon T. Unruh, M.D.

Anne K.I. Sonley, M.D., J.D.

Lois W. Choi-Kain, M.D., M.Ed.

Mentalization-based treatment (MBT; Bateman and Fonagy 1999, 2004) and good psychiatric management (GPM; Gunderson and Links 2014; McMain et al. 2009) are manualized treatments proven effective for borderline personality disorder (BPD). In this book, we are advancing the idea that GPM is a first-line "generalist" approach and that MBT is a "specialist" approach requiring greater intensity and precision by clinicians. This chapter summarizes points of theory and practice at which GPM and MBT overlap and diverge. A clinical vignette is presented to illustrate methods of sequencing and integrating GPM and MBT across various phases of an extended treatment course. The vignette highlights the typical sort of patient whom a clinician might consider referring to MBT after limited improvement with GPM.

GPM and MBT have a great deal in common: an ethic of optimizing treatment accessibility, an insistence on openly discussing the BPD diagnosis and providing psychoeducation, and an attitude toward flexibility in implementation. Their developers are good friends and share common values of pragmatism and empiricism. They both boil central ingredients of good psychotherapy down into a simple recipe, which in its basic foundation offers potential applicability beyond BPD.

The differences in GPM and MBT are quite modest. Their theoretical origins, their views concerning BPD's core phenomenology, the level of training required for adherent and effective implementation, and the degree of elaboration on techniques are divergent. Perhaps the central difference is that MBT is a psychotherapeutic approach and its techniques focus on process, whereas GPM is a case management approach designed to improve function with or without a concerted psychodynamic process.

Points of Overlap, Departure, and Elaboration

Theory

GPM's theoretical orientation is informed by the general medical and scientific literature on BPD, leading to its view of BPD as a disorder with neurobiological underpinnings, common psychiatric and medical comorbidities, and genetic vulnerability to a core phenotype of interpersonal hypersensitivity (Gunderson 2011). GPM explicates BPD's core phenomenology with a model of "interpersonal coherence" (see Appendix C, "Interpersonal Coherence Model"). This model explains how the symptoms of BPD oscillate according to shifts in the patient's level of interpersonal connectedness. These fluctuations are themselves caused by perceived or actual interpersonal stressors, such as rejection, separation, or withdrawal.

MBT's theoretical origins derive from psychoanalysis and attachment research. *Mentalization* refers to the ordinary imaginative activity of understanding mental states within oneself and others. This includes sorting out what one is feeling or thinking; considering how one arrived at any current experience and monitoring its impact on oneself and others; and considering the perspectives of others curiously and empathically rather than dismissively. The capacity to mentalize is either fostered or not through early attachment relationships. The developmental model for BPD includes three elements: 1) a constitutionally and environmentally mediated vulnerability to disruptions in mentalizing, triggered in response to interpersonal stress; 2) reemergence of nonmentalizing modes of experiencing self and others; and 3) the resultant painfully incoherent or extreme representations of self and others that are managed through adopting rigid views or taking destructive action toward self and others (Bateman and Fonagy 2004). Like GPM, MBT also contextualizes etiological factors from the biological and relational realms in transaction.

MBT thus usefully fleshes out two central elements of GPM's theory and practice. First, MBT extends GPM's phenomenology of BPD by elaborating how symptoms of interpersonal hypersensitivity are mediated by particular nonmentalizing *states of mind*, which emerge through an inability to modify and mitigate negative appraisals following stressful social interactions (Fonagy et al. 2017). These nonmentalizing modes become targets for clinical intervention according to specific MBT protocols. Second, MBT elaborates the conditions under which productive treatment relationships become possible. GPM refers to "corrective experiences" through the therapeutic relationship, but MBT expands on this. Informed by research on social cognition and learning, MBT requires that patients establish and maintain a belief in the trustworthiness of clinicians and in the personal relevance of what they communicate; this means that patients must experience clinicians as empathically recognizing their particular experience as individuals rather than addressing them as though from a textbook or protocol. This "epistemic trust" is considered a necessary precondition for new learning to take place. MBT thus offers more explicit instructions for molding meaningful interpersonal communication and dealing with typical barriers that arise. It considers how a patient with a personality disorder may first need to trust the source of information (the clinician) before being able to learn.

Goals and Mechanisms of Change

GPM's goals are informed by epidemiological studies of BPD's standard course without specialized treatment. Given the tendency for patients with BPD to symptomatically remit without functional recovery, GPM's primary goal is not "deep" personality change but rather "building a life worth living" by achieving a meaningful vocational role and a rewarding partnership. This "getting a life" is a "behavioral" target (the attainment of certain concrete goals thought to enhance quality of life) and an "intrapsychic" target (reaching these goals generally requires meaningful personality change). GPM firmly asserts that a stable and rewarding life itself is the best therapy.

Through its psychotherapeutic protocol, MBT more directly targets a specific intrapsychic vulnerability, unstable mentalizing capacity, which, in turn, is thought to underpin symptoms and functioning. MBT expects that the patient's relationships, behavior, emotional life, and sense of identity and functioning will secondarily improve as mentalizing stabilizes. GPM and MBT thus share ultimate aims of symptomatic remission and functional recovery, but MBT proposes that these are best targeted by stabilizing reflection about mental states within the context of an attachment relationship that challenges this capacity.

MBT is comparatively more "ambitious" than GPM in its aspirations to bring about greater "depth" of change, because improvements in mentalizing are considered fundamental building blocks and expressions of lasting personality change as well as symptomatic stability and functional growth.

Accessibility and Implementation

The impetus for systematizing GPM came from the public health imperative to equip generalist clinicians with the tools needed to deliver "good enough" treatment to the majority of patients with BPD because most patients can achieve remission and a better life without specialized care (see Appendix B, "Stepped Care Model"; see also Choi-Kain et al. 2016, 2017). GPM therefore emphasizes flexibility and adaptability for clinicians and patients in wide-ranging treatment contexts. MBT is more specialized and structured but shares a commitment to optimal access because it was developed in a public health setting and can be deployed in both private practice and insurance-based public health settings.

Training in MBT begins with attending a 3-day workshop and optimally continues with group or individual supervision. MBT training appears to have immediate positive effects on clinician attitudes and capacities. Both GPM and MBT trainings instill confidence for working with patients with BPD, overturn preexisting negative biases about BPD, and leave staff feeling that the material is highly applicable in a variety of clinical settings (Keuroghlian et al. 2016; Warrender 2015). Brief MBT training may even improve the mentalizing capabilities of novice therapists (Ensink et al. 2013).

Longer-term adherence has been studied more extensively for MBT than for GPM (Bales et al. 2017). Several adherence scales have been developed for clinician use (Bateman 2018; Karterud et al. 2013). Various versions of these scales have been used to monitor adherence in MBT replication studies (Bales et al. 2012). GPM expressly does not concern itself with adherence. As an approach that is founded on the idea that clinicians of any type can become well informed and follow a set of procedures such as diagnostic disclosure and psychoeducation, GPM does not require an adherence system but rather a simple checklist and a knowledge base quiz (Finch and Gunderson 2017).

Empirical Validation and Broadening Indications

MBT has been empirically validated as an effective treatment for BPD in two major formats: a day hospital program and an outpatient treatment with once-weekly individual and group components (Bateman and Fonagy 1999, 2001, 2008, 2009, 2013). Both formats are associated with reductions in suicidal and self-harming acts, hospitalizations, depressive symptoms, mental health service utilization, and medication use, as well as improvements in social and interpersonal functioning and employment.

Like GPM, MBT may have efficacy for a variety of other disorders beyond BPD. Benefits have been found for eating disorders and substance use disorders (Morken et al. 2017; Robinson et al. 2016). Modified forms of MBT have been proposed—but not yet empirically evaluated—for mood, somatoform, posttraumatic stress, and other disorders (Allen 2013; Bateman and Fonagy 2012, 2015; Luyten et al. 2012).

MBT has been shown to be helpful for treating personality disorders other than BPD. Perhaps MBT's most unique adaptation has been its application to antisocial personality disorder (Bateman et al. 2016). It has also been used to treat patients with BPD and comorbid personality disorders. In an 18-month trial of outpatient MBT, cases with more significant personality disorder comorbidity improved faster with MBT than with generalist treatments (Bateman and Fonagy 2013). Together, these data support a rationale for generalists to consider an MBT referral for particularly "hard-to-reach" patients with antisocial personality disorder or with more than one personality disorder who have not improved adequately with generalist treatment.

Structure of Treatment

Standard MBT is delivered by a team of clinicians as a structured package of psychoeducation, individual and group therapy, and peer supervision for team members. Like other specialist BPD treatments, MBT has a more extended process of "pretreatment," assessment, and formulation in contrast to GPM. GPM offers immediate clinical engagement, which is maintained if progress is made. MBT begins with assessment of a patient's mentalizing vulnerabilities and strengths, discussion of the personality disorder diagnosis, and an 8- to 10-week psychoeducation group blending didactic teaching about mentalizing and attachment with process-oriented interventions intended to foster mentalizing experiences.

As the main phase of treatment begins, an individualized MBT formulation is developed that integrates the patient's own description of presenting problems and goals with the clinician's assessment of the patient's attachment style and mentalizing vulnerabilities. This formulation is delivered and revised collaboratively with the patient using ordinary language. It is subsequently invoked and expanded throughout the treatment with a focus on keeping core relational patterns in view. As patients transition from the introductory psychoeducational group into longer-term mentalization groups, group members are expected to share their formulations with one another so that core difficulties remain actively "on the table" for mentalizing by the entire group whenever they emerge.

MBT's guidelines regarding the timeline of termination are relatively more specific than those in GPM. The duration of MBT offered by most established clinical programs is 1–1.5 years. When that initial treatment ends, some programs offer intermittent individual "check-up" sessions or an ongoing "maintenance" MBT group for an additional period of time that is focused on managing difficulties around optimizing vocational functioning and generalizing gains made during the main phase of treatment. GPM is an open-ended treatment, and termination is based on patient progress.

Unlike GPM, MBT does not systematically require patients to work. Some MBT programs, however, have operationally adopted this requirement as consistent with MBT's larger aims. Vocational endeavors are increasingly emphasized as treatment progresses.

MBT does not have specific pharmacological guidelines but refers to the United Kingdom's National Institute for Health and Care Excellence (NICE) guidelines for treating borderline personality disorder, which are more conservative about prescribing than GPM's suggestions of targeted, empirically guided medication management. The NICE guidelines recommend restricting prescribing to treatment for comorbidities (National Institute for Health and Care Excellence 2009). Both approaches share an attitude of conservatism about pharmacological interventions to maintain a focus on changes the patient needs to make for himself or herself, either psychologically or functionally.

Technique

GPM's technique eclectically combines psychoeducation; nonspecific BPD treatment ingredients (e.g., active listening, demonstrating concern); matter-of-fact problem solving and advice giving (consistent with supportive therapy and case management); confrontation of defenses (in the spirit of psychodynamic therapy); and emphasis on accountability and expectation of change (consistent with behavioral therapy). GPM clinicians assume a relatively more authoritative, less neutral, "wise uncle" stance that is organized around a clear vision of the patient's best interest in regard to what it takes to remit and recover from BPD. GPM clinicians are more likely to make directive recommendations and dole out practical life lessons. MBT employs a relatively less directive stance and attends more heavily to how here-and-now therapeutic interactions are experienced and interpreted by the patient. Expressly, MBT's developers endorse the idea that the desired destination *is* the mentalizing process, meaning the aim is not to get patients to think specific thoughts or in a specific way; MBT only aims to assist patients in being more reflective as they come up with their own ideas or decisions.

The main aim of MBT—reinstating and stabilizing reflection—is achieved in a systematic way. MBT therapists begin by continuously assessing for the emergence of mentalizing vulnerabilities. During this process, MBT therapists perform three tasks (Bateman and Fonagy 2016). First, clinicians assess for the presence of general signs of "good" mentalizing, such as curiosity and interest in others, self-reflection, cognitive flexibility, and perspective taking. They also assess for "bad" mentalizing, such as unrealistic certainty, concreteness, circularity, externalizing, and blaming. Second, clinicians probe the capacity to shift the patient's perspective in a balanced, flexible way across characteristic mentalizing dimensions, mapping out ways in which the scope of mentalizing becomes rigidly fixed and limited. Third, clinicians scan for the emergence of three prototypical nonmentalizing modes, which are known as *teleological mode* (when concrete realities become the sole vehicle for understanding or expressing mental states: "I had to cut to be understood after..."), *psychic equivalence* (when thoughts and feelings become conflated with reality: "Because I think it or feel it, it must be true"), and *pretend mode* (marked disconnection between aspects of experience within oneself or between clinician and patient).

MBT is anchored in a *mentalizing stance*. Core features of the mentalizing stance include a here-and-now focus on describing mental states (rather than merely recounting behavior or circumstances); active curiosity and interest in *how* patients sort out what is going on in their own and others' minds; and an "ordinary," nonexpert, "not knowing" approach in which clinicians eschew the guise of having privileged knowledge about what goes on in anyone's mind or what is happening in the therapeutic relationship. Instead, MBT clinicians seek to stimulate patients' own reflection on self and others, challenge areas of premature certainty, and elaborate implicit aspects of interpersonal interaction. The aim of the mentalizing stance is to help patients identify, question, and respond in a balanced way to a range of perspectives rather than collapsing into non-mentalizing, harmful modes of experience and behavior. MBT therapists share their own perspectives with patients in a "marked" way, highlighting where views differ or overlap and raising intrigue and curiosity to explore the origins of such discrepancies and concordances. MBT therapists are quick to admit that their own mentalizing process is fallible (e.g., "I'll have to think about why I said that," or "I wonder why I keep missing what seems obvious to you here"). This is done to model, and provoke, consideration of different perspectives within the self and between self and others.

As treatment unfolds, MBT adjusts interventions to ensure that the intensity and complexity of the interventions attempted do not outpace a patient's mentalizing capacity (i.e., what the patient can "take in" at any given moment). This requires MBT therapists to shift focus among supportive interventions when mentalizing is highly vulnerable; interventions to restabilize mentalizing when nonmentalizing emerges; and interventions to explore implicit relational dynamics within the therapeutic relationship. The type of intervention to be used at any one moment is calibrated by monitoring and managing levels of arousal and attachment activation. States of *attachment hypoactivation* are marked by insufficient interest, curiosity, or affective arousal to generate mentalizing, whereas states of *attachment hyperactivation* occur when perceived interpersonal threat or intensity of affective arousal is so high that it hampers mentalizing. The goal is to establish and maintain a level of emotional arousal and connectedness that is of ample intensity to sustain mentalizing but not so intense as to overwhelm it.

In summary, MBT techniques are designed to enhance reflective capacity, which is thought to undergird "deeper" change processes required to reduce BPD symptoms and to achieve greater interpersonal and vocational stability. The focus of MBT evolves from an initial emphasis on reopening social learning channels through facilitating basic mentalizing processes to later challenging and reexamining representational patterns using alternative perspectives generated by the individual therapist, group therapists, and fellow group members. The goal is eventual generalization of symptomatic, reflective, relational, and functional gains into the patient's social world (Fonagy et al. 2015). MBT's growing appeal is partly due to its compatibility with elements of psychodynamic and behavioral therapies (Swenson and Choi-Kain 2015). Mentalizing techniques can be readily integrated with most other approaches for enhanced mentalizing effect. Like GPM, MBT is flexibly multimodal and aims to combine with clinical resources that are realistic.

When to Consider Mentalization-Based Treatment

MBT is relatively more widely disseminated in Europe than in North America. Clinicians in regions where MBT is available can consider referrals to MBT when a generalist or specialist treatment has not achieved stabilization and function. In addition, MBT can be considered for the following:

1. Patients with multiple personality disorders
2. Patients who have gained some symptomatic stability through another BPD treatment but are motivated to work further on persistent problems in the interpersonal and identity domains of BPD psychopathology
3. Patients with unusually severe or challenging impairments in social cognition, such as particularly concrete interpersonal operations, pervasive difficulties with empathy, or profound alexithymia
4. Patients with a high degree of perceived malevolence or mistrust of others, especially mistrust of health professionals or government service representatives who assist with housing, education, and legal support

Case Vignette

The following case description includes decision points, each of which has several alternative responses listed at the end of the case. The reader will rate each alternative response in terms of its level of helpfulness. Discussions of responses follow.

This vignette illustrates shifting modalities between GPM and MBT over time in response to evolving difficulties in the treatment course.

> You are a first-year attending psychiatrist working in a hospital-based outpatient clinic. During residency, you received BPD didactics and supervision from a GPM trainer in your program who helped you gain solid experience with GPM, an interest in working with patients with BPD, and confidence that you can be helpful to most of them. During your final year as a chief resident, you also attended a 3-day workshop in MBT that left you intrigued by the differences between GPM and MBT. You have not yet gained any experience implementing MBT.

You receive a voicemail from a 24-year-old man named Evan requesting an urgent meeting. He sounds desperate but sympathetic and motivated. He tells you he used to work at a biotech company but has fallen down on his luck. He promises he will be a "good, hard-working patient" if only you will help him. You schedule an initial appointment, saying, "Let's see if I can be helpful."

Evan steps into your office, wide-eyed. He sits disquietedly and never stops intently scanning the room as though to ward off potential threats. He stares at you with doleful, pleading eyes as he tells you his main plight is failed romantic relationships. He blurts out woefully, "Why can't I get a woman to love me?" He then launches into recounting multiple failed courtships, including one engagement that ended after his fiancée became fed up with his going to electronic music festivals, using MDMA (3,4-methylenedioxymethamphetamine), and making out with other women. When you ask why he was surprised that his fiancée would not tolerate this behavior, he looks downward, appears frustrated, and quietly says, "I never would have had to do those things if she had really loved me."

While reviewing his general psychiatric history, Evan tells you that he once had "a small problem" with impulsive substance use, which he claims is behind him. You also discover he was recently charged with assault. The assault occurred when he caught a previous girlfriend cheating on him and he assaulted the man she was with. He says that because he was under the influence of substances at the time, he received only probation and was required to attend an anger management course. He says that if he would have been sentenced to prison, he would have killed himself before going there. He then tries to reassure you that he is not a suicide risk and does not manipulate people through making suicide threats.

Evan's prior psychiatric treatment consisted of 1 year of weekly psychodynamic psychotherapy with a psychology trainee. The trainee had recently become licensed, and Evan could no longer afford to see her. He now needs to use his insurance to access whatever treatment you recommend. About the prior psychotherapist, Evan said only that "she was nice and seemed to care about me, but nothing really changed."

You decide to begin seeing Evan once weekly within a GPM frame because he has not previously had any treatment targeting BPD. You give him the diagnosis of BPD based on deep-seated abandonment fears, relationships that careen between extremes of idealization and devaluation, impulsivity in the domains of substance use and seeking sex to manage feelings, recurrent suicidal statements and acts, and a deeply unstable sense of self.

You request a written autobiography from Evan. In his autobiography, Evan expresses a long-standing sense of being different and defective. You collaboratively set goals, including a return to work and reduction of substance use and suicidal behaviors (although he is not willing to commit to taking either off the table). You develop a crisis plan in which you offer your availability for emergencies but predict your support will be imperfect. You underscore that he will need to become a more reliable advocate for his own safety and sobriety over time.

You also suggest that Evan would be better off if he took time off from dating to focus on recommitting to his career and forming male friendships, which you predict will be less charged and more stabilizing. He agrees that returning to work is paramount, but he seems to pay only lip service to your suggestion of putting dating on the back burner.

You stay within a case manager role, at times utilizing both behavioral and psychodynamic interventions to shape his behavior in more adaptive directions and to call his attention to the connections between fluctuations in his emotional life and interpersonal stress. He seems interested in and reflective about these connections. However, his frenzied dating shows no sign of slowing down. You become increasingly matter-of-fact in pointing out what you see as obvious problems and increasingly directive in telling him the dating needs to stop if he wants to get better.

Six months into treatment, Evan is psychiatrically hospitalized while using LSD (lysergic acid diethylamide) at a rave after a disappointing second date. He tried to kill himself at the music venue by climbing up the speaker scaffolding and jumping down. Prior to doing this, he began calling and texting suicide threats to the person he went on the date with. On the inpatient unit, even while sober, he continues saying he is relentlessly suicidal because he cannot get over the thought that no woman will like him. Although you had hoped this hospitalization would be brief, his course is prolonged when, while out on a pass from the inpatient unit, he is found wandering near the subway tracks contemplating jumping. You are concerned and pause to review the past 6 months of treatment and evaluate your helpfulness.

Over the past 6 months, Evan had gained some behavioral control around his impulsive drug use and suicidality, seemingly in response to your efforts to educate, confront, and counsel him. His vocational functioning had improved, and he had kept his part-time "recovery job" at a cell phone retail store despite calling in sick several times when he felt "too pathetic as a person" after a failed date the night before. He has gotten himself back on track by reapplying to various biotech companies in the area. He is also more aware of the interpersonal context of his emotional problems, agreeing with you that dynamics of closeness prominently influence his sense of self and his behaviors.

Furthermore, significant interpersonal and identity problems have emerged that were not apparent at the outset of Evan's treatment. He continues to desperately seek a romantic partner, typically arranging "first dates" with up to five new women each week, and he is unsure why none of the relationships work out. You have come to see Evan's problematic interpersonal behaviors as reflective of serious and entrenched problems with social cognition. He seems to have a very inflexible understanding of how others' minds work. In his relationship with you, his boss, his probation officer, and other authority figures, he is highly mistrusting and quick to regard any interpersonal rupture as evidence of others' malevolence or his own "unlovability." He feels criticized by your plainspoken instruction about what to do differently and seems not to follow most of your advice.

You discuss with Evan your concerns that his treatment has plateaued, noting that he has made partial improvements but remains at high risk of long-term instability and suicide if he does not change at a deeper level. He replies that the prospect of giving up dating would be intolerable—although he sees that rejection sensitivity could sway him at any time to use substances or kill himself. He still seems to be genuinely overwhelmed and dismayed by how driven he is to find a woman and is despondent in his loneliness. Finally, he begins to cry and poses a now familiar question, as if it were for the first time: "Why can't I get a woman to love me?"

How could it be that what you have said to Evan so straightforwardly through the lens of GPM has not gotten through? You come to believe that a more specialized form of treatment might be more helpful. You ponder how to discuss this with him and what to recommend. As you begin presenting various options, he tells you he cannot imagine working with anyone else and begs you to stay on the case. [**Decision Point 1**]

You decide to educate yourself further about MBT in order to better target Evan's difficulties with understanding and managing what happens for him and others in the relationships he wants to sustain. You read the MBT treatment manual (Bateman and Fonagy 2016) and consider how to modify your GPM approach. [**Decision Point 2**]

Evan begins attending a mentalization group while you begin incorporating basic MBT techniques into your sessions. Over the next year, you and his group leaders consistently adopt a mentalizing stance to help him slow down and articulate how he comes to feel so misunderstood by romantic partners as well as figures of authority such as his boss. Together, you develop a more detailed shared understanding about how his mind works and how frequently and substantially his perspectives on social interactions differ from those of others.

MBT's focus on "understanding misunderstandings" helps Evan note instances of poor mentalizing in his relationship with you, with other members of the mentalization group, and with important others outside of treatment. He gains confidence in himself through controlling his suicidality, avoiding further hospitalizations, establishing longer sobriety, and avoiding legal problems. He also feels that he can handle working in his field again; he has maintained a high-paying job in a biotech company for the past 6 months. He considers how his perspectives on himself and others have led him to behave in ways that directly contribute to his difficulty with "finding a woman." He eventually gives up on serial dating and invests in a longer-term relationship that has now lasted 6 months. However, the relationship remains tenuous given that he is easily injured by his girlfriend and continues to seek the company of other women behind her back when he feels "unappreciated" and "unlovable."

Over the past year, Evan's BPD symptoms have lessened, his nonromantic relationships have stabilized, and his vocational functioning has improved—but he still has major identity issues and interpersonal difficulties manifesting in fraught romantic relationships and persistent loneliness. It is easy to imagine that an acute risk of suicide would reemerge if his relationship were to collapse and if he were to relapse on substances. You conclude that integrating MBT techniques with GPM has augmented the treatment's efficacy, but once again you feel Evan has reached a treatment plateau. You ponder what to recommend as a next step. [**Decision Point 3**]

You continue work with Evan and discuss in greater depth which aspects of MBT were most helpful for him. He names the mentalization group as most challenging and rewarding because it was there that he was shocked to discover that others' minds did not work the same way as his and later learned to check out his impressions of interpersonal interactions before trusting his immediate conclusions. He chooses to continue in a mentalization group for an additional year to retain some connection to the concepts he found helpful there.

You also incorporate more and more elements of MBT into your own therapeutic stance as you deepen your study of mentalizing techniques through self-directed reading and supervision from an MBT expert. You increase your attention to slowing Evan down and pushing him to examine exactly how his mind is working when he disagrees with you. You become adept at shifting as needed between GPM's doctorly, authoritative stance when Evan needs containment and MBT's "not knowing" stance when Evan benefits from more exploration. His romantic relationships remain a source of great pain for him, but with your help over the years he maintains his high-paying job, avoids catastrophic substance use, and has had no further charges for assault. Over the years, the frequency of your visits decreases to monthly. He has developed a healthy awareness of his own mentalizing vulnerabilities and how they lead to crisis and a useful appreciation of how your mind works, which he regularly channels to help himself slow down and sort through his difficulties.

Decision Points: Alternative Responses

Rate each response in terms of its level of helpfulness with a rating of 1 (will be helpful), 2 (possibly helpful, continuing reservations), or 3 (not helpful—or even harmful).

1. In your discussion with Evan about appropriate next steps toward more specialized treatment modality, you should

   A. Give Evan information about dialectical behavior therapy (DBT) and MBT, inviting him to choose which to pursue and empowering him as the best judge of which treatment is best for him.
   B. Ask Evan why he still thinks working with you can be useful beyond this point, telling him he would have to "make a good case" for you to keep seeing him, given your concerns about his stalled progress.

    C. Recommend that Evan try out a DBT skills group to evaluate whether a switch into a standard DBT program with individual skills coaching might be useful.

    D. Offer to keep working with Evan within a GPM frame while incorporating basic principles and techniques from MBT.

2. Which elements of MBT can you most easily incorporate into a GPM frame without full training in MBT in order to increase the efficacy of the treatment?

    A. Referring Evan to an adjunctive mentalization group to enhance his capacity to understand and manage the differences between his own and other people's perspectives.

    B. Providing psychoeducation about attachment styles.

    C. Focusing on the question of whether or not Evan is mentalizing. When he is not mentalizing, use MBT maneuvers to reinstate mentalizing.

    D. Employing a "not knowing" mentalizing stance.

3. After concluding that the augmentation of GPM with MBT has been successful but nevertheless limited in the scope of gains achieved, you should

    A. Insist that Evan move to live near a specialized psychiatric center where he can next receive a full package of insurance-based "adherent" MBT.

    B. Refer Evan to a psychoanalyst.

    C. Continue to incorporate within an overarching GPM frame the elements of MBT that have proven most helpful to Evan over the past year while improving your own facility with MBT techniques through further reading and supervision from an MBT expert.

Decision Points: Discussion

Numbers within brackets indicate level of helpfulness ratings.

1. In your discussion with Evan about appropriate next steps toward more specialized treatment modality, you should

    A. Give Evan information about DBT and MBT, inviting him to choose which to pursue and empowering him as the best judge of which treatment is best for him. [2] (GPM actively enlists patients in their own recovery, including by eliciting their own ideas about what they think should happen and why. This approach could provide useful data about what Evan thinks could work best, which may or may not align with what *would* likely work best. GPM is not shy about making doctorly recommendations based on what is known empirically about BPD and related conditions, but these recommendations are often focused on helping a patient think and make decisions with a broader view. However, asking a patient who is having severe interpersonal difficulties and reactive self-destructive behavior to choose between complex treatments is a tall order.)

B. Ask Evan why he still thinks working with you can be useful beyond this point, telling him he would have to "make a good case" for you to keep seeing him, given your concerns about his stalled progress. [1] (Stimulating a patient's reflectiveness on his own treatment goals and preferences is desirable in GPM. This response also emphasizes the point that treatment continues only if it is helping the patient get better. Being explicit about the problems in the treatment relationship vis-à-vis goals of treatment is compatible with both GPM and MBT.)

C. Recommend that Evan try out a DBT skills group to evaluate whether a switch into a standard DBT program with individual skills coaching might be useful. [2] (DBT skills groups in combination with case management can be helpful for BPD even in the absence of individual DBT therapy [Linehan et al. 2015] and are a frequent adjunctive approach used in GPM. Furthermore, the tight behavioral lens of DBT may seem a viable way of targeting Evan's ongoing high-risk behavioral problems, substance use, and suicidal acts. Evan would benefit from learning skills for regulating emotions and responding differently within relationships. Deeper change may ultimately require a more relationally focused approach that would focus on articulating the sources of his beliefs about what happens for him in relationships. There is some evidence to suggest that MBT in combination with DBT is more helpful than DBT alone for problems with social cognition and attachment security [Edel et al. 2017].)

D. Offer to keep working with Evan within a GPM frame while incorporating basic principles and techniques from MBT. [1] (This option makes good clinical sense because it incorporates an understanding of Evan's interpersonal hypersensitivity and his related impairments in interpreting motives of others—his entrenched mistrust and perceptions of malevolence, his concrete and unrealistic perceptions of the women he dates, and his general lack of understanding of how his own mind works.)

2. Which elements of MBT can you most easily incorporate into a GPM frame without full training in MBT in order to increase the efficacy of the treatment?

    A. Referring Evan to an adjunctive mentalization group to enhance his capacity to understand and manage the differences between his own and other people's perspectives. [1] (GPM has general guidelines for incorporating group treatments adjunctively. Groups are cost-effective and clinically effective tools for enhancing the effectiveness of individual sessions. This may be especially true when a goal is to foster greater awareness of differences between self and others. An MBT group specifically targets improving mentalizing and in Evan's case is preferable.)

    B. Providing psychoeducation about attachment styles. [3] (Delivering additional information about attachment styles is not likely to be helpful in and of itself for this patient at this juncture. Although Evan has heard your explanations of how his interpersonal hypersensitivity is tied to how his BPD symptoms evolve, it may be that he does not see the applicability of your advisement about romantic pursuits to his life.)

    C. Focusing on the question of whether or not Evan is mentalizing. When he is not mentalizing, use MBT maneuvers to reinstate mentalizing. [1] (Pattern recognition of particular nonmentalizing modes is likely helpful for any clinician who learns it. Evan's desperation in getting a woman to love him is difficult for him to give up. Helping Evan more steadily mentalize may help him see why his choices are problematic. Noting those moments where he is not mentalizing is the first step.)

    D. Employing a "not knowing" mentalizing stance. [1] (Employing a mentalizing stance is likely the single most helpful standalone MBT intervention that can be learned and implemented separately, without other MBT elements. The technique centers on just listening for and identifying any moments of certainty or important links in patients' reasoning that are not explicitly expressed, then using a stance of inquisitiveness to illuminate implicit mental state processes both within the patient's mind and between patient and clinician.)

3. After concluding that the augmentation of GPM by MBT has been successful but nevertheless limited in the scope of gains achieved, you should

A. Insist that Evan move to live near a specialized psychiatric center where he can next receive a full package of insurance-based "adherent" MBT. [3] (Asking Evan to pack up his life to pursue a further specialized treatment at this juncture, now that his symptoms and functioning have significantly improved, runs counter to GPM's prioritization of "getting a life." However, GPM clinicians can continue to deepen their integration of basic MBT principles and techniques within an ongoing generalist treatment frame.)

B. Refer Evan to a psychoanalyst. [3] (Your current assessment is that Evan has had a partially helpful course of GPM augmented by principles and techniques from MBT. Although psychoanalytic theory might be relevant to Evan and his difficulties, his mentalizing capacity may remain inadequate for this kind of intensive and unstructured intervention. Keeping in mind GPM's value on adaptation in the community, you also worry that prescribing further treatment specialization could set up the expectation that rarified treatment settings are the only place for him to be understood and work further on himself.)

C. Continue to incorporate within an overarching GPM frame the elements of MBT that have proven most helpful to Evan over the past year while improving your own facility with MBT techniques through further reading and supervision from an MBT expert. [1] (This approach continues to pragmatically distill the various elements that have worked for Evan thus far into an eclectic, integrative approach blending GPM and MBT. This is likely to be the most realistic and clinically effective option available. It also exhibits fidelity to the spirit of GPM, which contends that the essential ingredient of effective BPD treatment is a flexible "good enough" clinician interested in learning what works alongside his or her patient over time, through any tools available from a variety of modalities over time.)

Conclusion

MBT is a specialized treatment for BPD that can improve treatment efficacy for patients who do not adequately improve with GPM (see Appendix B). In theory, it can have some advantages in its focus on enhancing reflectiveness in interpersonally charged interactions. When delivered as a stand-alone treatment modality, MBT requires greater clinical training and precision, but GPM clinicians can readily augment ongoing treatments by adapting MBT's commonsense principles for managing areas of misunderstanding by exploring the perspectives of the patient with those of others. Patients who may particularly benefit from a referral to MBT or from the integration of GPM and MBT include those with multiple comorbid personality disorders, those with persistent interpersonal and identity-related disturbances, those with severely impaired social cognition, and those particularly mistrusting of others on whom they must rely for treatment or psychosocial services.

References

Allen JG: Restoring Mentalization in Attachment Relationships: Treating Trauma With Plain Old Therapy. Washington, DC, American Psychiatric Publishing, 2013

Bales D, van Beek N, Smits M, et al: Treatment outcome of 18-month, day hospital mentalization-based treatment (MBT) in patients with severe borderline personality disorder in the Netherlands. J Pers Disord 26(4):568–582, 2012 22867507

Bales DL, Verheul R, Hutsebaut J: Barriers and facilitators to the implementation of mentalization-based treatment (MBT) for borderline personality disorder. Pers Ment Health 11(2):118–131, 2017 28488379

Bateman A: Mentalization-Based Treatment Adherence and Competence Scale, 2018. Available at: https://www.annafreud.org/training/mentalization-based-treatment-training/mbt-adherence-scale. Accessed January 1, 2019.

Bateman A, Fonagy P: Effectiveness of partial hospitalization in the treatment of borderline personality disorder: a randomized controlled trial. Am J Psychiatry 156(10):1563–1569, 1999 10518167

Bateman A, Fonagy P: Treatment of borderline personality disorder with psychoanalytically oriented partial hospitalization: an 18-month follow-up. Am J Psychiatry 158(1):36–42, 2001 11136631

Bateman A, Fonagy P: Psychotherapy for Borderline Personality Disorder: Mentalization-Based Treatment. Oxford, UK, Oxford University Press, 2004

Bateman A, Fonagy P: 8-year follow-up of patients treated for borderline personality disorder: mentalization-based treatment versus treatment as usual. Am J Psychiatry 165(5):631–638, 2008 18347003

Bateman A, Fonagy P: Randomized controlled trial of outpatient mentalization-based treatment versus structured clinical management for borderline personality disorder. Am J Psychiatry 166(12):1355–1364, 2009 19833787

Bateman AW, Fonagy P: Handbook of Mentalizing in Mental Health Practice. Washington, DC, American Psychiatric Publishing, 2012

Bateman A, Fonagy P: Impact of clinical severity on outcomes of mentalisation-based treatment for borderline personality disorder. Br J Psychiatry 203(3):221–227, 2013 23887998

Bateman A, Fonagy P: Borderline personality disorder and mood disorders: mentalizing as a framework for integrated treatment. J Clin Psychol 71(8):792–804, 2015 26190067

Bateman A, Fonagy P: Mentalization-Based Treatment for Personality Disorders: A Practical Guide. Oxford, UK, Oxford University Press, 2016

Bateman A, O'Connell J, Lorenzini N, et al: A randomised controlled trial of mentalization-based treatment versus structured clinical management for patients with comorbid borderline personality disorder and antisocial personality disorder. BMC Psychiatry 16:304, 2016 27577562

Choi-Kain LW, Albert EB, Gunderson JG: Evidence-based treatments for borderline personality disorder: implementation, integration, and stepped care. Harv Rev Psychiatry 24(5):342–356, 2016 27603742

Choi-Kain LW, Finch EF, Masland SR, et al: What works in the treatment of borderline personality disorder. Curr Behav Neurosci Rep 4(1):21–30, 2017 28331780

Edel MA, Raaff V, Dimaggio G, et al: Exploring the effectiveness of combined mentalization-based group therapy and dialectical behaviour therapy for inpatients with borderline personality disorder: a pilot study. Br J Clin Psychol 56(1):1–15, 2017 27897326

Ensink K, Maheux J, Normandin L, et al: The impact of mentalization training on the reflective function of novice therapists: a randomized controlled trial. Psychother Res 23(5):526–538, 2013 23964813

Finch EF, Gunderson JG: General psychiatric management quiz: preliminary data and future directions. Poster presented at General Psychiatric Management Trainers Conference, Belmont, MA, July 2017

Fonagy P, Luyten P, Allison E: Epistemic petrification and the restoration of epistemic trust: a new conceptualization of borderline personality disorder and its psychosocial treatment. J Pers Disord 29(5):575–609, 2015 26393477

Fonagy P, Luyten P, Allison E, et al: What we have changed our minds about, part 1: borderline personality disorder as a limitation of resilience. Borderline Personal Disorder Emotion Dysregul 4:11, 2017 28413687

Gunderson JG: Clinical practice. Borderline personality disorder. N Engl J Med 364(21):2037–2042, 2011 21612472

Gunderson JG, Links PS: Handbook of Good Psychiatric Management for Borderline Personality Disorder. Washington, DC, American Psychiatric Publishing, 2014

Karterud S, Pedersen G, Engen M, et al: The MBT Adherence and Competence Scale (MBT-ACS): development, structure and reliability. Psychother Res 23(6):705–717, 2013 22916991

Keuroghlian AS, Palmer BA, Choi-Kain LW, et al: The effect of attending good psychiatric management (GPM) workshops on attitudes towards patients with borderline personality disorder. J Pers Disord 30(4):567–576, 2016 26111249

Linehan MM, Korslund KE, Harned MS, et al: Dialectical behavior therapy for high suicide risk in individuals with borderline personality disorder: a randomized clinical trial and component analysis. JAMA Psychiatry 72(5):475–482, 2015 25806661

Luyten P, Van Houdenhove B, Lemma A, et al: A mentalization-based approach to the understanding and treatment of functional somatic disorders. Psychoanal Psychother 26(2):121–140, 2012

McMain SF, Links PS, Gnam WH, et al: A randomized trial of dialectical behavior therapy versus general psychiatric management for borderline personality disorder. Am J Psychiatry 166(12):1365–1374, 2009 19755574

Morken KTE, Binder PE, Arefjord N, et al: Juggling thoughts and feelings: how do female patients with borderline symptomology and substance use disorder experience change in mentalization-based treatment? Psychother Res 17:1–16, 2017 28513339

National Institute for Health and Care Excellence: Borderline Personality Disorder: Recognition and Management. London, The British Psychological Society and the Royal College of Psychiatrists, 2009. Available at: https://www.nice.org.uk/guidance/cg78. Accessed June 23, 2018.

Robinson P, Hellier J, Barrett B, et al: The NOURISHED randomised controlled trial comparing mentalisation-based treatment for eating disorders (MBT-ED) with specialist supportive clinical management (SSCM-ED) for patients with eating disorders and symptoms of borderline personality disorder. Trials 17(1):549, 2016 27855714

Swenson CR, Choi-Kain LW: Mentalization and dialectical behavior therapy. Am J Psychother 69(2):199–217, 2015 26160623

Warrender D: Staff nurse perceptions of the impact of mentalization-based therapy skills training when working with borderline personality disorder in acute mental health: a qualitative study. J Psychiatr Ment Health Nurs 22(8):623–633, 2015 26148873

Chapter 15

Integration With Transference-Focused Psychotherapy

Richard G. Hersh, M.D.

Good psychiatric management (GPM) and transference-focused psychotherapy (TFP) are both empirically validated treatments for patients with borderline personality disorder (BPD) (Clarkin et al. 2007; McMain et al. 2009). Both were developed from distinctly different psychotherapeutic traditions but nevertheless share some core theoretical tenets. GPM's central aim—to equip clinicians with a "generalist" model for treating BPD—has a clear public health mission (Gunderson and Links 2014). This follows naturally from its roots in the American Psychiatric Association's (2001) "Practice Guideline for the Treatment of Patients With Borderline Personality Disorder"; this document's audience was a group of clinicians with heterogeneous orientations and training. TFP, in contrast, was developed by specialists attempting to adapt traditional psychoanalytic psychotherapy for a group of severely impaired patients shown to have limited response to the more classical psychoanalytic approach (Yeomans et al. 2015). TFP's developers were motivated by their dedication to psychoanalytic theory and technique; at the same time, they acknowledged the need for significant modification of standard interventions with patients with BPD. While GPM and TFP share some key elements—active therapist, open discussion of the BPD diagnosis, psychoeducation for the patient and family, and a focus on meaningful activity (work, studies), among others—their approaches are clearly different (Weinberg et al. 2011). The focus of this chapter is on the practical, clinical approach to using GPM and TFP together.

Although both GPM and TFP were developed over decades, with accruing support from rigorously conducted studies in the United States, Canada, and Europe, they remain relatively little known and understood by many clinicians and the general public (Clarkin et al. 2001; Doering et al. 2010; McMain et al. 2012). They are both far less well known and not nearly as proliferated as dialectical behavior therapy (DBT). That said, GPM and TFP training and practice can offer clinicians a valuable set of skills in the assessment and treatment of patients with BPD across the life cycle and along a continuum of disease severity.

The most likely use of GPM and TFP together would be a sequencing of treatment, beginning with the generalist approach of GPM and eventually transitioning to the specialist approach of TFP, when indicated. This type of sequencing is exemplified in this chapter's case vignette. The section "Vignette Summary" also touches on an alternative sequencing when the TFP therapist recommends a transition to GPM treatment. In addition, an exploration of integration of elements of TFP in GPM, and of GPM in TFP, which has been termed *technical eclecticism*, is advanced; this preliminary discussion grows out of educational initiatives offered by experts in both treatment modalities (Choi-Kain et al. 2016). This discussion of sequencing and/or integration of generalist and specialized treatments for BPD comes in the context of a broader controversy about how best to meet the challenge of providing treatment for the many patients with BPD without access to adequate treatment because of an insufficient number of trained clinicians, financial constraints, or both. Some experts in the field are concerned about the emergence of "silos" of expertise (Clarkin 2012; Gabbard 2007; Livesley 2012; Paris 2015). Both GPM and TFP trainings encourage clinicians to accept certain limitations inherent in their respective treatments and to maintain a degree of flexibility, to avoid doctrinaire thinking, and to best accommodate the needs and limitations of the individual patient. Moreover, in response to widespread educational and clinical needs, GPM and TFP thought leaders have moved beyond thinking exclusively about the traditional patient-therapist dyad. New endeavors aimed to introduce "applied" versions of GPM and TFP principles (e.g., in emergency departments, inpatient units, primary care treatment settings) complement continued refinement of the individual treatment modalities (Bernstein et al. 2015; Hersh et al. 2017; Hong 2016; Zerbo et al. 2013).

TFP and GPM were both first conceptualized as treatments for patients with BPD. The overarching mission of GPM's developers remains GPM's dissemination as a basic intervention for clinicians of many kinds for assessing and treating individuals with BPD. Although research on TFP has been limited to patients with BPD, TFP's application to a broader spectrum of patients with personality disorder pathology has been advanced in recent years. Specifically, the use of TFP's central elements in treating 1) patients with higher-level personality pathology and 2) a range of patients with narcissistic pathology has led to publications devoted to this subject, although there are still no TFP treatment trials for these populations (Caligor et al. 2007; Diamond et al., in press). Higher-level personality pathology describes those syndromes that are marked by significant elements of repression-based, as opposed to splitting-based, defenses. In general, these patients will be more stable, with elements of more consolidated identity, than those individuals with moderate to severe personality disorder pathology. In the current DSM-5 nosology (American Psychiatric Association 2013), patients with histrionic, dependent, or avoidant personality diagnoses might fall into this category. GPM clinicians, too, have begun to consider the utility of the therapy's central concepts and methods in work with patients beyond the distinct category of BPD, albeit in a preliminary way (for a discussion of GPM applied to another personality disorder, see Chapter 12, "Implementation of Good Psychiatric Management for Narcissistic Personality Disorder").

Goals, Assessment, Contracting, and Techniques

Goals

As described above, GPM and TFP have had distinctly different developmental trajectories. GPM has the goal of providing a "good enough" treatment for patients with BPD, factoring in an expectation that most patients with BPD will get better over time, with keen sensitivity about the risks of iatrogenically induced problems fostered by excessive (and ineffective) treatments for this population. GPM is a theoretically eclectic approach, borrowing from psychodynamic and cognitive-behavioral schools of thought. Driven by pragmatism, GPM prioritizes what works to help patients get a life. In contrast, TFP is a more purely psychodynamic intervention, one with a focus on the patient's experience in the treatment but not at the expense of attention to the patient's functioning, in multiple spheres, outside of the treatment.

The empirical validation of GPM and TFP rests on assessment of critical outcome measures. These measures include the following: a reduction in the frequency and quality of suicidal and self-injurious actions; a reduction in the frequency of emergency department visits and psychiatric hospitalization days; and an improvement in overall BPD symptoms. It makes sense that any treatment designed for individuals with BPD would prioritize these outcomes as targets. Moreover, TFP studies have identified a specific improvement in the patient's capacity for reflective functioning; this outcome measure is of particular interest as a general marker of psychological thinking within relationships as a result of psychotherapies.

The elements of empirical validation and overarching treatment goals of GPM and FTP may be overlapping, but they are not synonymous. The *goals* of these treatments differ, given their respective histories and contributors. Whereas GPM's focus is to impart to the patient an appreciation of the role of interpersonal hypersensitivity as an underpinning for a variety of maladaptive behaviors and to do so with guidance, direction, and support, TFP hews closely to a more explicitly psychodynamic hypothesis. TFP's overarching theory rests on a model of the fragmented and contrary experiences of self and others of the patient with PBD. This model postulates that the patient's experience of self and others alternates between a pattern of "all good" and "all bad" states, leading to dysfunction, chaos, and identify diffusion. The patient's move from fragmentation and splitting to identity integration rests on the patient's ability to take responsibility for thoughts, feelings, and actions that had been "split off" and are examined in the treatment via the patient's relationships with others, in particular with the therapist. It is important to remember that TFP rests on Kernberg's (1975) theory about the borderline *organization*, a broad and more inclusive category of psychopathology that includes BPD and extends to other personality disorder presentations with overlapping, but distinct, symptom constellations. TFP therefore will target patients with BPD, as GPM does, but also patients with comparable mid- and lower-level personality organization profiles, including those with narcissistic personality disorder, among others.

TFP and GPM also differ in their respective conceptualizations and management of aggression. The TFP therapist will highlight the way in which the patient's experience of himself or herself, and the patient's relationships with others, is impacted by often unconscious aggression. The GPM therapist will describe the way in which aggression can develop in the face of relational threats (e.g., a patient who becomes increasingly angry in the context of separation or rejection and then risks alienating others at a time when they might be most needed). This distinction between the two treatments can suggest that GPM is, by definition, a more supportive intervention, whereas TFP could be seen as a more confrontational one. That said, the TFP therapist will aim to explore the patient's aggression in a way that should feel supportive, with the structure and security of the treatment guaranteed by a rigorously defined frame.

Assessment

TFP differs quite significantly from GPM in its approach to diagnosis and to establishment of the aforementioned treatment frame. Quite literally, the GPM clinician may agree to begin treatment after the initial meeting, albeit with some provisos depending on details of the clinical situation. In contrast, the TFP assessment process requires at least two or three meetings and sometimes many more. The TFP assessment process rests on an understanding of the structural interview approach, as described by Kernberg (1981, 1984). Whereas the GPM clinician may proceed following a "medical model" assessment using a standard decision-tree delimitation of the BPD (and/or other disorder) symptom constellations, a clinician using the structural interview aims to include *both* a standard assessment approach utilizing DSM-5 nosological categories *and* an extension of the process to include exploration of multiple elements contributing to the patient's level of organization (Clarkin et al. 2018). Roughly speaking, a description of the patient's level of organization aims to establish how functional or how impaired a patient might be. The structural interview has the goal of describing both categorical and dimensional elements of diagnosis, akin to the current "Alternative DSM-5 Model for Personality Disorders" in Section III of DSM-5 (American Psychiatric Association 2013). The structural interview proceeds with a circular pattern, with a focus on areas of the patient's history that the interviewer finds confusing or vague, often guided by the interviewer's active monitoring of his or her countertransference. This would be different from a more standard medical model decision-tree approach of assessment. The GPM clinician, too, would surely assess the patient's level of functioning in key spheres, but the TFP clinician is compelled to do so, and the structural interview dictates investigation of six key areas with this goal—reality testing, aggression, defenses, identity consolidation versus diffusion, object relations, and superego functioning—easily recalled with the mnemonic RADIOS.

The TFP assessment process utilizing the structural interview will also investigate elements of antisocial traits in a particularly deliberate manner not necessarily expected in GPM. The TFP therapist will investigate, from the beginning, any deficits of moral values that might be marked, for example, by lying, cheating, stealing, or even more subtle parasitic exploitation. The structural interview goes beyond the DSM-5 nosology when investigating gradations of borderline, narcissistic, and antisocial pathology. In TFP, identification of significant superego deficits will cue the therapist about 1) the necessary rigor of the treatment frame and 2) the patient's prognosis. In general, the more prominent the antisocial traits, the more guarded a prognosis, and a more detailed and rigorous treatment frame is required. GPM instructs its practitioners that comorbid antisocial personality renders cases of BPD difficult to treat when treatment is pursued with compromised motives. (For example, patients who may agree to treatment only to placate concerned family members or school or court officials but who have little interest in marking changes in their behavior.) It does not, however, explicitly frame an approach to managing this comorbidity or assessing antisocial personality disorder.

The TFP therapist will not begin treatment posthaste, as a GPM therapist might. This distinction underscores the difference between GPM's place as a generalist's approach versus TFP's place as a specialized treatment. GPM assumes that its practitioners provide treatment for any patients with BPD who show up in an emergency department, inpatient service, and outpatient caseload. The TFP therapist, when contacted by a treatment system, family, or patient requesting an immediate transfer of care, would not reflexively accept the patient for an extended individual psychotherapy. The TFP therapist would either refer the patient to some kind of interim treatment situation or accept the patient while distinguishing between acute care services offered and the prospect of a more extended psychotherapy process, educating those involved about the deliberate process of assessment and treatment contracting required in TFP that can take weeks, sometimes even months, before that psychotherapy would begin.

As noted, the extended assessment process in TFP will take time. After the clinician has accumulated sufficient material to make a diagnosis, the clinician will then spend time sharing with the patient (and often the patient's family) the clinician's diagnostic impression, as would be done in GPM. TFP does not dictate a more full discussion of etiology, genetics, and prognosis, as would be done in GPM, but such psychoeducation would certainly be consistent with TFP theory. Because TFP's assessment process includes personality pathology as reflected in borderline personality organization, including but not limited to BPD, the TFP clinician would also discuss with a prospective patient other possible primary or co-occurring personality disorder diagnoses. In particular, TFP's growing consensus that patients with narcissistic pathology should and do benefit from an understanding of their diagnosis, even if the clinician does not necessarily use DSM-5 terminology, would compel the TFP clinician to convey to the patient the essential elements of alternating fragility and grandiosity. The GPM clinician might be open to discussion of the contribution of narcissistic pathology if this topic arises organically during the course of treatment, but the TFP clinician will *initiate* this discussion if indicated.

This discussion thus far has explored the goals for GPM and TFP treatments in a number of ways. These include 1) goals defined by empirical studies and measurements of treatment efficacy and 2) goals informed by clinicians' overarching theoretical hypotheses. Working with patients to define *their* goals for treatment is another aspect of both GPM and TFP treatments, although the two interventions have somewhat different approaches. The GPM therapist could agree to go forward with treatment even if the patient's initial goal of the treatment is limited to *identifying* personal and treatment goals. In contrast, in TFP the elucidation of the patient's personal goals and treatment goals are understood to be anchoring processes. The therapist's clear understanding of the patient's personal goals and treatment goals justifies the establishment and maintenance of the treatment frame. The TFP therapist encountering the patient who is unable (or unwilling) to articulate goals would not be able to initiate a standard TFP treatment; in such cases, the therapist could continue an even more extended evaluation process or consider a preliminary period of supportive psychotherapy. This distinction between the two treatments may reflect the scope of the respective treatment's ambition; GPM is more likely to accept most patients "where they are," whereas TFP would require some evidence of the patient's desire for and motivation to change.

Contracting

TFP's deliberate assessment process and discussion of diagnosis are followed by an extended contracting phase that will include a meeting with spouse, parents, or others when the patient has any significant active dependence on this other party or parties. (This would include, for example, the patient whose treatment is paid for by another party or the adult patient who is living with family.) Whereas GPM may be open to family involvement, TFP will stress family involvement in cases as described. The contracting phase is another essential element of TFP that is not part of the GPM approach. The contracting process is considered a "dress rehearsal" for the TFP treatment; in the contracting phase, the clinician expects to identify important elements of transference patterns that are likely to emerge during the course of the treatment. Contracting in TFP is not the same as the clinician sharing with the patient his or her office policies. The contracting process should facilitate exploration of the patient's emerging experience of the therapist. Is the patient overly agreeable or overtly confrontational? Does the patient exhibit suspiciousness about the agreement with the therapist or an unrealistic acceptance of the contract's stipulations that might suggest an early idealizing stance? The therapist will begin to consider the patient's dominant experience of the therapist during this process. GPM is notable for its flexibility and accommodation; TFP is defined by its structure as reflected in the extended contracting phase and detailed treatment contract elements. In this respect, the different goals of the two interventions inform the nature of their respective treatment frames. GPM aims to be elastic and accommodating; TFP aims to establish a frame that will allow essential transference elements to emerge over time.

The TFP contracting process will include discussion about many varied aspects of the prospective treatment. This process is designed to be extensive, even belabored, and therefore, it obviously contrasts with GPM's priority of accommodation and flexibility. TFP's contracting process has two overarching goals: 1) establishing a treatment situation that will feel safe for both patient and therapist and 2) establishing a treatment frame that will facilitate emergence of critical transference elements than can then be examined over time. A complete discussion of the TFP contracting process (see Yeomans et al. 1992) is beyond the scope of this chapter; the following are representative examples of elements of the TFP contract, which are compared with aspects of standard GPM practice:

- TFP is a twice-weekly treatment, estimated to last 1–3 years. The fixed frequency and expected duration are in marked contrast to GPM's flexibility about frequency and duration. TFP's twice-weekly, relatively set duration of treatment correlates with the overarching goal of gradual integration of aspects of behavior that are understood to be split off and therefore responsible for the chaos and identity diffusion seen in patients with BPD.

- The TFP contract will require, rather than just recommend, that a prospective patient allow the therapist contact with prior treaters and/or individuals on whom the patient is dependent. Whereas GPM does stress the benefits for the therapist conferred by such contacts, TFP will make it a requirement for treatment.
- The TFP contract would not convey the kind of openness regarding contact between sessions that is expected in GPM. In TFP, the therapist will delineate what constitutes rare "emergency" situations but will review at length in advance an algorithm for emerging suicidality or other crises between sessions. The TFP therapist will distinguish between emergency services available in the community (e.g., hospital emergency departments) and the therapist's relative inability to accommodate patients outside of scheduled meetings.
- In TFP, the creation and maintenance of the treatment frame will inevitably lead to exploration of the negative transference. For example, the patient who had in the past regularly managed intersession anxiety or suicidality by reaching out to his or her therapist may feel that the TFP contract limiting intersession contacts leads to an experience of the therapist as disengaged or indifferent. This element of the negative transference would then be a central area of exploration. The GPM therapist, by contrast, might allow for intersession contact, but the reality of the limits of his or her availability could, nevertheless, lead the patient to feel disappointed or abandoned at times. Such a situation could then be used as an opportunity for the patient to learn that it is unwise to depend too much on anyone to manage safety. This lesson is learned in GPM as a reality of the treatment dyad and in TFP as an exploration of a projection.
- Although the TFP therapist is open to adjunctive treatments (e.g., pharmacotherapy, 12-step programs, couples counseling, DBT skills groups), the contracting phase will underscore the centrality of the treatment relationship in TFP in a way that is not done in GPM. For example, whereas the GPM therapist will routinely support a patient's ongoing participation in a DBT skills group without reservation, the TFP therapist would endorse simultaneous psychotherapy modalities only under certain circumstances and then only after exploring the risk of splitting with all parties involved. Again, GPM's hallmark flexibility will differ from TFP's relatively prescribed course.
- Although GPM strongly stresses the need for a patient's embrace of meaningful activity, TFP makes it a requirement for treatment. In the

TFP contracting phase, the specific details of the required paid work, volunteer work, or studies are reviewed at length. Whereas the GPM therapist might make such engagement a near-term goal of treatment, TFP considers it a requirement.

Techniques

The GPM handbook (Gunderson and Links 2014) describes specific attitudes and interventions understood as helpful for the therapist to 1) form a useful working alliance with the patient and 2) convey an expectation for change. The GPM therapist will aim to translate the patient's experiences outside of the treatment and with the clinician in a way that links the model of interpersonal hypersensitivity with the material shared by the patient. The GPM therapist may not always begin the session but will not allow extended periods of silence when the patient does not spontaneously speak. GPM is an amalgam of psychodynamic, behavioral, and case management interventions; what the therapist says and does can vary throughout a session or from session to session. TFP, in contrast, is a relatively fixed set of interventions. The key TFP interventions include the following:

1. Establishing at the beginning the patient's responsibility to speak freely during sessions
2. Focusing on the three channels of communication: what the patient says, how the patient acts, and how the therapist feels
3. Tolerating the confusion that is inevitably part of the early stages of treatment with a patient with moderate to severe personality pathology
4. Identifying the patient's dominant affect displayed in words or actions
5. "Naming the actors" or articulating the patient's experience of himself or herself, the dominant affect, and the patient's experience of another at a given time
6. Identifying the dominant object relation in evidence at a given time, often suggested by the process of "naming the actors"
7. Identifying role reversals or ways the patient may behave that suggest the patient may display behaviors he or she reflexively ascribes to others
8. Consideration of ways particular object relations dyads defend against other dyads (most prominently when a patient's pattern of focusing on perceived lack of caring or exploitation as coming from the therapist alternates with the patient's own uncaring and exploitative behaviors and serves to protect the patient from the vulnerability of closeness and dependence he or she may wish for)

9. Use of systematic clarification (asking for more information), confrontation (bringing to the patient's attention material that is somehow confusing or discrepant), and eventual interpretation (offering a hypothesis about conflicting motives and defenses) as part of the steps described above

As mentioned, the GPM approach is an eclectic one; the therapist's technique, or what he or she says during a session, will draw on different approaches. The GPM therapist may explore elements of the emerging transference or offer interpretations (essentially a hypothesis about motivation and associated defenses), which would be consistent with a TFP approach. On the other hand, the GPM therapist would also freely give advice, act as a case manager to help the patient with nuts-and-bolts projects, or assign homework such as a standard cognitive-behavioral therapy chain analysis—all techniques that would not fit with a TFP focus.

Summary

This review of the differences and commonalities of GPM and TFP puts into context a clinician's decision making about how and when to employ these treatment modalities. There are three possible approaches: 1) to follow the standard recommendation, if indicated, of referring a patient who has been treated with a generalist's model (GPM) to one offered as a specialized treatment (TFP), 2) to consider a recommendation for GPM for those patients who seem unable to benefit from TFP (or perhaps any other specialized treatment) and may have an unremitting presentation that is unresponsive to treatment, or 3) to integrate of elements of GPM and TFP, described as *technical eclecticism*, which could incorporate elements of both (and possibly other) modalities, reflecting the genuine logistical requirements of a particular case, or a clinician's personal preferences and orientation, or both.

What are the clinical situations that might dictate a recommendation for a change from the generalist's GPM approach to the specialist's TFP treatment? One useful first question is the following: Did the patient benefit from GPM, and if not, why not? Consider the subgroup of patients who do not progress as hoped using the GPM model. One consideration may be the clarity of the patient's diagnosis. GPM was designed specifically as an intervention for patients with BPD. What about the patient who may meet DSM-5 criteria for BPD but who also exhibits prominent elements of narcissistic or antisocial personality disorder? The TFP assessment process and the development and maintenance of its specific frame may allow for exploration of these co-occurring elements in a way that GPM would not. (The development of transference-focused psychotherapy–extended (TFP-E) aims to build on TFP's empirical evidence for patients with BPD, to work with those patients with other primary or co-occurring personality disorders; Caligor et al. 2018).

A second consideration would be the patient with BPD whose unintegrated aggression interferes with functioning in major spheres of his or her life. This patient may require a treatment modality that has such exploration as a specific goal, with a frame tailored accordingly, in ways that GPM's more supportive and pliant approach would not. TFP is set up to facilitate exploration of the negative transference; the treatment frame and the therapist's stance of technical neutrality invite such exploration in a way that GPM's more directive and encouraging approach does not.

A third possibility would be the patient who *does* find GPM beneficial but who may want "more" for certain reasons. For example, the patient who is stabilized by GPM treatment but wants improved capacity for self-regulation and increased self-understanding might be motivated to access a more intensive treatment of longer duration. A familiar scenario is the patient who may have benefited from GPM with adjunctive DBT skills and managed to curb certain patterns such as recurrent self-injury or impulsive behavior. This patient may no longer meet DSM-5 criteria for BPD but may be motivated for additional treatment to address barriers to functioning in work, friendships, and romance.

It might seem counterintuitive to consider recommending a shift from a specialized treatment for BPD to a generalist one, but there are certainly cases where this would be appropriate. Choi-Kain et al. (2016) outline this possibility, stressing situations when the patient's presentation reflects chronic, unchanging symptomatology. When such cases tax a system's limited resources, referring the patient to a less-intensive, less-change-oriented intervention might be the best course of action. This thinking is echoed in Kernberg's writings about particularly challenging patients and the decision some clinicians might be forced to make to move away from a change-oriented expectation to one that prioritizes protection for those in the patient's orbit (Kernberg 2007). There are also many situations when moving from TFP to GPM might be dictated by logistical realities, such as a patient's inability to come to a twice-weekly treatment because of finances or his or her travel schedule. The TFP therapist considering such a transition will do so after giving full consideration to the possibility that the patient or the therapist or both might be avoiding some kind of important but challenging exploration by this move.

The possibility of integration of GPM and TFP elements may accurately describe the actual work done by many clinicians who are not compelled by adherence to a study protocol but, instead, borrow those ideas from the various treatment choices they have been exposed to in training. Using TFP elements outside of a sustained twice-weekly individual psychotherapy would fit with the fledgling "applied TFP" movement, describing use of TFP principles in public mental health systems, inpatient and consultation-liaison psychiatry services, and general pharmacotherapy practice (Hersh 2015; Hersh et al. 2017; Lee and Hersh 2018; Zerbo et al. 2013). GPM's handbook strongly endorses the integration of TFP concepts, serving as a model for technical eclecticism, meaning "permission" to borrow from whatever school of thought might be useful (Gunderson and Links 2014).

Case Vignette

The following case description includes decision points, each of which has several alternative responses listed at the end of the case. The reader will rate each alternative response in terms of its level of helpfulness. Discussions of responses follow.

The vignette underscores the evolving challenges faced by the patient with BPD and the ways these changes inform decision making about treatment choices over time. This case describes a patient who is best served by a supportive case management–focused treatment (GPM) for an extended period but then displays specific symptoms and describes particular personal goals resulting in a referral to an extended exploratory psychotherapy (TFP).

> Sandra is a 28-year-old graduate student in a 2-year program at a competitive university located about 2 hours from her hometown. When Sandra started graduate school, she had already had treatment on and off since her junior year of high school. Sandra's difficulties began in her late teens at the time of her parents' divorce. She entered into a period of intense moodiness, often arguing with her mother. Sandra began cutting herself superficially on her thighs to relieve anxiety. Following a breakup with her boyfriend on the night of prom, Sandra took an overdose of Tylenol, leading to an emergency department visit and a referral for treatment to a local treatment team. Sandra and her mother remained confused by the diagnoses conveyed by the therapist and psychiatrist she saw because they did not see Sandra's condition improving with the counseling and medications offered and, in fact, saw Sandra's behaviors escalating, including continued nonsuicidal self-injury and occasional threats of suicide. Sandra's mother accompanied Sandra to one appointment with the providers

to ask, "How come Sandra isn't getting any better? My friend's daughter was diagnosed with depression and in 3 months on Prozac she was back to normal, while Sandra is still suicidal after a year." The therapist responded, "Treatment-resistant depression can require multiple medication trials before the doctor gets the right cocktail." Despite Sandra's persistent symptomatic state (affective instability, weekly binge-purge activity, continued self-injury), she planned to move farther away from home after graduating from a local college to attend a paraprofessional graduate program. She had a vague plan to continue treatment after her arrival.

Sandra did not follow through with her plan to seek treatment after arriving at graduate school but came to the university counseling center just before midterm exams during her first semester. The counseling center was able only to refer Sandra to area clinicians and could not offer on-campus treatment anytime soon. At that time, she was becoming increasingly preoccupied, anxious about both her academic obligations and her concerns about the fidelity of her fiancé who was overseas with the military. She had not taken the medications prescribed for her by her psychiatrist and had not gone for follow-up meetings, concerned about weight gain from the medications compounding that from her high-calorie dorm diet. Sandra was evaluated by an intake coordinator and referred immediately to a community-based "DBT-informed skills and mindfulness group" with a focus on "facilitating attention and wellness." Sandra's mother searched online and identified mindfulness as a key element of DBT, described as a treatment developed for individuals with borderline personality pathology. Sandra asked the intake coordinator about the reason for the referral to the mindfulness group and was told that the group could help Sandra with "depression, attention problems, and stress." When Sandra asked if the group was for individuals with BPD, the group leader demurred and stated, "DBT has been shown to help with lots of things like depression, addiction, and attention problems."

Sandra found the mindfulness group of little use; in fact, she found the DBT skills to be "insulting, infantile exercises" better suited for someone younger, and she dropped out. As final exams approached for the first semester of graduate school, she became increasingly erratic, prone to explosive outbursts when speaking on the phone to her mother, frequent binge-purge activity, and occasional excessive drinking to manage her distress about her strained relationship with her boyfriend. Sandra did manage to pass her exams, but her despairing state and vague threats of self-harm prompted her dean to refer Sandra directly to a private mental health group practice to ensure that Sandra would have more consistent treatment in place as she began the following semester.

When you are assigned to work as Sandra's therapist at the beginning of her second semester of graduate school following the Christmas holiday break, you are struck by the familiarity of Sandra's clinical course and treatment history and reflect on certain points stressed during the 1-day GPM course offered the preceding year at the annual meeting of your state's psychological association. (You took this course because of your wish to have more skills for assessing and treating BPD in the clients you see. You had come to appreciate that you and your colleagues in your group practice had mixed feelings about diagnosing BPD, due to concerns about the capacity to manage these cases and fears that making and conveying a BPD diagnosis would be unduly and unfairly stigmatizing to a client.) You approach Sandra's treatment with the key elements of GPM in mind (sharing the BPD diagnosis, psychoeducation) and find that over the year she is under your care she is generally responsive to the treatment. You assume a case manager role at times, helping Sandra find a support group for bulimia, setting up a schedule for studying and exercise, and eventually helping her with job applications.

You refer Sandra to a psychiatrist in the community who frequently works with clients in treatment with practitioners in your group practice; she has seen her approximately quarterly during the course of her treatment with you. This psychiatrist is familiar with the GPM approach to pharmacotherapy and works with you to avoid problematic polypharmacy, especially during Sandra's crisis episodes. Despite this, the psychiatrist has prescribed antianxiety and sedative-hypnotic agents at times for Sandra to take during periods of heightened distress when her calls to you for support are only somewhat helpful. You periodically review Sandra's course with this psychiatrist, specifically Sandra's positive response to antidepressant treatment for the target symptom of her bulimia.

During her year of treatment with you, Sandra has a significant lessening of suicidal thoughts and behaviors; however, she remains challenged by romantic intimacy and expresses self-doubt about her ability to transition from student to employee. At one point during discussion of Sandra's plans for graduation about 5 months in the future, she becomes so overwhelmed that she shares her fantasy of applying for disability based on her psychiatric condition so that she would not have to face the pressures of an entry-level job in her field. As Sandra moves toward completing her degree, you begin the process of evaluating the optimal course going forward: you start to wonder whether continuing with a GPM treatment, making additional adjustments to her treatment plan, or identifying a different treatment would be the best alternative. Just as you are considering the options to share with Sandra at the 1-year mark of your treatment, you also check in with her psychiatrist to get her assessment of Sandra's progress. [**Decision Point 1**]

You set a date with Sandra to review her treatment course thus far and possible treatment course following graduation. You discuss with Sandra her symptoms of BPD that seem to have improved significantly over the past year (binge-purge activity, self-injurious behavior and threats of suicide, and intense anger) and those that have persisted (identity confusion, particularly regarding her career path; unstable relationships; and marked sensitivity to rejection). You note that despite Sandra's gradual improvement in functioning over the past year, she has continued to have brief but intense periods of distress that make stopping treatment altogether seem like a bad idea. You discuss with Sandra what the next steps in her treatment might be, given her history, her preferences, and the resources available in your locality. You review a variety of treatments that might be available, and because of your knowledge of colleagues who offer TFP, you encourage Sandra to consider TFP as one of a few viable options for treatment. [**Decision Point 2**]

Your are aware that Sandra has about 5 months left in her graduate program as she begins the second semester of her second year. Although she has intermittently continued to raise the prospect of applying for disability, she has, nevertheless, used this last semester to successfully apply for jobs. As part of your tentative planning for discharging Sandra from your practice, you invite Sandra to include her mother at your next meeting; Sandra agrees this would be a good idea. You had met with Sandra and her mother early in her treatment, and you now feel that the focus of your meeting should be on the next step in Sandra's treatment. In this meeting with Sandra and her mother, you review Sandra's history, review her positive response to GPM, and clarify the symptoms Sandra and her mother identify as persistent. Sandra's mother expresses her concerns: "I think she is much better, but I worry about how she'll manage when she has a full-time job. She has told you she has been looking online about disability benefits, hasn't she? On top of that, her boyfriend will be discharged from the service soon, and when he's around, Sandra can get distressed pretty quickly." When describing TFP you sense that Sandra and her mother both feel she could benefit from a more in-depth treatment; in fact, Sandra's mother becomes notably excited by the prospect of this different intervention and exclaims, "That skills group I paid for was a bust, but maybe this could turn her around!" Sandra is particularly motivated to explore her patterns of difficulty that might interfere with the new job she has secured and her ambivalence about her long-term romance. Sandra feels that exploration of these difficulties through the prism of interpersonal hypersensitivity has been helpful only up to a point. You identify a TFP-trained clinician who is available to evaluate Sandra for treatment. As part of this process, you reach out to Sandra's psychiatrist to prepare for this possible transition. [**Decision Point 3**]

After Sandra graduates she begins her evaluation for TFP with Dr. Hines, a local psychologist. Sandra moves off campus, begins an entry-level job in her field, and continues with her psychiatrist as planned. You hear from Dr. Hines that he and Sandra have concluded their evaluation phase and have had a meeting together with Sandra's mother, but there are significant conflicts in the process of establishing a treatment contract. You hear from Sandra that she has developed an instant dislike of Dr. Hines and at the same time has soured on her bulimia support group, feeling she no longer can tolerate "hearing about everyone else's problems." You start to have misgivings about having referred Sandra for this treatment, wishing Dr. Hines would bend the frame to accommodate Sandra's wishes and feeling irritated with Sandra that she is undermining her treatment. [**Decision Point 4**]

Decision Points: Alternative Responses

Rate each response in terms of its level of helpfulness with a rating of 1 (will be helpful), 2 (possibly helpful, continuing reservations), or 3 (not helpful—or even harmful).

1. As Sandra begins her last semester of graduate school, you should do the following as the primary therapist in charge of her care:

   A. Invite Sandra to consider whether continued work with you in a GPM model can still be useful.
   B. Discuss with Sandra her treatment options going forward, acknowledging the likely limited resources available in your community.
   C. Consider supporting Sandra's investigation of disability benefits, given her persistent difficulties even after years of treatment.
   D. Stress the need for Sandra to identify paid work as soon as possible after completing her studies.
   E. Encourage Sandra to transfer her care to an expert psychopharmacologist.

2. In your meeting with Sandra to discuss the next step in her treatment, you convey to her the following:

   A. Having had GPM over the past year makes her a poor candidate for other evidence-based treatment interventions.
   B. She should wait to consider a treatment such as TFP until she finds herself in a crisis situation.
   C. You are skeptical about Sandra's ability to tolerate a treatment such as TFP because you worry that it may be insufficiently supportive for her.
   D. You assure Sandra that she could identify a TFP therapist and begin a twice-weekly psychotherapy whenever it would be convenient for her.
   E. You stress the value of revisiting her personal goals and her treatment goals as she contemplates this transition.

3. In meeting with Sandra and her mother, you stress the following as part of your efforts to help her with decision making about her plans that include choices about her treatment:

A. You caution that because Sandra found the DBT skills groups objectionable, she may also have complaints about TFP.

B. You agree with Sandra's mother that TFP may be the intervention that "turns her around."

C. You explain to Sandra and her mother that you cannot guarantee that TFP will be a good fit and that Sandra should expect to participate in an extended evaluation process before starting the therapy.

D. You make it clear that you are committed to working with Sandra if it turns out that she chooses not to go forward with TFP.

E. You report that you have recently been in touch with Sandra's psychiatrist and that you both agree that given Sandra's improvement, she should work to limit her use of as-needed medications.

4. Following your phone call with Dr. Hines about Sandra's evaluation for TFP, you should consider doing the following:

A. You should reach out to Sandra and let her know that you do not think TFP is going to be the right treatment for her at this time.

B. You should call Dr. Hines back and suggest that he make accommodations for Sandra by allowing for intersession contact, given your experience of the benefits of such coaching during her treatment with you.

C. You should call Dr. Hines back and let him know that you would be open to continuing treatment with Sandra if they are unable to agree on a treatment contract acceptable to both of them.

D. You should think twice about future referrals for TFP given Sandra's negative reaction to Dr. Hines.

E. You should check to make sure that Sandra's psychiatrist and Dr. Hines are in touch.

Decision Points: Discussion

Numbers within brackets indicate level of helpfulness ratings.

1. As Sandra begins her last semester of graduate school, you should do the following as the primary therapist in charge of her care:

A. Invite Sandra to consider whether continued work with you in a GPM model can still be useful. [1] (The GPM therapist will consistently check in with a patient about the utility of an on-going treatment. If a treatment does not seem to be effective in addressing a particular complaint or symptoms, the therapist would then question the advisability of continuing.)

B. Discuss with Sandra her treatment options going forward, ac-knowledging the likely limited resources available in your com-munity. [1] (This process would model GPM's collaborative approach and would educate Sandra about treatment resources, including evidence-based interventions like DBT or TFP, if they are available.)

C. Consider supporting Sandra's investigation of disability benefits, given her persistent difficulties even after years of treatment. [3] (Such a recommendation would be unhelpful. GPM's focus on "getting a life" would understandably be undermined by encour-agement to seek disability benefits, and TFP's meaningful activ-ity requirement would be inconsistent with such an intervention as well.)

D. Stress the need for Sandra to identify paid work as soon as pos-sible after completing her studies. [1] (Stressing Sandra's need to identify paid work after graduation would not be an absolute requirement of either GPM or TFP, but it would be an optimal outcome.)

E. Encourage Sandra to transfer her care to an expert psychophar-macologist. [3] (This would not be a helpful intervention; GPM's emphasis on accepting the limitations of pharmacotherapy in the treatment of personality disorder symptoms is also a part of TFP's overarching approach.)

2. In your meeting with Sandra to discuss the next step in her treat-ment, you convey to her the following:

A. Having had GPM in the past year makes her a poor candidate for other evidence-based treatment interventions. [3] (Although GPM is a "gateway" intervention that is likely to be "good enough" for many individuals with BPD, there will be a subset of patients who may want a more intensive treatment such as TFP or who may respond only partially or not at all to GPM but might benefit from treatment in another format.)

B. She should wait to consider a treatment such as TFP until she finds herself in a crisis situation. [2] (You may feel that Sandra would do well to try to manage without continued treatment, but she should know that specialized treatments are not often available and can take many weeks to access when actually sought.)

C. You are skeptical about Sandra's ability to tolerate a treatment such as TFP because you worry that it may be insufficiently supportive for her. [2] (Although you do not want to actively dissuade Sandra from investigating TFP, you do want to be frank with her about the specifics of the treatment.)

D. You assure Sandra that she could identify a TFP therapist and begin a twice-weekly psychotherapy whenever it would be convenient for her. [3] (Clinicians offering evidence-based treatments for BPD are in short supply even in major metropolitan areas, and Sandra should know that finding one trained in TFP would be rare.)

E. You stress the value of revisiting her personal goals and her treatment goals as she contemplates this transition. [1] (Having Sandra revisit her personal and treatment goals will likely be beneficial. Sandra should know that any continued treatment is premised on an expectation for change.)

3. In meeting with Sandra and her mother, you stress the following as part of your efforts to help her with decision making about her plans that include choices about her treatment:

A. You caution that because Sandra found the DBT skills group objectionable, she may also have complaints about TFP. [2] (This is true. Sandra may become uneasy in any treatment situation that is not as flexible as GPM. It is not your goal to encourage her unease, but it could be helpful to explore her concerns before starting this new treatment.)

B. You agree with Sandra's mother that TFP may be the intervention that "turns her around." [2] (It is probably helpful to convey some optimism about this new opportunity, but it would be important not to support an unrealistic idealization of the new treatment or treater.)

C. You explain to Sandra and her mother that you cannot guarantee that TFP will be a good fit and that Sandra should expect to participate in an extended evaluation process before starting the therapy. [1] (Communicating with honesty and sharing realistic expectations is good modeling.)

D. You make it clear that you are committed to working with Sandra if it turns out that she chooses not to go forward with TFP. [2] (You want to remain flexible, as would be consistent with the GPM approach, but at the same time you want to give Sandra a chance to evaluate this new treatment. TFP treatment is not as accommodating as GPM would be, so offering Sandra a backup plan makes sense.)

E. You report that you have recently been in touch with Sandra's psychiatrist and that you both agree that given Sandra's improvement, she should work to limit her use of as-needed medications. [1] (Sandra should know that her treatment team members are in contact. Using as little medication as is possible should be a goal of whatever treatment for BPD she chooses to access.)

4. Following your phone call with Dr. Hines about Sandra's evaluation for TFP, you should consider doing the following:

A. You should reach out to Sandra and let her know that you do not think TFP is going to be the right treatment for her at this time. [3] (This may be true, but you should let Sandra's evaluation for TFP go forward.)

B. You should call Dr. Hines back and suggest that he make accommodations for Sandra by allowing for intersession contacts, given your experience of the benefits of such coaching during her treatment with you. [3] (Sandra may have benefited from these contacts, but it would not be useful for you to pressure Dr. Hines to change his approach. It may be that Sandra decides she will not go forward with a treatment that precludes such contacts, but you should let the evaluation process run its course.)

C. You should call Dr. Hines back and let him know that you would be open to continuing treatment with Sandra if they are unable to agree on a treatment contract acceptable to both of them. [2] (While this communication may be reassuring to Dr. Hines, you run the risk of inadvertently conveying that you do not think Sandra can work within the constraints of TFP. It is probably too early to conclude this, and this would be Dr. Hines's and Sandra's call to make.)

D. You should think twice about future referrals for TFP given Sandra's negative reaction to Dr. Hines. [3] (TFP's evaluation process and contracting usually elicit a patient's negative transference, which becomes the focus of exploration for the treatment. Sandra's negative reaction to Dr. Hines would be expected, at least at the beginning of the treatment.)

E. You should check to make sure that Sandra's psychiatrist and Dr. Hines are in touch. [1] (It is important that the members of Sandra's team stay in close contact. Your role may be critical during this transition period, and ensuring that all the parties involved are working together is a valuable intervention.)

Vignette Summary

This vignette describes the case of a patient who benefits from GPM treatment for symptoms of her BPD but has some persistent challenges and expresses motivation for a more intensive treatment. Sandra's story captures the complex calculus that would be part of a change in treatment modalities, in particular a change from GPM to TFP. The GPM therapist remains aware that facilitating a change in treaters could cause a patient anxiety about perceived rejection but focuses on the possible additional benefit that a different approach could add to what has already been offered in GPM. In this vignette, Sandra's therapist is deliberate in this process, remaining mindful of potential pitfalls; referring a patient for a more specialized treatment can reflect a clinician's frustration with a particular patient and/or can reflect collusion with a patient's expectations for "rescue" by an idealized treater or modality, both of which the clinician would like to avoid. Sandra's therapist remains realistic and practical in this process, again modeling for Sandra "thinking before acting" and thoughtfulness.

As mentioned earlier, although it stands to reason that a more typical course would be a referral from a generalist intervention such as GPM to a more specialized treatment such as TFP, there are cases when the TFP therapist might recommend a transition to GPM. These situations often fall into two categories: 1) patients who have logistical obstacles that prevent the recommended twice-weekly extended treatment and 2) patients who for whatever reason are not able to use TFP and its contract-focused strategy. Clearly, with the first group the therapist would want to make sure that the obstacles raised are, in fact, genuine and not a reflection of an emerging negative transference that is acted out by the patient through avoidance of the treatment. Avoiding such exploration could risk engaging in an enactment that reinforces the patient's unconscious concerns that the therapist finds the patient unlikable or unworkable. The second category of patients also presents multiple challenges. (For example, the patient who refuses to engage in either work or studies or who finds the expectation that he or she speak freely to be too challenging.) Usually after extensive exploration of the meaning of the patient's inability to adhere to the treatment contract, the therapist will have to determine how best to proceed. It may be required in certain cases to move from a TFP treatment to a more flexible and supportive intervention such as GPM, with the proviso that should the patient's motivation change, then there would be an opportunity to resume TFP with its well-defined expectations.

Conclusion

The development and study of evidence-based treatments for BPD have ushered in a new period of optimism. The era of undue pessimism and resignation about the course of BPD has passed. Clinicians now face new and different concerns: how to help patients with BPD when resources are often limited and when specialists are in short supply. Added to these issues is the dilemma about how to choose which intervention is best suited for the patient. GPM borrows some important elements from TFP theory, but TFP has a significantly different approach and philosophy when practiced in its pure form. An appreciation of the utility of sequencing treatment—moving from GPM to TFP, for example—is still limited to case reports. Yet the prospect of increased awareness about BPD, increased grass-roots activism, lessening of stigma, and a greater emphasis on well-studied and well-conducted treatments promises a better understanding of what works best.

References

American Psychiatric Association: Practice guideline for the treatment of patients with borderline personality disorder. Am J Psychiatry 158 (10 suppl):1–52, 2001 11665545

American Psychiatric Association: Diagnostic and Statistical Manual of Mental Disorders, 5th Edition. Arlington, VA, American Psychiatric Association, 2013

Bernstein J, Zimmerman M, Auchincloss EL: Transference-focused psychotherapy training during residency: an aide to learning psychodynamic psychotherapy. Psychodyn Psychiatry 43(2):201–221, 2015 26039228

Caligor E, Kernberg OF, Clarkin JF: Handbook of Dynamic Psychotherapy for Higher Level Personality Pathology. Washington, DC, American Psychiatric Publishing, 2007

Caligor E, Kernberg OF, Clarkin JF, Yeomans FE: Psychodynamic Therapy for Personality Pathology: Treating Self and Interpersonal Functioning. Washington, DC, American Psychiatric Association Publishing, 2018

Choi-Kain LW, Albert EB, Gunderson JG: Evidence-based treatments for borderline personality disorder: implementation, integration, and stepped care. Harv Rev Psychiatry 24(5):342–356, 2016 27603742

Clarkin JF: An integrated approach to psychotherapy techniques for patients with personality disorder. J Pers Disord 26(1):43–62, 2012 22369166

Clarkin JF, Foelsch PA, Levy KN, et al: The development of a psychodynamic treatment for patients with borderline personality disorder: a preliminary study of behavioral change. J Pers Disord 15(6):487–495, 2001 11778390

Clarkin JF, Levy KN, Lenzenweger MF, et al: Evaluating three treatments for borderline personality disorder: a multiwave study. Am J Psychiatry 164(6):922–928, 2007 17541052

Clarkin JF, Lively WJ, Meehan KB: Clinical assessment, in Handbook of Personality Disorders: Theory, Research, and Treatment, 2nd Edition. Edited by Lively WJ, Larstone R. New York, Guilford, 2018, pp 367–393

Diamond D, Yeomans FE, Stern B, et al: A Clinical Guide for Treating Narcissistic Disorders: A Transference Focused Psychotherapy. New York, Guilford, in press

Doering S, Hörz S, Rentrop M, et al: Transference-focused psychotherapy v. treatment by community psychotherapists for borderline personality disorder: randomised controlled trial. Br J Psychiatry 196(5):389–395, 2010 20435966

Gabbard GO: Do all roads lead to Rome? New findings on borderline personality disorder. Am J Psychiatry 164(6):853–855, 2007 17541040

Gunderson JG, Links PS: Handbook of Good Psychiatric Management for Borderline Personality Disorder. Washington, DC, American Psychiatric Publishing, 2014

Hersh RG: Using transference-focused psychotherapy principles in the pharmacotherapy of patients with severe personality disorders. Psychodyn Psychiatry 43(2):181–199, 2015 26039277

Hersh RG, Caligor E, Yeomans FE: Fundamentals of Transference-Focused Psychotherapy: Applications in Psychiatric and Medical Settings. Cham, Switzerland, Springer, 2017

Hong V: Borderline personality disorder in the emergency department: good psychiatric management. Harv Rev Psychiatry 24(5):357–366, 2016 27603743

Kernberg OF: Borderline Conditions and Pathological Narcissism. New York, Jason Aronson, 1975

Kernberg OF: Structural interviewing. Psychiatr Clin North Am 4(1):169–195, 1981 7232235

Kernberg OF: Severe Personality Disorders: Psychotherapeutic Strategies. New Haven, CT, Yale University Press, 1984

Kernberg OF: The almost untreatable narcissistic patient. J Am Psychoanal Assoc 55(2):503–539, 2007 17601104

Lee T, Hersh RG: Managing the clinical encounter with patients with borderline personality disorder in a general psychiatry setting: key contributions from transference-focused psychotherapy. Br J Psychiatry 2018 doi.org/10.1192/bja.2018.63

Livesley WJ: Moving beyond specialized therapies for borderline personality disorder: the importance of integrated domain-focused treatment. Psychodyn Psychiatry 40(1):47–74, 2012 23006029

McMain SF, Links PS, Gnam WH, et al: A randomized trial of dialectical behavior therapy versus general psychiatric management for borderline personality disorder. Am J Psychiatry 166(12):1365–1374, 2009 19755574

McMain SF, Guimond T, Streiner DL, et al: Dialectical behavior therapy compared with general psychiatric management for borderline personality disorder: clinical outcomes and functioning over a 2-year follow-up. Am J Psychiatry 169(6):650–661, 2012 22581157

Paris J: Stepped care and rehabilitation for patients recovering from borderline personality disorder. J Clin Psychol 71(8):747–752, 2015 26189972

Weinberg I, Ronningstam E, Goldblatt MJ, et al: Common factors in empirically supported treatments of borderline personality disorder. Curr Psychiatry Rep 13(1):60–68, 2011 21057901

Yeomans FE, Selzer MA, Clarkin JF: Treating the Borderline Patient: A Contract-Based Approach. New York, Basic Books, 1992

Yeomans FE, Clarkin JF, Kernberg OF: Transference-Focused Psychotherapy for Borderline Personality Disorder: A Clinical Guide. Washington, DC, American Psychiatric Publishing, 2015.

Zerbo E, Cohen S, Bielska W, et al: Transference-focused psychotherapy in the general psychiatry residency: a useful and applicable model for residents in acute clinical settings. Psychodyn Psychiatry 41(1):163–181, 2013 23480166

PART IV

Conclusion

Chapter 16

Conclusion

THE FUTURE OF
GOOD PSYCHIATRIC MANAGEMENT

Lois W. Choi-Kain, M.D., M.Ed.

More than 5 million people are living with borderline personality disorder (BPD) in the United States alone. There are more than 120 million worldwide. Considering the total package of treatment that DBT entails, a single practitioner working full time for 40 hours could at most take 32 individual clients per year if they ran one 2-hour skills training group and attended a 2-hour team consultation. This estimate does not include time for writing notes, speaking to insurance companies, eating lunch, or taking coaching calls. Both transference-focused psychotherapy

(TFP) and mentalization-based treatment (MBT) would require slightly less clinical face time, but at most under the same pressed conditions, practitioners of these psychodynamic evidence-based treatments could only see 20–35 patients, maximum, in 40 hours of clinical face time. Although DBT, TFP, and MBT embody the enormous progress made in the treatment for BPD, they will remain highly specialized in the sense that only a small fraction of mental health practitioners will ever receive the training and support necessary to implement them. This absence of training and support is even more relevant for the providers at the front lines of care, the primary care and mental health practitioners who see the majority of patients who interface on the basic level available with health care services.

About 25,250 psychiatrists are practicing in the United States (Bureau of Labor Statistics 2017). Using the previously stated figure of 5 million people with BPD in the United States, every psychiatrist could have as many as 200 patients with BPD in his or her individual catchment area (Lenzenweger et al. 2007), assuming that all individuals with BPD seek treatment. This ratio tilts to be more extreme in emerging economies. For example, India has an estimated 2 million people with BPD (Gupta and Mattoo 2012) for only 4,000 psychiatrists (Mohandas 2009). This means that a psychiatrist in India could have as many as 500 patients in his or her individual catchment area, assuming a conservative BPD prevalence estimate of 0.15% (Gupta and Mattoo 2012). Although the specialized treatments for BPD are elegant and comprehensive, they are clearly not a public health solution.

Having not only learned from but also trained many professionals in the best of the best psychotherapies the BPD world has to offer, I deeply appreciate the sophistication and coherence that can optimally characterize psychotherapies and what they can offer: treatments that heal the core of serious mental illness. However, as I have described elsewhere, they are only one facet of care in a stepped care model (see Appendix B, "Stepped Care Model"; Choi-Kain et al. 2016). Effective generalist care of burgeoning and mild symptoms of BPD can be addressed by *good* and *general* care. Psychoeducation, prompt diagnosis, and functional support, paired with practical assistance to live life with an illness, constitute just plain good medical care. That is what GPM embodies—good general medical care. Perhaps it is primary care for the psychiatric management of BPD.

Ultimately, GPM practitioners can be like the old-fashioned primary care doctor before the rise of administrative medical bureaucracy and the fall of humanistic holistic care of patients (Tingley 2018). Like the traditional primary care or family doctor, the GPM practitioner could know you all your life, know your whole family, and with broad strokes know the life you have lived. He or she may refer you to specialists as any primary care provider would do, for consults and discrete episodes of care, but would then resume care to help you live the optimal life you can in sickness and in health. As described in several chapters in this book, there is a synergy between GPM and DBT (Chapter 13), MBT (Chapter 14), and TFP (Chapter 15). Ideally, patients go to these treatments when they experience failure in *general* care, and they come back to *general* care when the most life-threatening symptoms stabilize so they can again be outpatients and resume life in the real world. While we, the authors of this book, advocate for short-term use of these BPD treatments for addressing public health needs and limiting the identity that those with BPD develop as patients, a long-term health maintenance application of GPM seems appropriate.

BPD is no different from any other medical entity. This is why GPM incorporates the term *psychiatric* rather than *psychological*. BPD's acute episodes resolve with added support, and its chronic vulnerabilities are best managed by patients between office visits. Importantly, GPM medicalizes BPD as an illness rather than as an amalgam of psychological traits. When any illness is detected earlier, intervention can be less intensive and can prevent treatment delays and sequelae of a more advanced disease process. In this book, the GPM model has been applied to narcissistic personality disorder, for which no evidence-based treatments have been established. This basic recipe of *general* care can be applied to all psychiatric diagnoses and still constitute *good* care. It can be utilized in any setting to medicalize chronic and recurrent problems, which allows patients and health care professionals to view personality disorder features as symptoms of the illness for which they seek treatment rather than as character flaws.

As our friend Glen Gabbard has written in the *American Journal of Psychiatry* (Gabbard 2007), "many roads lead to Rome" when it comes to treatment for BPD. The "horse race" of building better and better treatments is subsiding, and now we can focus on making all the good treatments that we know work more available, realistic, and practical (Choi-Kain et al. 2017). Although GPM's empirical profile could be enhanced with another large randomized controlled trial, the decision to commit all our academic time and energy to testing something we know works against so-called treatment as usual seems on some level irresponsible. The field would benefit from someone doing that, but in this era of competitive grants and ever-shrinking research budgets, I believe we will best advance treatment for patients with BPD by proliferating what we know to all the places that want to learn it. Ultimately, we accept that this is *good enough general* care, because it is particularly valuable to address the still-growing need for basic services. For now, we will operate on the idea that what we have here is *good enough* to spread as far as we can to all the patients who need care but cannot find it and all the clinicians who want to do better but cannot become specialists.

References

Bureau of Labor Statistics: Occupational Employment Statistics, May 2017. 29-1066 Psychiatrists. Washington, DC, U.S. Department of Labor, 2017. Available at: https://www.bls.gov/oes/current/oes291066.htm. Accessed July 17, 2018.

Choi-Kain LW, Albert EB, Gunderson JG: Evidence-based treatments for borderline personality disorder: implementation, integration, and stepped care. Harv Rev Psychiatry 24(5):342–356, 2016 27603742

Choi-Kain LW, Finch EF, Masland SR, et al: What works in the treatment of borderline personality disorder. Curr Behav Neurosci Rep 4(1):21–30, 2017 28331780

Gabbard GO: Do all roads lead to Rome? New findings on borderline personality disorder. Am J Psychiatry 164(6):853–855, 2007 17541040

Gupta S, Mattoo SK: Personality disorders: prevalence and demography at a psychiatric outpatient in North India. Int J Soc Psychiatry 58(2):146–152, 2012 21177705

Lenzenweger MF, Lane MC, Loranger AW, et al: DSM-IV personality disorders in the National Comorbidity Survey Replication. Biol Psychiatry 62(6):553–564, 2007 17217923

Mohandas E: Roadmap to Indian psychiatry. Indian J Psychiatry 51(3):173–179, 2009 19881044

Tingley K: Trying to put a Value on the doctor-patient relationship. The New York Times, May 16, 2018. Available at: https://www.nytimes.com/interactive/2018/05/16/magazine/health-issue-reinvention-of-primary-care-delivery.html. Accessed July 17, 2018.

Appendix A

Additional Resources

Online Trainings for Clinicians

McLean Borderline Personality Disorder Training Institute's Course on Good Psychiatric Management

- *Website:* http://hms.harvard.edu/BPD

The McLean Borderline Personality Disorder Training Institute continuing education online course offers training in good psychiatric management (GPM) through Harvard Medical School Continuing Medical Education (HMS CME) Online. GPM, an empirically supported treatment approach, has been demonstrated to match the effectiveness of dialectical behavior therapy in treating patients with borderline personality disorder (BPD; McMain et al. 2009). The course, offered free until 2021, will teach mental health professionals and primary care clinicians what they need to know to become competent providers who can derive satisfaction from treating these patients.

Through lectures, case vignettes, and interactive decision points, the course covers management strategies that incorporate practicality, good sense, and flexibility. Techniques and interventions that facilitate the patient's trust and willingness to become a proactive collaborator are described. The course reviews guidelines for handling the common and usually most burdensome issues of managing suicidality and self-harm (e.g., intersession crises, threats as a call for help, excessive use of emergency departments or hospitals). Furthermore, it describes how and when psychiatrists can usefully integrate group, family, or other psychotherapies.

Cost: FREE until 2021

Continuing Education credits will be available for physicians, psychologists, social workers, licensed mental health counselors, and nurses

Other Resources

National Alliance on Mental Illness (NAMI)

- *Website:* www.nami.org
- *Information:* Can find BPD under the topic "Learn More" (click on "Mental Health Conditions"); provides information about etiology, comorbidities, treatment, self-harm, and medications
- *Links:* Information on treatment modalities for BPD, substance use disorders, self-injury, mental illnesses discussion groups; also National Education Alliance for Borderline Personality Disorder and National Institute of Mental Health websites
- *Referral source:* For state and local affiliates that provide support, education, information, referral, and advocacy

National Education Alliance for Borderline Personality Disorder (NEABPD)

- *Website*: www.borderlinepersonalitydisorder.com
- *Information:* Provides information about BPD for clients, families, Family Connections leaders, and professionals; also includes information on GAP (Global Alliance for Prevention and Early Intervention for BPD) and podcasts

- *Links:* To national organizations, research, and treatment
- *Referral source:* None; has a "Looking for Treatment" page with suggestions on finding the right treatment and professional
- *Lists:* Recommends publications, books, a library of articles, and the NEABPD journal; a media library including conference presentations and course/workshop videos

New York-Presbyterian BPD Resource Center

- *Website*: www.nyp.org/bpdresourcecenter
- *Information:* Provides information on diagnosis and treatment, instructional DVD to demonstrate different treatment modalities for BPD, message center and hotline monitored by mental health professionals
- *Links:* National organizations, research, and resources on personality disorders
- *Referral source:* Database of clinicians, agencies, and facilities located nationwide with experience treating BPD and co-occurring disorders
- *Lists:* Recommended books on BPD for laypeople and professionals alike

Personality Disorder Awareness Network (PDAN)

- *Website:* www.pdan.org
- *Information:* Provides information on personality disorders, including BPD, and has a blog, online parenting programs, and webinars
- *Links:* To national and international organizations; various websites
- *Referral source:* Links to Theravive, a network of mental health professionals in the United States and Canada
- *Lists:* Recommended books, including some for children

Treatment and Research Advancements for Borderline Personality Disorder (TARA4BPD)

- *Website:* www.tara4bpd.org
- *Information:* Provides information and many resources about BPD, including neurobiology, comorbidities, and different treatments, for clients, families of clients, and clinicians

- *Links:* To science-related resources such as science magazines, lectures, and online webinars and resources, but they are not specific to BPD
- *Referral source:* Provides helpline to refer people to clinicians specializing in BPD treatments and to various support groups, meetings, research, information, and advocacy efforts
- *Lists:* Recommends a wide variety of books; limited in recommending articles

Reference

McMain SF, Links PS, Gnam WH, et al: A randomized trial of dialectical behavior therapy versus general psychiatric management for borderline personality disorder. Am J Psychiatry 166(12):1365–1374, 2009 19755574

Appendix B

Stepped Care Model

The stepped care model outlines an approach to managing BPD depending on the patient's clinical stage. Figure B–1 illustrates the stepped care model.

Preclinical Stage

Early detection is the optimal intervention for burgeoning symptoms of borderline personality disorder (BPD; Chanen et al. 2017). The early signs and symptoms of BPD overlap with those of mood disorders in youths (Chanen et al. 2016). At this early point in time, psychoeducation for patients and families is essential. Although diagnostic clarity may be difficult to attain in the rapidly evolving developmental phase of adolescence and young adulthood, teaching patients and families what BPD is, in ad-

---

Appendix B has been adapted from Choi-Kain et al. 2016.

Severity	Definition	Potential interventions
5 Chronic persistent Unremitting disorder Unresponsive to intervention	Unresponsive to interventions from previous stages, due to severity and complexity, or nonadherence to treatment recommendations	GPM (low frequency, e.g., weekly, monthly, or quarterly) Supportive therapy Case management (e.g., state/public services)
4 Severe Remitting and relapsing	+ Severe self-harm + Potentially fatal suicide attempts	GPM (+ medication management) PLUS Higher level of care Integration of EBTs OR Change EBT (rarely available)
3 Sustained moderate Sustained threshold-level symptoms	Unresponsive to basic treatment + Self-harm + Suicidal gestures	GPM (+ medication management) PLUS DBT skills, MBT, or STEPPS group when available
2 Early mild First episode of threshold BPD	+ Self-harm − Suicidality	GPM Case management DBT skills, MBT, or STEPPS group when available; self-help if relevant
1 Preclinical Subthreshold	Interpersonal hypersensitivity Rejection sensitivity Emotional dysregulation	Psychoeducation and health literacy Focus on problem solving and supportive counseling addressing interpersonal hypersensitivity and rejection sensitivity

FIGURE B–1. Stepped care model.

BPD=borderline personality disorder; DBT=dialectical behavior therapy; EBT=evidence-based treatment; GPM=good psychiatric management; MBT=mentalization-based treatment; STEPPS=Systems Training for Emotional Predictability and Problem Solving; TFP=transference-focused psychotherapy.

Source. Adapted from Choi-Kain LW, Albert EB, Gunderson JG: "Evidence-Based Treatments for Borderline Personality Disorder: Implementation, Integration, and Stepped Care." *Harvard Review of Psychiatry* 24(5):342–356, 2016.

dition to defining other disorders related to patients' presentations (e.g., mood, anxiety, trauma-related, eating, and substance use disorders), helps patients and families recognize the experience they may suffer and provides a nonpejorative medical language with which to provide help.

A large study on diagnostic assessments demonstrated that even one symptom of BPD increases likelihood of suicidality, depression, and hospitalization (Zimmerman et al. 2012). Identifying these symptoms early on as signs or early symptoms may allow patients to utilize resources to treat problems when they are generally easier to solve. General mental health literacy—focusing on good mental health habits that help most, such as regular sleep, avoidance of substances especially during critical stages of brain development, regulated eating, and steady self-care—helps reduce risk for any population. The challenge of this task is that these directives are antithetical to the habits of many teens and young adults. Generic help with problem solving and thinking through decisions by a well-meaning, mature advisor can be helpful if he or she can broker a productive alliance with both patient and parents.

Early Mild Stage

When a patient meets at least five criteria for BPD, especially when self-harm occurs, the full syndromic disorder is already set in motion. Good psychiatric management (GPM) can start as an entry-level treatment, with active case management optimally assisting patients to stay in the game of life outside treatment. When young people with BPD fall off a usual developmental trajectory of being in school, this eliminates essential sources of structure, learning, socializing, and identity building around which individuals with BPD are already more handicapped. If a patient needs a medical leave, being in a dialectical behavior therapy (DBT) skills training group would be ideal, but in the absence of that, any type of BPD-focused group (e.g., psychoeducation, mentalization-based treatment [MBT], Systems Training for Emotional Predictability and Problem Solving [STEPPS; Blum et al. 2002]), or self-help (e.g., Alcoholics Anonymous, Narcotics Anonymous) if those are unavailable, allows a continuous socialization forum for growing adults who are sensitive to being alone.

Sustained Moderate Stage

When patients do not improve adequately from these earlier stages of interventions, it is always important to assess why this might be the case. Socioeconomic, cultural, or familial issues may conflict with the patient's follow-through or utilization of treatment. In these situations, case management might actively address obstacles to improvement. However, when the level of contact and intensity of care is insufficient, despite patients' follow-through and motivation, an increased complexity of intervention is called for; this might require adding medications to GPM plus a BPD-specific group therapy such as DBT, MBT, or STEPPS. When available, an increase in the level of care to partial hospitalization or residential treatment can help, allowing the patient a fuller immersion in treatment and a more intensive holding environment while still assuming the patient will need to manage his or her own safety and impulse-control difficulties. Another intensification of treatment can occur if a relatively adherent full-package evidence-based treatment such as DBT, MBT, or transference-focused psychotherapy (TFP) is applied when available.

Severe Stage

If problems persist despite steady alliances, adequate motivation, follow-through with treatment agreements, and active efforts to problem-solve life's challenges through case management, then residential or hospital level of care is essential for containment. Such placements are rare and not to be used in a repeated or lengthy way. Safety can be achieved only with higher levels of containment when self-destructive risks are high and productive treatment alliances are not intact. Ideally, these levels of care provide patients with active assistance in their preparation to reenter life, rather than escape as an emotional solution to overwhelming problems. These levels of care can become addictive havens for patients, so attention to following productive protocols for BPD as illustrated in Chapter 2, "Inpatient Psychiatric Units," is indicated. If the patient is in a highly specialized environment where multiple different evidence-based treatments are offered (i.e., McLean Hospital, Lausanne Centre for Interventional Psychiatry, New York-Presbyterian Hospital, De Viersprong National Institute of Personality Disorders), a consult to determine the specific impasse in the treatment, followed by consideration of switch to a different evidence-based treatment, is a rare and expensive option.

Chronic Persistent Stage

If for any reason a patient is unresponsive to interventions from previous stages of this model, he or she may need a lower level of intensity of care. The expectations, resources, and interpersonal interactions involved in more complex treatments may be too much for a patient with very severe

BPD to make use of at any given time. The ability of a patient to make use of intensive treatments can be subject to change. When more complex treatments prove to be too much for patients, low-level frequencies of GPM or supportive therapy are indicated, as often as weekly if the patient is making good use of the contact to stay outside of an inpatient unit or as infrequently as monthly to quarterly depending on the patient and the system's resources. Case management for these patients might involve application to disability or other services as a last resort. Importantly, patients and their clinicians should leave the subject of frequency of treatment open for reconsideration. A few patients go to a state hospital, reconstitute, and resume more active levels of treatment over time.

References

Blum N, Pfohl B, John DS, et al: STEPPS: a cognitive behavioral systems-based group treatment for outpatients with borderline personality disorder—a preliminary report. Compr Psychiatry 43(4):301–310, 2002 12107867

Chanen A, Berk M, Thompson K: Integrating early intervention for borderline personality disorder and mood disorders. Harv Rev Psychiatry 24(5):330–341, 2016 27144298

Chanen A, Sharp C, Hoffman P: Prevention and early intervention for borderline personality disorder: a novel public health priority. World Psychiatry 16(2):215–216, 2017 28498598

Choi-Kain LW, Albert EB, Gunderson JG: Evidence-based treatments for borderline personality disorder: implementation, integration, and stepped care. Harv Rev Psychiatry 24(5):342–356, 2016 27603742

Zimmerman M, Chelminski I, Young D, et al: Does the presence of one feature of borderline personality disorder have clinical significance? Implications for dimensional ratings of personality disorders. J Clin Psychiatry 73(1):8–12, 2012 22054015

Appendix C

Interpersonal Coherence Model

Interpersonal hypersensitivity is a core feature of borderline personality disorder (BPD). Figure C–1 and Table C–1 illustrate the interpersonal coherence model of BPD. The model helps provide a framework around which patients can develop self-awareness of their behavioral patterns and how these are affected by interpersonal events.

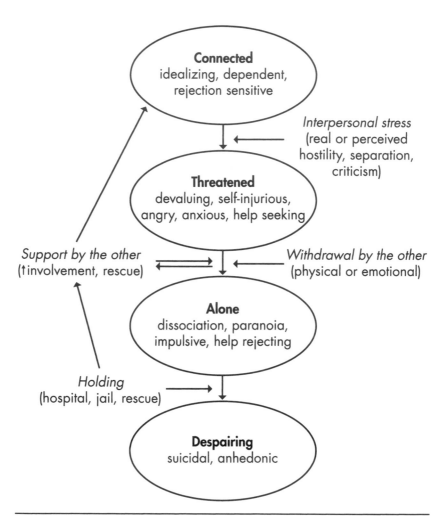

FIGURE C–1.   Interpersonal coherence model.

Source.   Adapted from Gunderson JG, Links PS: *Handbook of Good Psychiatric Management for Borderline Personality Disorder.* Washington, DC, American Psychiatric Publishing, 2014, p. 14. Copyright © 2014 American Psychiatric Publishing. Used with permission.

TABLE C–1. **Interpersonal coherence model**

	Phenomenology
Connected	The patient feels "held" and contained by an idealized relationship. In this connected state, the patient is collaborative, dependent, and rejection sensitive.
Threatened	The patient encounters real or perceived hostility, rejection, or abandonment, resulting in more aggressive behaviors toward others and oneself (e.g., anger, self-harm).
Alone	If the patient's behavior elicits withdrawal, the patient becomes more distressed, dissociated, and help rejecting. At this stage, the patient is more difficult to reach or influence.
Despairing	Without a containing relationship, when truly alone, the patient becomes anhedonic and more seriously suicidal.

Note. The *holding environment* refers to the calming influence of a relationship that the patient feels he or she can depend on. When others show concern, consistency, and responsiveness, the patient develops a belief that someone cares about him or her. When threatened, the aggressive behaviors may succeed in gaining the attention from the desired caregiver. When the caregiver provides rescue or increased involvement, the patient calms down and goes back to a connected state. When the patient devolves into aloneness and despair, an external container (e.g., hospital, jail) provides containment where the patient may encounter caregivers or sources of support that relieve the sense of loneliness. See Gunderson and Links 2014, pp. 13–14.

Reference

Gunderson JG, Links PS: Handbook of Good Psychiatric Management for Borderline Personality Disorder. Washington, DC, American Psychiatric Publishing, 2014, pp. 13–14

Index

Page numbers printed in **boldface** type refer to tables and figures.